# Winds Against The Mind

Based on True Stories

## LOLA BAMIGBOYE L.L.B, B.L, MSN, RN

Printed in the United States of America by Building Towards Success L.L.C.
P.O. Box 275, Brentwood, Tennessee, 37024.

Original cover designed by Ken Strickland

ISBN: 9780981753706

Books are available at quantity discounts when used to promote products or services. For information, please write to marketing division, Building Towards Success L.L.C, P.O. Box 275 , Brentwood, TN 37024.

DISCLAIMER
The names of the people used in the stories are fictitious. The stories were slightly modified to disguise and to protect the identity and the confidentiality of the real people in the stories.

NOTICE
Attempts were made to trace the copyright holders for borrowed materials in the publication of this book. If anybody has been inadvertently overlooked, we express our sincere apology, and all necessary arrangements will be made to correct the oversight at the first available opportunity.

Second Edition

# Dedication

*In memory of my parents, Joseph and Catherine Omotomilola. Thank you for bringing me into this world; thank you for your unconditional love, your giving and caring, and your honesty. Thank you for living your lives as a language that everybody could read "by example." You were kind and served others without expecting anything in return. Thank you for teaching me to put my trust in God and not to rely on my own strength and understanding. Thank you for teaching me the importance of striving in life to serve others and to think of how I can contribute constructively to my presence here on earth. You both left a good legacy, and you touched many lives in positive ways. I pray to be able to walk in your footsteps and to do even more in my journey here on earth.*

*To my wonderful husband, Babajide, the greatest blessing that God gave me here on Earth, I say thank you. Your inspiration, patience, dedication, and support are unparalleled. Your unconditional love, belief in me, and encouragement have helped me to fulfill my dreams. I love you very much and thank God for you every day. I feel very fortunate to be your wife.*

*To my children, Tosin, Buky, and Samuel, thank you for bringing so much joy into my life. You are caring, giving, and loving. Thank you for always being there for me and for always wanting to know what you can do to make things easier for Mom. I thank God for blessing my life with the three of you.*

# Table of Contents

# Introduction

The human mind has been a mystery for ages and man is constantly inquisitive and desiring to know more about the mind. Despite all the information that we have out there, it is amazing that we uncover new information everyday. We are still thirsty and searching for more understanding, knowing fully well that there is still a lot to learn about the human mind. Whether we admit it or not, the way our mind functions has a strong effect on our total well-being.

*Winds Against The Mind* takes us on a journey into the human mind and how our mind affects our body. In this book, the in-depth understanding of the human mind is made more comprehensible and easily understandable to the everyday person, without necessarily requiring any special academic qualifications. The information is very straightforward and written from a voice of advocacy and compassion. The book encourages individuals and families to access resources and restore balance and health into their lives. The stories are captivating and real, something we can all relate to.

Each chapter opens with a short story about a person or family member facing the challenges of a specific disorder (depression, bipolar, schizophrenia, substance abuse, Alzheimer, anorexia nervosa, bulimia nervosa, autism etc), followed by the factual information about the causes, symptoms, presentation, description, treatment options, prognosis, resources, and closes with a message of hope regarding the particular illness.

The book furnishes substantial information about the complexity of the human mind, and how a disturbed mind affects our body and total well-being. *Winds Against The Mind* focuses on solutions, taking responsibility for our health, and moving toward total wellness. The importance of the psychological, medical and spiritual resources to our mental health is strongly emphasized.

Collectively, we have to continue to move away from the stigma and bias that views mental health problems as a sign of weakness, evil, or character flaws. The mention of the words "mental illness", "mental health problems", "mental health disability", or "mental health difficulties" often evokes fear, shame, and anxiety in many people. This view or perception must change because we can learn a lot about our body by knowing a lot about our mind.

The good news is science has provided us with the knowledge about the naturally occurring chemicals in the brain called neurotransmitters and how they function. When these chemicals malfunction, they can seriously affect our mental health. *Winds Against The Mind* simplifies the understanding of the effects of these chemicals on our thinking. Factors in our environment and our life experiences can also affect the way we think and view our body.

To live a healthier life and experience total wellness, we need a more in-depth, unbiased knowledge about our mental health, and not define total wellness by physical fitness alone. We have to continue to increase public understanding about mental health issues through ongoing open dialogue. If we can talk freely about diabetes and hypertension, we should be able to talk freely about depression and not be judged as weak. More open dialogue is our only hope of removing the stigma and shame attached to mental health related problems. *Wind Against The Mind* promotes this dialogue through the narration of the struggles with the human mind in the first person format by allowing the reader to empathize, visualize and experience this journey with the person in the story.

We owe it to ourselves to improve the world view on mental health issues. Collectively we can have a better world with healthier minds and bodies. The more we know the better off we are because in knowledge there is power.

## PART I

# HOW HARD IS THE WIND BLOWING?

# HOW HARD IS
# THE WIND BLOWING?

**M**any people perceive mental health problems as something that happens to other people but not to them. Unfortunately people's lives can be impaired or even devastated by some of the common mental health problems that they live with on a day-to-day basis, especially if they don't know that these illnesses are treatable. Mental health disorders affect people at different levels, but if they are not educated about these illnesses, they may not know what they are up against. My purpose in writing this book is to increase public awareness of mental health related problems, so that these disorders can be recognized, accepted without stigma, and managed.

Most societies invest in and promote physical wellness and external beauty; the truth is that complete wellness encompasses both the body and the mind working together in harmony and unity. True beauty includes both inward and outward beauty. A physically or an externally beautiful woman could be secretly dying inside from a constant battle with the eating disorder of binge eating and purging (bulimia). A handsome man with enormous physical strength could be secretly dying inside from continuous flashbacks of a traumatic experience from a war (post traumatic stress syndrome). What use is the external beauty and physical fitness when the mind feels like a troubled field with a strong tornadic wind blowing against it?

Mentally ill people are sometimes thought of as crazy people locked up behind the four walls of a mental institution. They are pictured as banging their heads on the walls, screaming and yelling at one another. This image, however, is not accurate, and the truth is that the majority of common mental health problems are the day-to-day battle of the common person within his or her own mind. Further, many people with mental health problems are unaware that they have these problems; they sincerely believe they are supposed to be like that for the rest of their lives. Why? They have no understanding about mental illness. Unfortunately, people around them misunderstand or despise them for their actions and behavior. Some sufferers are aware but are afraid to get help because they feel ashamed.

Part of the goal of writing this book is to open the eyes of the reader to these common mental health problems, with the hope that more people will seek help, once they have a better understanding of what they are dealing with.

These are the words of a divorced woman about her ex-husband; she had no knowledge about bipolar disorder or mood swings when she left her ex-husband.

*"I thought he was just wicked and crazy; he would go very quickly from very sad to very happy, from 'I love you' to 'I hate you,' and from gentleness and kindness to viciousness and rage. For a long time, I thought I was the problem, and if I would just try a little harder, then everything would be all right. I finally got to the point that I could not handle him anymore; I had to let him go. I was tired of his emotional ups and downs and the endless roller coaster. Now his illness has a name; it is called bipolar or mood disorder. He is in treatment and is now very stable and is functioning very well. What he needed when I left him was not a divorce; he needed psychiatric help. Unfortunately I did not have the information that I have about bipolar now. I am now re-married and he is now re-married, but we could still be one happy family now if I had known then what I know now about his mood swings."*

Talking about mental illness is usually an unpleasant or uncomfortable topic to discuss in many societies. Some cultures view mental illness as a weakness of the mind, and people who suffer from mental illness are seen as weak people. Others see it as a "taboo", a "curse", or a "punishment for evil". Some cultures attach terrible stigmas to mental illness, and people feel very uncomfortable around anybody perceived or believed to have mental illness.

Most of these negative public reactions to mental illness are due primarily to the lack of in-depth knowledge about it. The brain which controls the mind is an organ of the body, just like the liver, kidney, or pancreas. When people have diabetes, something could be wrong with the pancreas, and they probably would not feel ashamed to ask for insulin to control their blood sugar. Likewise, people with hypertension or high blood pressure may have a kidney that is not pumping water out of the body effectively. They probably would not be ashamed to request water pills to control their blood pressure.

However, when the brain, an organ of the body, is not functioning well, just like any other organ of the body, people may find it difficult to tell those close to them or their doctors that their minds do not feel right, or that they feel as if they are losing their minds. They may be afraid of voicing how they feel because of the negative reactions they might receive from the people around them.

Mentally ill people may not always enjoy the same public accommodation and sympathy that those with diabetes or hypertension may receive. Many people find it difficult to tolerate people with mental illness, whether it is mild, moderate, or severe. Again, the low tolerance and frustration could be due to lack of knowledge about the illness. For instance, most people are not likely to divorce their spouses because they have hypertension or diabetes, but divorce is far more likely to occur when mental illness is involved if the spouse of the mentally ill person is not knowledgeable about the illness. With the help of education regarding this type of illness, these statistics may improve because the majority of these illnesses are treatable.

These are the words of a man who divorced his wife who was suffering from flashbacks of a childhood sexual molestation experience (post-traumatic stress syndrome).

> "She told me about her childhood sexual abuse, but I thought she should be over it by now. I could not understand why a grown woman would be hiding under the bed in the middle of the night. I found this behavior very strange, and I could not continue to put up with it, so I asked her for a divorce. I now understand what was behind her actions. When she was a child, she would hide under the bed to protect herself from her abuser, although she was still dragged out from under the bed and was repeatedly raped for years. Whenever the memories came back to her, she would re-live the experience again and would try to hide from the perpetrator by hiding under the bed. I did not know how to help her at that time; I was too ashamed to discuss what I considered a strange behavior with anybody outside of my home. So I finally left her. If I had known then what I know now about post-traumatic stress disorder, I would not have divorced her."

## *Winds Against The Mind*

Most mental illnesses are usually not self-inflicted. The people suffering from the mental illness are usually victims of their dysfunctional minds or their environments, among other factors. People do not choose to be mentally ill, and mental illness is not a character flaw. The majority of the people who suffer from mental illnesses are not dangerous, evil people who deserve to be locked up by the government because they are out to hurt innocent, hardworking people.

The majority of the mild to moderate mental illnesses and traits of mental illnesses that are seriously affecting many people are primarily the day-to-day problems of the people that we love and are constantly surrounded with. They are the day-to-day problems of our children, spouses, parents, relatives, co-workers, schoolmates, friends, associates, elected officials, law-enforcement agents, teachers, actors, actresses, singers, doctors, nurses, engineers, pharmacists, accountants, philosophers, electricians, professional drivers, the homeless man standing under the bridge begging for money, and many other people from different walks of life.

These are the words of a couple who were not well informed about addiction and drugs, and who consequently ended up losing their only son to a drug overdose.

*"We live in a very good neighborhood, and we sent him to a private school, so we thought we were safe. This is the best neighborhood in the city. We never looked for the signs of drug problems in our son because we thought it could never happen to us. It did not cross our minds even once that he could have access to drugs, not to mention overdosing on drugs."*

For some people, their first real exposure to mental illness takes place when it touches them personally. There are many sources of information about mental illness available to the public, but most people seek information only when they have a tragic experience. The media, schools, and the community as a whole should help to increase the public awareness and educate the general public about mental illness. Americans are familiar with the media's coverage of HIV/AIDS (Human Immuno Deficiency Virus) and cancer; programs and more publicity should be targeted against misunderstandings about mental illness as well.

Part of the purpose of the book is to bring hope to people who suffer from mental illness, to help educate the public about mental illnesses, and to discourage negative attitudes towards the mentally ill. It is hoped that the readers will have a more sympathetic understanding of what the mentally ill are going through. The book is designed to remind the public that those who are "well" should take care of the "sick," especially those who are too sick to ask for help. It is to emphasize that some people who do not have insight into their mental problems can be dangerous because their minds have deceived them, and they must never be ignored for public safety. It is also meant to awaken people who have knowledge of their mental illness to the fact that they are responsible for their recovery; if they can realize that mental illness as an illness is not so scary, they can get help from the professionals whose knowledge and insights can improve their lives.

We cannot afford to remain in ignorance about mental illness, or to talk about it in whispers. It is everywhere. Forewarned is forearmed: the National Alliance on Mental Illness (NAMI) informs us that one in four adults in America will experience a mental health disorder in a given year, and that one in ten American children have a serious mental or emotional disorder.

Many of the victims of mental illness are fighting for their lives, and again, the battleground is the mind. Whether or not we want to accept it, the wind is blowing against a lot of minds. The question is, how hard is the wind blowing? And how hard are we going to let it continue to blow before we do something about it? Are we going to continue to watch from a distance and to stay in denial as long as we are not personally affected? Or are we going to get involved and help to increase the awareness to the reality of this debilitating illness?

Everyone can do something to minimize the way the wind is blowing against the minds of many victims out there, instead of sitting and watching the wind get stronger. People can donate money to increase the research into the study of mental illnesses, volunteer to participate in mental health research, give charitable contributions into improving mental health related problems, volunteer their time to relieve families who are taking care of mentally ill people round the clock such as Alzheimer patients, and just do something, no matter how small, to help improve the fate of the people suffering from mental illness. Love, acceptance, and support must be shown to those against whom the wind is blowing. To know how you can help, please see the lists of contact information and website addresses of National Alliance on Mental Illness (NAMI) for different states on page 365. The state organizations will help you to get in contact with your local NAMI organization.

When reading these stories, you may see traits you recognize in yourself or traits in someone you know. The goal is for all of us to get to the point where we will no longer be ashamed to talk about mental illness. Success stories and failures are discussed in the book. The reality about mental health is this: there will always be successes and failures. We do not always fail, and we do not always succeed in the treatment and management; we struggle daily in the field of mental health to understand and to manage the illness better. We hope that the day will come when we would always succeed and never have to fail again. The stories told describe the everyday experiences of real people who struggled or are struggling with mental illnesses or traits of mental illnesses that have compromised their lives. Their identities have been disguised, and the stories slightly modified to enhance the reader's understanding of the illness and its symptoms. These stories are all of our stories. One of the stories is the story of the writer. The stories reach across the divides of age group, gender, race, and socio-economic class.

If we start to pay more attention to some of the behaviors that frustrate us in our dealings with other people on a day-to-day basis, we may start to realize that such annoying behaviors could be symptoms of a mental illness not dealt with or properly diagnosed. The more understanding we have, the more we can recognize the early signs and symptoms of mental illnesses, and the more we can seek professional help for ourselves or for others.

The title of the book is taken from a poem written by a very bright schizophrenic woman, who expresses her thoughts through poetry. She does not like to talk much; her favorite phrase is, "Don't talk to me; read my poems, and my poems will talk to you about me". She wrote:

*"I am not mean, I am not evil, I am sorry if I hurt you,*
*I don't mean to hurt you; it is this voice inside my head,*
*This voice won't go away no matter how much I try to make it go away,*
*I tell the voice to go away; I even beg it to go away,*
*The voice won't listen to me, but I have to listen to the voice,*
*Forgive me if I hurt you, it is not my fault, it is the wind,*
*This voice is the wind; it is the wind that will never stop blowing,*
*It is the wind that is constantly blowing against my mind,*
*Teach me how to make the wind stop, and I will be grateful to you forever,*
*Please don't judge me; what I need from you is help,*
*Help me to make the wind go away and I will be your friend forever,*
*Help me to stop the wind from blowing against my mind,*
*And I will never hurt you again."*

Everyone can read this book, readers may choose to read some of the sections of the book that interest them, or read the entire book from start to finish. It is also intended to serve as a quick-learning resource or a reference book for students and professionals in the field of medicine, nursing, psychiatry, psychology, social work, or any mental health related field. It is also written for an international audience, because mental illness is a universal illness. Mental illness affects human beings in every race, culture, and civilization. It may be better diagnosed in some parts of the world than others simply because of more public education and awareness in certain parts of the world.

Each chapter addresses the issues in a major mental illness. First, the reader encounters the stories of the people who lived with or are still living with the illness. The true stories are followed by quotations of encouragement to the readers. The quotations were taken from *The Best of Success*, a motivational book that has been useful to the author in her clinical practice. The quotations and statements attributed to "LB," the author, are her own extrapolations from the ideas originally presented in the collections of quotations from *The Best of Success*. The third section of each chapter is a discussion of the particular illness that was portrayed in the stories.

The goal of the book is to bring an understanding of common mental illnesses to the general public. The more understanding we have, the better our intervention and outcome in the management of these illnesses will be. Again, we have to take mental illness seriously because it is the fate of the common human being, those people we run into at the grocery stores, sit next to on a plane or a bus, sit next to at the football field, and or even at home at night eating dinner. The goal is for us not to give up; we have to continue to tap into every resource available to us, including medical, psychological, and spiritual resources. We have the responsibility to strive to calm down the wind that is constantly blowing against the minds of too many people. The reality is, mental illness touches every household and every family, directly or indirectly. If you see yourself or someone you know in the book, don't feel alone or ashamed. Instead, take the next step and get help for yourself or the person you know. Remember that it is okay to have mental illness, but it is not okay to let mental illness have you. We must all remember that if we all put our resources together and act quickly, we can prevent many tragedies and have healthier mind, bodies, families, societies and nations. Reflect on the stories, and if they sound familiar to you, pursue the solutions. I hope the book is a blessing to you or someone you know.

*Winds Against The Mind*

## PART II

# COMMON PROBLEMS RELATED TO MOOD: MAJOR DEPRESSION

## Major Depression:

# MR. CONWAY'S STORY

Nancy and I had been working together for over five years and I knew her well enough to be convinced of her good character. I had been thinking of talking to Nancy about what was going on in my marriage, but I was ashamed of the situation. I had been raised in a very conservative home, and my mother had always told me that the first rule for keeping a marriage intact is not to discuss your marital problems with anyone. I have carried this burden around for over a year and could not take it anymore. I finally convinced myself that I had to talk to somebody about it before I lost my mind. I concluded that I could trust Nancy.

We were on lunch break one day at a restaurant, and I broke down in tears. Nancy was shocked because that was unlike me; I have always presented myself as a very strong person. I told Nancy that I had a very deep secret that I have been reluctant to share with anybody for the past year. She was shocked because nothing has changed in my demeanor or attitude at work to make anybody suspicious that any serious problem could be troubling me. I told her that there had not been any physical intimacy in my marriage for more than a year. Nancy was shocked and asked me if I was saying what she was thinking. Relieved to be able to express this to someone, I confirmed to her that my husband has not been willing to have sex with me for over a year now. Nancy asked me how I have been dealing with the situation emotionally, and I told her that I have focused my energy on taking care of the children.

Nancy jumped up from her seat and said, "I know exactly what is going on; it must be another woman!"

## Winds Against The Mind

I told Nancy that I had secretly followed him for six months with a rental car and found no evidence or trace of another woman. Nancy suggested that we hire a private investigator and have my husband professionally investigated.

To our surprise, the private investigator came back with the same result that there was no other woman. Nancy then suggested that I should create more excitement into my marriage—buy more sexy nightgowns, use enchanting fragrances, and plan more romantic dinners. I took Nancy's advice and tried all of the above, but nothing worked. In fact, my husband found ways to avoid going to a formal dinner outside of the house, or even having a special dinner with me at home. I was determined not to have an extramarital affair, so I planned to put all I could into our marriage and to ask for a divorce only if nothing worked.

Suddenly, I realized that I was primarily preoccupied with my own emotional neglect and feelings of rejection by my husband, and was not taking into consideration the totality of the picture of what was going on with him. I started paying more attention to some of the changes in my husband that I had refused to acknowledge.

My husband has always been generally very interested in his environment; he has always been the handyman around the house and has never believed in being idle or doing nothing when at home. Lately this same man was finding it difficult to do anything around the house. Even changing a light bulb was a challenge for him. He used to be an early riser, but gradually he had started sleeping longer, and now he was having trouble getting up in the morning or arriving at work on time. Thank heaven he has a flexible schedule; otherwise he would have lost his job.

Then I began noticing that he was gradually deviating from his usual routine, like watching the evening news and calling his family members at a certain time of the evening, especially his parents. He did not want to receive or make any phone calls, unless compulsory or an emergency. He started getting out of taking the kids to their activities, like soccer, basketball, and piano lessons. He used to be a fun dad with a lot of energy. He would wrestle on the floor with the kids, play in the yard with them, and take them to the park. Eventually he completely stopped playing with the children, who could not understand why Daddy was not spending time with them. He would be 'spaced out' at times, like he was in a different world. Essentially he was becoming completely disengaged from those around him; I was far from an isolated exception.

It was the last straw when he decided that we had to take our laundry to the dry cleaners. (One of the qualities that attracted me to my husband was his cleanliness and the fact that he always liked to do the laundry and ironing. I like to cook, but I was not too crazy about the laundry part of the domestic chores. I thought it would work out perfectly if I cooked and he cleaned.) I threw the worst temper tantrum and told him that we could not afford to take huge laundry loads to the dry cleaners with our already very tight financial budget. My husband responded in a sweet, low voice that he just did not have the energy to do the laundry anymore. It finally dawned on me that something was very seriously wrong.

In a panic-stricken state, I mentally considered a range of possible maladies. Maybe he has cancer? I hurriedly scheduled a complete physical examination with our primary care physician and also went to the appointment with him. To my surprise, the doctor mentioned that he has been calling the office a lot, complaining of discomfort and pain in different parts of his body, but he never kept any of the appointments that were scheduled for him. The doctor did a thorough work-up on him and also decided to assess him for depression. The doctor said that some of his complaints fit the perfect picture of a depressed person. The doctor gave him some questionnaires to fill out to assess him for depression. The conclusion was that he was severely depressed. He was immediately started on some medications, and the doctor also referred us to a psychiatrist for counseling and follow-up care. He went to some of the counseling sessions alone, and the psychiatrist suggested that I attend some with him.

I was shocked at some of the facts that came out during our sessions together with the psychiatrist. My husband mentioned that he had considered suicide several times when he felt so down and depressed. He said he could not go through with the suicide plan because of his family. He described his battles with feelings of grief and worthlessness inside and of not wanting to live. He said he thought he could beat it, only to realize that it was getting worse daily. He was able to share about how difficult it was to perform his daily hygiene such as showering and getting dressed for work, and how hard it was to make it through every single day at work. The only thing he wanted to do was to stay in his bed and sleep. He told the psychiatrist that he found himself drained emotionally all of the time, and he finally got to the point where he did not feel like living anymore. I had not realized the magnitude of the guilt and grief he was carrying because he could not live up to his own expectations as a father and a husband. Little did I know how close I had been to becoming a widow; he had made a suicide plan to shoot himself in the head.

He also stated that he felt like a failure in his professional life because he had not been functioning too well at work. He found it difficult to complete new assignments or to take on new projects, and he was terrified of losing his job and thus forfeiting his stable means of making a living. He worried about the financial and psychological damage of losing his job, especially on his family. He stated that some of the routine work he had been doing for years was easier to manage, but any new assignment was literarily impossible for him to accomplish. Some of his co-workers had compensated for his deficiency because of the good working relationship they have all established over the years. The co-workers had also noticed that he had not been himself, but they hadn't known what to do.

We started the long road to therapy. The doctor suggested that if there was no improvement with medication and counseling, we should consider ECT (electroconvulsive treatment) or shock treatment. ECT usually helps to relieve the incapacitation symptoms of severe depression when all other types of treatment fail. Thank heavens for all the medical knowledge; my husband's story would have been a tragic story. He has had two major relapses since the first diagnosis, but he is functioning very well with medications and therapy. He had the shock treatment once, and it was very helpful.

My husband later revealed to me that two of his extended family members committed suicide when he was younger, but they were not formally diagnosed with depression. He said he never told me about it because he was ashamed, and the family was upset and embarrassed in their community because of such losses. In all of our years of marriage I had never been told about these events by any of his family members. With his newly gained insight, my husband now recognizes that his family members who ended their own lives were experiencing similar symptoms of severe depression, but sadly, were never diagnosed and treated.

Thankfully, we have our lives back now. We still have room for improvement, but what we have now is much better than what we had with the untreated illness, and our lifestyle is getting even better every day. He is not suicidal anymore; his ability to function daily has greatly progressed. Consequently, the intimacy in our marriage has been restored, and we have a wonderful love life again.

Having gone through this illness with my husband, I cannot but wonder how many people out there are facing a similar problem and how many lives have been lost to undiagnosed depression. I am very grateful for a second chance, especially since our family has a success story. The children are much happier now that their dad is more involved in their lives. He is at the children's school for the Father's Day breakfast, he goes on field trips with them, and he is on the sidelines cheering for them when they play sports on the weekends.

All of us tend to think of mental illness as someone else's problem; we do not want to believe it could happen to us. For my family, getting medical help was a lifeline. If our family story resembles yours, do something about it before it is too late. There are many helpful resources available to you, but help may not look for you unless you look for help.

# Quotes of Encouragement...

As the wind blows harder and Mr. Conway's story sounds familiar to you, remember the following:

*"Picture yourself vividly as winning, and that will contribute immeasurably to success."*

~ *Harry Emerson Fosdick*

If you believe you can never fail, you already maximize your chance of winning; if you indeed fail, you can always try again until you succeed because your mind is already set on success. Never, never give up! Don't lose the battle to depression; declare yourself the winner by tapping into every resource available for help until you beat the blues. Tell yourself over and over again that you can do it, seek the necessary help, and do whatever it takes to fight for your life; you deserve a life sentence with happiness and freedom, not a death sentence under six feet. *(LB)*

*"He who does not hope to win has already lost."*

~ *José Joaquin Olmedo*

No matter what you are feeling or facing, don't give up; see your life as worth fighting for because you only have one chance at living. If you believe you can, you will. Believe you have won the battle against depression and you will find yourself pursuing the help you need to beat the blues. *(LB)*

*"The first step towards getting somewhere is to decide that you are not going to stay where you are"*

~ *John J.B. Morgan & Ewing T. Webb*

Don't give in to depression or it will never go away; you have a choice to not live with it by taking a positive step toward getting help and working toward recovery. Don't stay where you are; that place of hopelessness and helplessness is not a good place to be. Depression will deprive you of the joy of living and will keep you in a place of despair and sadness. Tap into the resources available to you and fight to beat this illness. *(LB)*

*Winds Against The Mind*

## Major Depression:

# MRS. ANDERSON'S STORY

Mom was very active, full of energy, and always on the go. She kept the family together, cleaned the house, helped with our homework, went to all of our school events, planned family vacations, and took us to church every Sunday, just to mention a small part of Mom's routine when we were growing up. She was so much fun and had such a natural sense of humor that we never had a boring or dull moment in the house. Mom would make us laugh all the time. We all adored her, especially my dad.

We all grew up to be very successful, well-balanced adults with successful careers; and on top of that we all have wonderful families. We children always knew that Mom and Dad were proud parents. As much as they doted on us, they always stayed busy. Both of our parents worked until they reached the retirement age; Mom retired five years after Dad.

We started noticing the changes in Mom after we all left home; she was not as happy as she used to be. We would tease her about suffering from empty nest syndrome because all the children were grown and gone. When we were in college, she was devastated if we took a summer job away from home. Through the years after college, we all kept moving farther and farther away from home in pursuit of greater opportunities.

Our moving away from home had a profound effect on our parents, especially Mom. She was always her old self all over again whenever we all came home on major holidays such as Christmas, Thanksgiving, and Easter. We were all married with children, and we looked forward to getting together during the holidays. She would feel very sad after we left, and Dad would encourage her to take on more volunteer work in the community, especially since she no longer had a career on which to focus. Mom would complain that she was not seeing her grandchildren enough, but we could not help the situation much because we all lived very far away from home. I was the closest to home, and my house was at least a nine-hour drive away from our parents.

We would encourage Mom and Dad to come for visits to spend some time with us, but unfortunately, Mom had a phobia of flying, so she would not get into a plane unless it was a life-and-death situation. Unfortunately, long-distance driving became more difficult as they grew older. We also noticed that it was getting more difficult for Mom and Dad to keep up with maintaining the house and the yard. We suggested a retirement home, but they were not receptive. We then hired a maid to clean the house, and Dad contracted out the lawn maintenance. For a while the arrangement seemed to work well for everyone.

Our father's frequent phone calls were the first red flag that something was not quite right with our mother. He always told us that he was calling us privately without letting Mom know. He expressed great concern about her because she was always sad and was not herself anymore. We suggested that she see the doctor, but she adamantly refused, telling us that nothing was wrong with her. My siblings and I decided to take turns calling the house every night and also to have the grandchildren talk to our parents. Despite all of our efforts to stay more in touch with our parents, Dad still continued to call us privately, saying that Mom was always sad and she was getting less and less interested in things that she loved to do. We all made more frequent trips home and noticed that our presence was not even making Mom feel better. We did not know how to fix the problem because Mom refused to acknowledge the existence of a problem.

I was getting ready to go to work one day when I received a frantic call from my mom. She was greatly distressed and told me that Dad had just had a heart attack. I took the next plane home to be there for them. My other siblings also came home almost immediately. The doctor said that Dad needed surgery. Fortunately, the operation was successful, and Dad was able to go back home. We were unhappy to see that Mom's sadness worsened after Dad's surgery, because she was preoccupied with the fear that Dad might die.

Unfortunately, nine months after our father's surgery, her worst fear became reality; Dad died in his sleep. The entire community rallied around Mom, especially the church family. All of us children also took turns staying with her for a few weeks. After several months, everybody moved on with their lives, and she had to face the reality of losing her beloved husband on her own. We were all very devastated and were quite worried about how our mother would be able to cope with such a loss, knowing how close they had always been. Mom and Dad had been married for forty-eight years, and they were each other's best friend.

As we had feared, Mom was completely lost without her husband, and her depression took a worse turn. She had a very hopeless, helpless outlook on life, and gradually she took herself away from the few activities in which she was involved. We brought up the issue of a retirement home again, but Mom bluntly refused to go. She was stuck in her ways. When any of her children (myself included) invited her to come for a visit, she would agree to come, but would call at the last minute to say that she had changed her mind.

On one occasion after a very persuasive conversation on my part, she finally agreed to come on the bus to visit me. It seemed that she would really come this time, and we were all quite excited. She told all her neighbors that she was going to be out of town for few weeks to spend time with her son and his family. As usual, she called us at the last minute to say that she was not coming. Unfortunately, all of her neighbors and her church members thought she was actually away this time, and they stopped checking on her.

Mom stopped going out of the house; she stopped eating and completely neglected her hygiene. She was living in a filthy environment. The pets were not fed, and she answered her phone less and less. Whenever we finally did reach her, she gave us different excuses as to why she had not been able to come to the phone. By the tone in her voice, we knew that even when she did answer the phone, she did not want to be bothered.

The last straw was the time when one of us tried to reach her continuously for two days, but she did not pick up her phone. We panicked and called her neighbors to go and check on her. They were shocked when they got to the house and found her there, because Mom had told them that she was traveling to see her son for few weeks. Subsequently, I received a telephone call from a kind woman, asking me to come down immediately and to see the situation with my own eyes. I was shocked to see my mom when I got home. She had lapsed into major depression. She was wasted, filthy, and unkempt. All of the food in the freezer and the refrigerator had expired. I was dumbfounded to see my mother, whom I had always thought of as a perfect homemaker, living in such squalor, but my greatest surprise was to discover that Mom had empty bottles of liquor and beer all over the house; apparently she had been self-medicating with alcohol to treat her depression. I was especially shocked by this because Mom had never seemed to care too much about alcohol in her younger years. Her drinking had been restricted to social events and special holidays.

Mom was immediately hospitalized on a medical floor to stabilize her medically, and was later transferred to a psychiatric floor. She was formally diagnosed with major depression, and the doctor talked to us about shock treatment or ECT (electroconvulsive treatment) if she did not respond to medication management. Fortunately, she did well with medications and therapy; she did not need ECT. Finally, Mom was convinced during a family session with all of her children present that she could not go back home. It was a very painful decision for her, especially parting with her pets. We adopted the pets and promised to bring them by to see her. Arrangements were made for her to go to a retirement center.

Watching all these events unfold, it was very difficult for us to watch Mom go through such a difficult time, especially knowing how energetic and bubbly she had been in her younger years. I now know this illness called depression, when undiagnosed and untreated, is horrible. You hear about it, but you sometimes don't know the seriousness of it until it touches you personally. As educated as we were, we knew something was amiss, but it was difficult for us to accept that the mom we knew could suffer from major depression. We thought she was strong and could handle any situation, but we were wrong. It was a different mom then and a different mom now. She reluctantly adjusted to the retirement center, and although she did have an additional hospitalization while she was living in the retirement center, she is doing very well now. With medication and follow-up counseling, she is holding on well and is close to her old self, the mom we used to know.

My siblings and I count our blessings every day; we realize how close we were to losing Mom to depression, which would have meant losing both of our parents within a short period of time. Many elderly people battle with undiagnosed depression daily and the symptoms are often mistakenly attributed merely to old age.

If your story or the story of somebody you know sounds like my mom's, don't give up hope. Depression is real. It is not a sign of weakness. Situations in life can trigger it as well as a natural or genetic predisposition for it. There is treatment for depression, and it would be sad not to do anything about it. Please get help before it is too late; it is worth it to give life a second chance.

# Quotes of Encouragement...

As the wind blows harder and Mrs. Anderson's story sounds familiar to you, remember the following:

*"This inner speech, your thoughts, can cause you to be rich or poor, loved or unloved, happy or unhappy, attractive or unattractive, powerful or weak..."*

*~ Ralph Charel*

Depression will sneak into your mind, disguising itself as your thoughts. Recognize its tricks and get help; don't allow it to germinate in your mind from a seed to a giant tree and to become the inner speech that will eventually destroy you on the outside. *(LB)*

*"Your living is determined not so much by what life brings to you, as by the attitude you bring to life; not so much by what happens to you, as by the way your mind looks at what happens."*

*~ John Homer Miller*

Let your mind search for the good in every bad situation, and you will surprisingly discover many things for which to be thankful. Your mind can dwell on all your losses or all your gains, on all the good or all the bad; what are you allowing your mind to dwell on? And what direction is your mind taking you? Make a U-turn and fight to stay in the positive lane. The negative lane will lead you into depression. *(LB)*

*"Sooner or later comes a crisis in our affairs, and how we meet it determines our future happiness and success. Since the beginning of time, every form of life has been called upon to meet such crisis."*

*~ Robert Collier*

Don't allow a crisis to push you around; see it as another tide in the ocean that will eventually calm down; look for the inner strength to keep going, and the crisis will surely pass. *(LB)*

## Major Depression:

# MOLLY'S STORY

Molly was a little overweight as a child, but not obese. She was a beautiful, happy baby. As parents, we were not concerned about her chubbiness, and we always thought she would outgrow the baby fat as she grew older. To Molly's great frustration, she retained a lot of her baby fat and continued to be chubby. By the time she was five, she was already coming home crying that other kids were making fun of her at school for being overweight. We always told her that she was beautiful and that God did not intend for everybody to be thin.

Molly was brilliant and an especially talented musician. By the time she was in middle school, she could play three musical instruments fluently. We reinforced her efforts and praised her for her academic achievements and musical talents, but unfortunately, the pressure outside of the house about her weight made it difficult for her to accept the compliments. Molly did not believe that she could be good at anything.

By the time she was ten, we noticed that she was socially withdrawn. She complained that she did not have any friends because she was overweight. She slept a lot, became irritated easily, and cried often. Molly's grades started dropping; she hated going to school and looked for every excuse to miss school. As her parents, we tried to be very supportive, thinking this was a phase she would work through.

As a family routine in the house, we talked at the dinner table about the events of the day and other issues affecting our lives inside and outside of the home. Molly constantly talked about popularity issues at her school, and described how some kids were classified as popular, and some were classified as unpopular losers.

## Winds Against The Mind

Molly was classified as unpopular, and she was treated very badly by her schoolmates because she was overweight. She was called terrible names, and she was teased a lot. When she was in high school, she broke down one night because somebody wrote a cruel poem entitled "Molly the Fat Mama," and pasted it on her school locker. Several kids read it before she saw it on her locker and could remove it. Everybody was laughing and joking about it all day long in school. We suggested the possibility of transferring to another school, but Molly was reluctant to change schools.

The following school year she broke her arm and had difficulty carrying her school bag, and no one would help her because they did not want to be seen with a fat girl. Molly got more depressed and got a little paranoid and suspicious of others; she was always thinking that other people were talking about her weight. She woke up in the night with nightmares and felt hopeless, helpless, and worthless. She talked negatively about herself all the time. She saw the world as a horrible place. The bullying and the teasing continued, and we finally decided to talk to the principal and the guidance counselor of the school, against Molly's advice. The principal was honest with us and said that such behavior was common in the school, but promised to talk to some of the students involved with the teasing and the name calling. The school principal's conversation with these unkind students worsened the situation for Molly; she was called a 'mama's girl' and 'a whiner' and was treated worse than before.

At the end of that school year, we decided to change Molly to another school against her wishes. As parents, when your child is hurting and unhappy, you share the pain and anguish and desperately want to fix the problem. Unfortunately, the new school was not any help either; the shadow quickly followed her from her former high school. Within a few days in the new school, she was approached by another set of unkind teens; they laughed in her face and told her they had already heard that she was the biggest loser in her old school. The problem continued, and we watched Molly get worse by the day, without knowing how to help our precious daughter.

Molly tried to use humor to cope occasionally. She would crack jokes at times that she would need her bedroom at the family house forever because no man would want a fat woman. One winter evening Molly came home and burst into inconsolable tears. Apparently another student had put a sticker on her jacket with some "fat" jokes written on it, and she had been the laughing stock of the school all day long. She had noticed that people laughed each time she had walked by, but she had not understood why they were laughing. Molly was so accustomed to being teased that she hadn't pursued it further. When she finally took off her jacket at home, she saw the sticker with the jokes on the back of her jacket and was utterly devastated. We thought of pulling her out of school completely and homeschooling her, but we were worried about isolating her even further.

We also noticed that she ate a lot when she was at home in order to cope with her emotional pain. Food became a medication and a comfort for her, which, of course, became a vicious cycle because she ballooned and gained more weight.

Molly was always cautious about eating in school around other students. Some of these cruel schoolmates watched her plate at mealtime to see how much food she would eat, so that they could make fun of her. She would hide her food and sometimes go to the bathroom to eat. She was tortured daily just because she was overweight.

Molly was an enthusiastic football fan, and she tried not to miss any of her school's football games. One night she went to watch the championship game, the biggest game of the year, and Molly had been especially looking forward to it. During the game, one of the students cracked a joke that the huge football players with their enormous football pads weighed less than Molly, and everybody started laughing at her. She tried to ignore the laughter at first, but after a while Molly could no longer tolerate the teasing. Somehow this was the last straw for her.

She came home and locked herself in her room, telling us that life was not even worth living. We got really scared and talked to her, but she assured us that she was fine, that she just wanted to be alone.

My husband has a long history of clinical depression, and because he was overweight in younger years, he faced some of the same issues with teasing as Molly. My husband's depression was not as severe as Molly's; he was not picked on as much as Molly. He was able to survive both high school and college, where we met. After college my husband was diagnosed with clinical depression, and he was well managed on medication. Although my husband has a strong family history of clinical depression on both sides of his family, somehow it did not occur to us that Molly could be suffering from clinical depression, apart from the situational-induced depression she was suffering from in the hands of the school bullies. We certainly weren't ignoring her pain, but we truly thought that solving the bully problems at school would help improve Molly's mood, so we focused our efforts on the situation at school.

It finally dawned on us that Molly might also be battling clinical depression, and if so, adding situational depression to it would be a double jeopardy. We decided to seek a professional help for Molly immediately. We knew then that our parental support alone could not take care of the situation.

We scheduled an appointment with a psychiatrist for the following week, and in the meantime we decided that Molly should take some time off from school until after her appointment with the psychiatrist. Unfortunately, Molly never made it to her appointment. My husband and I went to work one morning and left her in bed to sleep late. We called the house several times later in the afternoon to check on her, and at first there was no answer. Later on, she answered the phone and told us that she had gone for one of her usual long walks to reflect on some issues. We came home from work and knocked on the door to her room to see if she was all right, she answered and said that she just needed some time alone. When it was time for dinner, she did not come out to eat dinner, which was unlike Molly; she always looked forward to sitting down and venting her frustrations to us at dinnertime.

My husband grew suspicious and broke into her room. We found Molly cold, stiff, and with no pulse; she had overdosed on pills. We called 911 the emergency service; they did everything they could do to revive her, but it was too late—Molly was dead. Molly left a note, telling us she was sorry. She wrote that she had decided there had to be a better place other than this world. She also left a note for the schoolmates who drove her to her death, saying that she hoped she would be their last victim and that they would not drive another overweight child to her grave like they did to her. She also stated in her note that they must not come to her funeral or her ghost would haunt them.

Our daughter's story did not have a happy ending, and it really hurts. My husband and I spent time trying to figure out if Molly died from situational depression, or if she had clinical depression coupled with situational depression. Our greatest regret was that we did not seek professional help for Molly early enough. Our efforts with the school principal and guidance counselor had ended in such failure as we were trying to handle the situation on our own.

We thought about what we could have done differently, such as relocating to a new environment just to save our child. We were busy with details of our own lives, especially with our jobs, and we never thought Molly could get depressed to the point of killing herself. We felt as though we failed Molly, and we went through a lot of self-blaming. Therapy helped us to work through the difficult days, especially the days when we did not feel like waking up the next day.

We hope Molly's story will serve as a wake-up call for other parents. Whether it is situational or clinical depression, the most important point is to take any sign of depression in your child seriously. We did the best we could with our limited knowledge, but in hindsight, we know we definitely could have done more by seeking professional help for her sooner. We completely ignored Molly's genetic predisposition to be depressed, despite the fact that we know that depression runs very strongly in my husband's family. Perhaps because Molly was a child, we just didn't consider the possibility of such an illness at her young age. We focused on the situational factors only. A possible undiagnosed clinical depression probably made the situational depression more unbearable and probably pushed Molly to the edge.

We will never find out what made Molly's depression worse, whether it was situational, genetic, or both. Whatever the case may be, depression is depression, and there is not a good type of depression; any signs of depression must be taken seriously. We have learned that it is very common for adults to overlook the fact that a child could be depressed due to a chemical imbalance from a genetic predisposition. Now we know that the goal is not to take anything for granted; we cannot assume that children can always beat their emotional problems.

Some of the schoolmates who drove Molly to her grave wrote us letters of apology, claiming they did not understand the extent of the psychological damage they had caused Molly with their jokes. They thought they were just being "funny." To us, as Molly's parents, it will always be sad; it will never be funny because Molly will never come back home again. We will never hear our daughter laugh again on this earth.

We allowed something good to come out of Molly's death. We volunteered to talk with school children about depression and about the devastation of bullying and teasing other kids, especially when they have an attribute that can distinguish them as being "different." We also organized parent conferences to educate families on the passive signs and symptoms of depression in children that can be easily ignored. We emphasized the need for parents to educate their children to be responsible with their jokes and to be tolerant of others. Unkind comments made at the expense of someone else are not funny—they are cruel. We should never underestimate the impact that such remarks might have on someone. In Molly's case, they caused her death, and a bright, talented young girl was lost. With more parental involvement and tougher standards and consequences from the school authorities, the bullying situation could be kept under control. Our hope is that another child will not have to lose his or her life to mental torture and depression like Molly, be it clinical or situational depression. If Molly reminds you of your child or a child that you know out there, do something before it is too late.

*Winds Against The Mind*

# Quotes of Encouragement...

As the wind blows harder, and Molly's story sounds familiar, remember the following:

*"The greatest power that a person possesses is the power to choose."*

*~ J. Martin Kohe*

Remember to make wise choices. Do not allow the situation or circumstance to choose for you; choose life instead of death; you must not give anybody enough power to drive you to your grave. You have only one chance to live; hold on to your life; whatever situation you are facing, you can change it only when you are alive. *(LB)*

*"These then, are my last words to you, be not afraid of life, believe that life is worth living, and your belief will help create the fact."*

*~ William James*

You cannot afford to trade your life for death; it is a one-way transaction; once dead, the transaction is completed and irreversible. Choose life. *(LB)*

*"No one can make you feel inferior without your consent."*

*~ Eleanor Roosevelt*

Love yourself for who you are; you are not a mistake of God's creation. You are the apple of His eye; you are uniquely created, wonderfully put together; He made you exactly the way He wants you to be. God is the greatest artist; His creativity and love of variety can be seen everywhere around us. Celebrate your uniqueness with pride; if what you look like bothers anybody, let it be their problem, not yours. *(LB)*

43

## Major Depression:

# BASIC FACTS & UNDERSTANDING

M r. Conway, Mrs. Anderson, and Molly all suffered from major depression. *Depression* is a mental illness that affects our mood. A depressed mood may manifest in the form of prolonged sadness, with the individual giving up on life. Victims of depression may feel totally discouraged about everything, wearing a sad facial expression called a *flat affect.* They may lack the ability to derive pleasure in things that were formerly pleasurable to them. This is referred to as *anhedonia.* Such activities may include sports, family functions, eating out, going to the movies, going to church or work, gardening, cooking, sex, working around the house, watching television, and many other enjoyable pursuits.

Anxiety is also very common in depression. Victims may be fearful, full of dread, sweat, have palpitations (racing heartbeat), anticipate danger, have a rapid pulse, complain of chest pain and of having butterflies in their stomach. Changes in appetite could manifest as eating too much (overeating) or eating too little (anorexia). Changes in bowel habits are also very common; they could complain of feeling constipated or having frequent diarrhea.

Sleeping disturbance is one of the major symptoms of depression; the victims may report having difficulty falling asleep and then struggling with turning and tossing all night long. Others may report waking up frequently in the night, having horrible nightmares and feeling very tired in the morning. As a result of the sleeplessness, they may have difficulty in getting out of bed in the morning.

Depressed people usually feel tired (*anergia*), despite the fact that they have not engaged in any strenuous or difficult activity. They may state that they feel "beaten up" or "run down," and they have a tendency to believe that these feelings are caused by a serious illness or something terminal that would eventually kill them. They may be perceived as very lazy by the people around them who have no knowledge or understanding of what major depression is. Feelings of fatigue or tiredness can make small tasks difficult, such as brushing the teeth, showering, and other general grooming or daily hygiene.

Problem solving skills may diminish. Judgment may be very poor, and a lot of indecisiveness may be observed — they may not be able to make up their minds on what to do in any situation. They may feel like their mind is slowing down on them (called *slow thought process*), and speech may be slow. Their gaze may be fixed — you may see them staring at the same point for hours. Their action and reaction time could be slow, and the body movement could be very slow as well. This feeling of everything slowing down in the body is referred to as *psychomotor retardation*. On the other hand, a depressed person may experience what is called *psychomotor agitation*, which is manifested as a sense of restlessness, feeling fidgety or tense. The person just cannot relax. Psychomotor agitation is very common in the elderly people experiencing major depression, causing them to be very combative and physically aggressive at times.

A depressed person may feel inadequate in everything; she may blow every mistake she makes out of proportion and be extremely self-critical. She may need constant reassurance and continuous reinforcement to feel good about her achievements. Some depressed people experience serious difficulty concentrating. Watching television, sitting through a movie, reading a book, or sitting through a lecture in a classroom may become very difficult. They may not be able to follow a general conversation; they may have difficulty remembering things and may find it difficult to pay attention to their environment. Feelings of worthlessness and low self-esteem are common in depressed people; these feelings and traits can pose a big problem at school or at work.

Feelings of hopelessness and helplessness are also very common with depressed people. The future may seem doomed; their cup is always seen as half-empty and never seen as half-full. They can never see the light at the end of the tunnel. As a result, they may turn to drugs and alcohol to self-medicate in an effort to try to get rid of the feelings of doom and severe sadness that they are experiencing.

46

Suicidal thoughts or strong desires to kill themselves are very common in severely depressed people, and some may eventually carry out the suicide plan if there is no quick or adequate intervention. Some people are at a higher risk for suicide when their depression is lifted; this may be because the depressed person's outlook to life is still very negative, and gaining enough energy provides just enough of a lift to carry out the suicidal plan.

*Somatic* complaints (which are frequent complaints of not feeling well with no documentation of a verifiable medical problem by a physician or a clinician), may be a sign that a person is depressed. The victim may confuse the depressed feelings with physical problems. Frequent visits to the doctor's office with complaints such as headaches, chest pain, constipation, back ache, muscle pain, stomach ache, heartburn, and shortness of breath are very common. All medical examinations, laboratory studies, X-rays, and diagnostic tests always come back negative, showing that there is nothing wrong with the client medically. Lack of organic or medical reasons for the illness is usually a red flag for primary care physicians or other health care providers to evaluate the comprehensive history more thoroughly and to rule out other factors that may cause frequent somatic complaints of pain everywhere. Once it is confirmed that there is no medical basis for these somatic complaints, the physician or the clinician can then look into the possibility that the client may be experiencing major depression.

*similar to schizophrenia.*

A depressed person may be *psychotic* (sense of losing one's mind or losing touch with reality). He may experience *auditory hallucination* (hearing voices that are not there), or *visual hallucination* (seeing things that are not there). *Paranoia* is also common, which is a strong belief or feeling that somebody is trying to hurt him or come after him. He may be *delusional*, which is usually manifested in irrational beliefs, and it may be difficult to convince him that his belief is not rational. For example he may have the irrational thought that he is being punished by God for something he has done in the past, and this is why he has to suffer from depression.

A person experiencing major depression may not necessarily experience all of the symptoms already discussed, but may experience the majority of the symptoms for an extended period of time. Some people also suffer from a milder to a moderate form of depression. They may be able to function and still experience some of the symptoms discussed above but to a milder degree. Some may also suffer from *dysthymia,* which is a very low grade of depressed feeling extending over a long period of time. Some people may experience seasonal depression, which may come on in the colder time of the year such as the winter time, and their depression may lift in the warmer time of the year such as the summer time. Major depression affects people in most societies; it is believed that more people are affected in colder climates. Major depression also affects both males and females, irrespective of their ethnicity, race, income, and education.

Depression is believed to be more common in women, and this is partly attributed to their monthly cyclic changes or menstruation. Another form of depression that is gaining more attention lately among women is called *postpartum depression*, which usually happens shortly after the birth of a baby. It has a similar classic picture with major depression. The victim could be *psychotic* (sense of losing one's mind or losing touch with reality) or *delusional* (a fixed false belief that is held to be true by an individual experiencing the belief despite evidence to the contrary; the belief is not shared by the rest of the culture or the community). If postpartum depression is not quickly recognized and carefully treated, the consequences could be fatal. In very severe cases, the victims may have a nervous breakdown. They may be extremely suicidal. The psychosis and the delusions may also lead them to commit suicide and even to kill their children. Women experiencing postpartum depression may require immediate hospitalization.

One of the most important causes of major depression is the biological theory called the *neurotransmitter theory*. The brain is made up of many tiny cells called *neurons*. These cells are in continuous communication with one another. The communication between the cells or the neurons is like the big network of a complex wiring system, working around the clock whether we are awake or asleep. Messages are sent between the cells by some chemicals that are naturally produced in the brain called *neurotransmitters*. The messages are sent by what is called *electrical impulse*. When these chemicals are found in abnormal level, either too much or too little, or there is a dysfunction or a problem in any of the communication pathways between the cells, or a malfunction within the cell itself, people may show signs of mental illness. With major depression, some of the neurotransmitters are believed to be at an abnormally low level in the brain. When the neurotransmitters occur in the right amount and the communication system of the brain is working together in harmony, a person would appear stable, and the mind will function normally.

*causes: hereditary, bio-factor/neurotransmitters, environment, situational/ life events, genetic predisp.*

Major depression could also be *hereditary* (meaning passed down from one generation to the next, or from a parent to a child through the gene). Twin studies support the view that both identical twins are likely to have major depression as compared to fraternal twins. One of the fraternal twins may have major depression, and the other twin may not. Generally, identical twins are expected to have the same genetic code or be a mirror image of each other as opposed to fraternal twins who may not even look alike. Hereditary factors could also be strong in fraternal twins; it is just believed to be stronger in identical twins because of the mirror image and same gene similarities. People with major depression always have a strong family history with family members suffering from, or having suffered from, major depression in the past.

Life events may also trigger major depression; this may be particularly worse for a person with a *genetic predisposition* (that is, depression runs in the family and has been passed down from one generation to the next) to be depressed. Depression triggered by an unfortunate life event is called *situational depression* (that is, the depression was brought about by an unfortunate life event that happened to the person at that particular time in his or her life). A good example would be the death of a spouse or a child. A stressful life situation or personal stress can trigger changes in the composition of some of the naturally occurring chemicals in the brain called *neurotransmitters.* This may in turn affect the victim's feelings, causing him or her to be depressed. If a depression is strictly triggered by a life stressor, when the trigger or the stressor is removed or resolved, the person may return to normal functioning level. For example, losing a job of thirty-five years may trigger depression; finding a better job with more pay, better working conditions, and more benefits may resolve the depression.

Environmental factors may also contribute to major depression. Being surrounded with negativity all of one's life can affect the person's outlook on life, producing feelings of hopelessness, worthlessness, and doom.

*dx*

Diagnosis and treatment of major depression must be made by a licensed clinician with sufficient medical knowledge, training, and certification in the area of psychiatry, medicine, psychology, or nursing, or any other properly licensed clinician who is qualified to make such a diagnosis in the sufferer's community. A lot of factors are considered in making the diagnosis; these may include but are not limited to the client's health history, family history, psychological and social history, duration or length of the problem, and environmental history.

A combination of treatments is used in the management of major depression. These include medication management, individual therapy, group therapy, and rehabilitation. There are several medications used for the treatment of major depression; the type of medication that is appropriate for each person must be strictly determined by a licensed clinician based on the person's history.

It is very important to assess a depressed person for suicide. Appropriate action must be taken to prevent suicidal clients from killing themselves. A suicidal person's thinking is usually irrational; the individual may be too sick or too depressed to make a sensible decision and the only solution or relief they can see to solving the problem is death. People in these circumstances have convinced themselves that death would put an end to their pain, suffering, and feelings of doom. It must be taken very seriously if a suicidal person has a plan to carry out a suicidal act, such as having a loaded gun. A suicidal person may require hospitalization. *Psychosis* (sense of losing one's mind or losing touch with reality) must be taken seriously in a depressed person who is suicidal. As mentioned earlier, extra caution must be taken with a person suffering from postpartum depression and also suicidal as well. A depressed person may respond to an *auditory hallucination* (hearing a voice or voices that are not there), telling the person to take his own life or the lives of others.

*Electroconvulsive treatment (ECT)* or shock treatment is used as a last resort when a person does not respond to medication treatment. It could also be used in addition to medication to produce a better result in severely depressed people. People who are allergic to medications may also receive only shock treatment or ECT for the treatment of their depression. In administering ECT, a very mild electric shock is passed to the brain through a special electrode to induce a mild, artificial seizure in the person. The seizure activity in the brain in turn helps to normalize or correct the imbalance in the quantity of some of the neuro-transmitters (the naturally occurring chemicals in the brain serving as messengers between the cells or the neurons) that have been produced in abnormal proportion (too low or too much), causing the person to be depressed. Clients may suffer from mild, temporary forgetfulness called *amnesia* after ECT, but they usually have their memory back in a very reasonable and short period of time. ECT does not require hospitalization; it can be done as an outpatient treatment. It is not recommended that one drive immediately after ECT, especially because of the mild forgetfulness. ECT is relatively safe; many people are scared and discouraged about ECT because of what they have seen in the media, especially on

TV and movies. ECT has gone through years of scientific, technological modification and reform, and it is not the scary procedure as is sometimes portrayed by the media. A clinician will thoroughly explain and educate clients and their families before recommending ECT or shock treatment. ECT is strictly done by a licensed physician who is trained to administer ECT.

Individual therapy is also helpful in the treatment of depression. This is a one-on-one therapy with a clinician. It can be a short or long-term treatment. The therapist usually helps the clients identify, examine, and resolve the conflicts affecting their lives and their thinking during the depressed period. The therapist also helps the client to explore positive ways to look at life, cope with unpleasant situations, and make wise decisions.

The importance of group therapy cannot be overemphasized in the treatment of major depression. Group therapy provides a great deal of support for the clients. Clients are able to realize that they are not alone and that other people in the world are suffering from depression just as they are. There is mutual understanding of a common struggle in the group. Members of the group openly discuss their problems and describe their individual styles of dealing with their depression. People are able to learn new social skills, improve their self-esteem, form positive bonds, and have a sense of community in the group setting.

A family support group may also be beneficial for the family members of depressed people. Listening to other people living with someone with this illness will provide better insight into the problems. Families can also rely on one another for support and understanding. As mentioned earlier, people suffering from depression can be perceived as lazy and not motivated. The family members may not understand why the person is feeling this way and why they cannot just "beat it" or "shake it off." Attending a family support group can help the family in learning how to support the depressed person and one another without becoming enmeshed and feeling sorry for the depressed person and one another to the point of having an unhealthy family relationship or family dynamics. Such an unhealthy family dynamic is called *codependency*.

Other types of treatment for major depression include light therapy, which is used mainly for people with seasonal depression. People with seasonal depression are usually depressed in seasons of shorter days and longer nights, which occur more in the colder time of the year in the very cold climates. The goal is to expose them to several hours of bright artificial lights during the days of shortened sunlight. Light therapy has produced good results with seasonal depression.

Exercise is recommended in the treatment of major depression because of its profound effects in reducing stress. Healthy eating habits are also recommended in the treatment of major depression. Balanced, healthy nutrition will help the body to function better. As mentioned earlier, depressed people may consume excessive alcohol to self-medicate, use illicit drugs, or eat excessively to ease their pain. Some may just quit eating. As a result, the body will be deprived of the appropriate nutrients or the body will be provided with excessive nutrients in case of overeating. Unhealthy eating habits are self-destructive and are obviously not helpful to depressed people. This is why a very healthy, balanced nutrition plan must be incorporated into the treatment plan.

Having major depression is not a sign of weakness or something to be ashamed of. Not doing something about depression is the sign of weakness. Depression is one of the most common and one of the most undertreated mental illnesses. A lot of people do not seek help for major depression, especially males in certain societies where men are expected to be strong and never show any sign of weakness or emotion. Some people experiencing depression are also clueless about what is going on within their minds. They know something is not right, but they cannot figure out exactly what is wrong with them. They cannot put a name to what is causing this unusual feeling. Some people also believe that depression is something they can overcome on their own, and they struggle daily to make it go away. With appropriate intervention, prescribed medication, therapy, support group, and all of the suggested treatment approaches discussed, a person diagnosed with major depression can have a normal life. If reading about depression is telling you something about yourself, or others that you know, do not ignore it, get help and help others as well.

PART III

# COMMON PROBLEMS RELATED TO MOOD: BIPOLAR OR MOOD DISORDERS

# Bipolar:

# ANGELA'S STORY

My memories of growing up in my home are not happy. Living with my mother could sometimes be compared with living in hell. I did not know that what my mom was experiencing all those years was mood swings or *bipolar disorder*. Mom had some moments that she would cook, clean, mop the floor over and over again, work in the garden, quilt, sew, repair things around the house and she would keep going for hours without taking a break. This happy, elated, energetic movement would go on for days; Mom would require little or no sleep or food; she would sew and quilt throughout the night. Sometimes she would wake all of us up by singing very loudly during the night. In her happy mood, she would tell us how much she loved us and would give us frequent treats and rewards for every little effort on our part.

At the end of this time of heightened happiness, called a *manic phase*, Mom would lapse into her depressed phase. She would get angry with us for no obvious reason. She would overreact to every little mistake we made and would whip or beat us. She would curse at us and call us bad names, telling us she regretted ever bringing us into this world. Mom required more sleep during her depressed or down phase. She would go through a period of sadness mixed with anger, and she would stay in bed for days and totally neglect us. We were always happy when she had low energy and slept for days after exhausting herself. This was because she left marks on our body from beating us when she was cranky, and it was always a relief when she was too tired to beat us.

We were very confused growing up; we could not predict which side of the bed our mother would wake up on from day-to-day; nor could we predict what her behavior would be toward us each day. I was the oldest of five children. I have three brothers and a sister. Our dad worked in the factory. He left very early in the morning and came back very late at night. Dad had no clue about what was going on in the house most of the day. Being the oldest, I had to grow up very quickly. When Mom was in her depressed phase, we were totally neglected. I had to get up very early in the morning, get my younger siblings ready for school, and prepare breakfast for all of us so that we could wait outside for the school bus. This is the story of our lives, growing up in the midst of confusion. We did not realize that Mom's up and down cycle was an illness. We just prayed that Mom would have more good days than bad days. Occasionally when Dad was home and Mom was having her usual bad days, she would make his life miserable, pick a fight with him, and even threaten to divorce him. Dad was very patient with her. He was equally clueless about Mom's illness. Dad did not have much education; he was a very quiet, laid-back man. The family accepted Mom for who she was; we all assumed that other moms were like her, too. We all believed that this was how mothers were supposed to be because this was the only life we knew. We grew up in a very chaotic environment.

With all the confusion and dysfunction, I was able to survive, but little did I realize that I had inherited Mom's gene. As a teenager, I would work two jobs, make a lot of money, and go on a spending spree to spend it all. I was having up and down days just like Mom. I called in sick at work a lot on my down days, because I was too tired to get out of bed, but I was a very hardworking employee on my up or manic days. I was so super efficient on my manic days that my employers would literarily overlook my calling in sick when I was depressed or down. I was very hypersexual as a younger adult, and I went from one boyfriend to another. I would date two or three boys at the same time in order to meet my insatiable sexual appetite on my manic days.

Despite my mood swings, I was able to make it through college and earn an accounting degree. I got a lot done with my school work on my up days to compensate for my down days. I met my husband in college; he majored in business administration. We both got high-paying jobs after college, and got married a year after graduation.

I thought I would finally be able to settle down. I blamed all my previous hypersexual and frivolous behavior on the "girls just want to have fun" ideology. I rationalized and justified my behavior as going through the youthful phase of my life. I called it what teenagers do and what college kids do, and thought I would be different as soon as I settled down and was happily married.

Unfortunately, some of my earlier behavior still continued after I got married. In my manic phase, I would have an insatiable sexual desire and would beg my husband to call in sick at work so that we can both stay home and have sex. I would have a lot of grandiose ideas such as wanting to start a new business or to change my profession. I would go on shopping sprees, and run up our bills. My husband and I had several talks about my spending sprees, and I would apologize and try to justify my actions. Finally, I volunteered to take on a second job to offset some of the bills I ran up. In no time, I found myself having extramarital affairs because my husband could not meet my insatiable sexual desire during my manic phase. I would even shoplift at times, but I was never caught.

During my depressed or down phase, getting up in the morning would become a problem just as it was in my teenage and college days. I would brew dark, thick coffee and drink several cups, just to get enough energy to get myself on my feet and make it to the office and back for the day. I found myself living my mom's life all over again and picking fights with my husband for no reasonable purpose. I also spent a lot of time sleeping in my down phase, just like my mom. Fortunately, we did not have any children at present; I probably would have put them through a miserable life like my mom did to us. I could sense the frustration in my husband, but he loved me very much and just believed that his unconditional love would pull us through and would help me to change. He thought it was a maturity issue, and I needed more time to make the transition from a college kid to a married adult.

My husband finally took control of our finances, which was very frustrating for me. I then came up with another plan, which was to manipulate figures and embezzle money at my job. I started initially with embezzling little amounts of money, and gradually increased it because I was getting away with it. I would buy things and hide them. Whenever my husband found out, I would tell him a bogus story about the bonus I always got because of my productivity at work. I made up the story that the bonus was an incentive that was built into my work, and it was separate from my salary. My husband knew I was lying, but he could not prove it. He would demand to see the bonus check, and I would get into a big fight with him for not trusting me.

Finally, I was caught at work for stealing and embezzlement, and found myself facing criminal charges with the possibility of going to jail. My employer worked out a deal with me because everybody loved me and valued my productivity. I was put on probation, allowed to keep my job, and required to pay back the money.

I was also advised to seek professional help. I was referred to a psychiatrist. During my appointment with the psychiatrist, I broke down and talked about these uncontrollable up and down feelings I have been dealing with all of my life. He asked me several questions and concluded that I suffered from bipolar or mood disorder. Now I have a diagnosis; I have been suffering from bipolar disorder or mood swings all these years. I now understand that what Mom was experiencing was bipolar disorder, and that I had inherited it from her.

Many issues came out during my counseling sessions, and I wondered how I had even made it this far. My husband and I also had couple counseling. I did not realize how much pain I had caused him, to the point that he had contemplated divorce several times. He said he could not make himself go through with the divorce because he loved me very much. It really hurts to realize how much I had put my husband through, and how close I was to destroying my marriage and career. Two of my brothers are always having run-ins with the law and are usually in and out of the jail system. Now I know what their problems are; they have bipolar disorder that is undiagnosed and untreated. I am working hard to get help for them.

My dad died suddenly during my final year of college, and my mom died two years later. My dad always took care of my mom. I believe Mom probably died because she could not take care of herself during her severely manic or depressed phase. I am doing well with medication and therapy, and I am thankful for the blessing of having a second chance to live a functional life. Reflecting on my life makes me wonder how many people in the world are dealing with similar issues and are walking around with absolutely no insight as to why they are behaving the way they are.

Bipolar disorder is such a devastating illness that it takes over your life. The sad thing is you may not even know that you have an illness. Who wants to complain when they are happy? The manic phase of the illness is like getting high without the influence of drugs. You enjoy the happy feeling and want to keep it that way forever, if possible. The depressed phase is the only time you hate who you are and sometimes want to die. If your story sounds like mine, or you see a reflection of yourself or someone you know, please get help. Do not allow this illness to destroy you or your loved ones. Help is available, and it is never too late to get help. Nobody should be living with bipolar; please do something about it.

# Quotes of Encouragement...

As the wind blows harder and Angela's story sounds familiar to you, remember the following:

*"We lie loudest when we lie to ourselves."*

~ *Eric Hoffer*

Denial is a powerful ingredient in bipolar disorder; victims of this illness always believe that they can handle it. They do not want to give up the manic phase because of the heightened happiness; the first step to success is to accept the illness and then to move to the next step of getting all necessary help towards stabilization and recovery. *(LB)*

*"Success... my nomination for the single most important ingredient is energy well directed."*

~ *Louis B. Lundborg*

The heightened energy during the manic phase could be self-destructive or self-improving; direct your energy to self-improve and allow something good to come out of a bad situation. *(LB)*

*"History has demonstrated that the most notable winners usually encountered heartbreaking obstacles before they triumphed. They won because they refused to be discouraged by their defeats."*

~ *B.C. Forbes*

You can win only when you do not give up; you may fumble along the way, see it as a growth process and do not be discouraged. Stay the course until you get it right and take advantage of every resource for improvement, until you improve. *(LB)*

# MR. LADSON'S STORY

It happened that my husband had to go to a conference in Las Vegas, and I was so concerned, knowing the problems he has with gambling and spending sprees that I talked him into letting us use the trip as a family vacation. I have always taken my marriage vows very seriously, including when I said, "for better or for worse." I struggled over the years to keep this marriage together, but the struggles seemed to have no end. I wanted to raise our children in a home with both parents, and our religion frowned upon divorce. Several times I wrestled with making a choice between getting a divorce or ending up as homeless with the children one day just because of my husband's out-of-control spending during his manic phase (heightened happiness). My only purpose for going to Las Vegas was to keep an eye on our family money. I love Las Vegas, but a Las Vegas vacation was not at the top of my list!

We got to Las Vegas, and I tried very hard to monitor my husband's movements and spending. As usual, he found a way to max out all his credit cards in order to keep gambling. Four days into our vacation, he asked me to sign documents to set up an equity line of credit on our house so that he could cash out some money to gamble. He was frantically trying to convince me that he would win some money, pay back all the debts, plus win some extra money for us to spend.

We got into the biggest fight, and I refused to sign the papers. I threatened a divorce and told him that I would sign divorce papers if he could make them as readily available as the papers he had produced to take out an equity line of credit for gambling.

I worried all the time about how much longer I could stay in this marriage because he did not seem to understand the seriousness of our situation or the implications of his behavior on the family. No matter how much I tried to explain to him how irresponsible his behavior was, he would still repeat it. My husband would go through this manic phase of buying expensive things that we could not afford.

He would buy expensive gifts for me as well, knowing that our budget could not accommodate them. I had to take items back to the store for a cash refund on numerous occasions. He bought a gold wrist watch for me one time as a Valentine's Day gift. It was beautiful, but if I had kept it, we would not have been able to pay our bills for three months. I had to return it and begged the jewelry store to take it back from me. They were reluctant to do so because they had some strict conditions for their jewelry purchases. I was relieved when they finally took it back.

He would come home and try to convince me to accept different payment plans that he had arranged for large purchases. I always wondered how he planned to meet the conditions for the multiple payment plans that he took out all the time. I am grateful to live in a country where you can return purchases if you change your mind and get your money back. I remember another day when he came home with a brand new car. He said when he read about the car, he knew it was a must for us to have as a family. I was so upset because we were already struggling to pay two car payments. Why did we need another car with another payment to go with it? I went through hell to convince the dealer to take back the car. I was living every day in fear and anxiety, not knowing what he was going to do next.

The problem was not limited to his gambling; he would go for nights without sleep, and he would be extremely restless. He would get agitated very easily and would also become incoherent. He would sometimes say things that would not make any sense, and he would appear to be talking to himself. I later found out that those episodes were probably *psychotic episodes*, which are periods of time in which a person loses touch with reality, but at that time I had no idea why he was behaving in such odd ways.

He would get into fights in public places, which caused numerous embarrassments for the family. He would go to the children's sports activities like soccer, football, or basketball games and would pick fights with the coaches or the referees. The children always begged him not to come to their games because they feared what he might do to embarrass them.

One summer, we went on a family vacation to a large, popular amusement resort. We planned this vacation for three years, and the children looked forward to it. While we were there, my husband got into a physical fight at the park over something inconsequential. The police and the security guards had to arrest him.

On other occasions, he would snap at the children for no reason, and he would get violent and slap me sometimes in the presence of the children. The next minute, he would be apologetic, and would even cry for forgiveness. For every "up" moment for him, there would always be a "down" moment. He would be the most loving, caring, and generous husband in his manic phase, and then would switch to be the meanest, evil, uncaring person, using every vulgar curse word you could think of.

He would go through a phase where he would need a lot of sleep, and would struggle with getting up in the morning to go to work. Several mornings he left for work with poor personal hygiene—without brushing his teeth or combing his hair. His clothes would be wrinkled, but if you tried to suggest cleaning up a bit, he would snap and scream at you. During his depressed phase, he went straight to bed after work without having dinner, and slept until the next day.

As a working mother, I struggled to balance work and family, but having to deal with the mood swings of my husband drained me emotionally. I talked to the minister in our church, who suggested that we go through marriage counseling. My husband would promise by heaven and earth that he was going to change, but he would go right back to his old ways. When he was being mean, evil, and unkind, I thought he was doing so by his own choice. I did not realize that he had an illness. I had no understanding about bipolar or mood disorder at that time. I just thought he could change if he wanted to, and he must not want to change.

Some people later suggested that we seek professional help from a psychiatrist, but he bluntly refused to go, calling it a sign of weakness. He believed he could handle the situation. I reached a point when I knew I could not go on living with him. It was becoming a codependent relationship rather than a marriage. I found myself constantly trying to save him and to keep the problem within the family, away from the public as much as possible.

Finally, I summoned the courage to file for a divorce. It was a very difficult decision for me, and it upset me to divide our family, but I was left with no other choice. The children were devastated because they still loved their father in spite of his unpredictable behavior. The children would always have a wonderful time with him during his happy or elated mood. He changed jobs frequently during our marriage because he was always getting into fights at work. He was able to get another job very easily because he had a marketable skill that was highly in demand. He was completely taken by surprise that I would go through with the divorce. He never thought I could leave him, because I had threatened to leave several times and never left.

His life completely fell apart after the divorce because of lack of family support. I insisted on his getting a professional help as part of the divorce settlement if he wanted to be involved with the children. He finally did, and he was formally diagnosed with bipolar or mood disorder. We attended family counseling together after the divorce because of the children. The divorce was very difficult for the children. It was during one of the therapy sessions that I learned a lot about his illness (bipolar or mood disorder). Instead of the anger and resentment I had struggled with during our marriage, I felt very sorry for him. I left open a possibility of reconciliation if he would follow through with therapy and medication management. Deep inside me, I have a secret fear that he may not be sincere about his promise to follow through with professional help. He has told me a few times that he likes the happy phase of his illness. I will have to wait and let time tell if he was sincere about making changes with medication and therapy. I still love him very much, but I am not willing to go back to him unless I see a changed man, and complete sincerity on his part to stay on medications, go to therapy, and also follow all professional advice. He must be willing to take responsibility for his illness. If your story sounds like my family story, please get help. My husband may remind you of yourself or someone you know; it is never too late to do something about this illness. Many families have experienced the pain of divorce because of this illness, but with treatment this does not have to happen. Bipolar disorder is treatable if there is a desire to get better.

# Quotes of Encouragement...

As the wind blows harder and Mr. Ladson's story sounds familiar to you, remember the following:

*"Take a look at your natural river. What are you? Stop playing games with yourself... where's your river going? Are you riding with it? Or are you rowing against it?... Don't you see that there is no effort if you are riding with your river?"*

*~ Carl Frederick*

Bipolar will toss you up and down if you do not confront this illness and do something about it; do not give up; be a fighter; do not feel powerless; feel empowered; make every effort to get the appropriate help; do not be a victim; be a victor. *(LB)*

*"Whatever failures I have known, whatever errors I have committed, whatever follies I have witnessed in private and public life have been the consequences of actions without thought."*

*~ Bernard M. Baruch*

Bipolar can make you impulsive during the manic phase, and you do a lot of things without thinking through them; the truth is, consequences of your impulsivity will not be excused by society. If you go on spending the money that you do not have, you still have to face the consequences of paying back the money; when you are manic and you feel out of control, take a step back to think of the future consequences of your actions when the manic phase passes and you are in control. *(LB)*

*"We have forty million reasons for failure, but not a single excuse."*

*~ Rudyard Kipling*

No excuses. Do not just articulate your problems; articulate the solutions. Do not hide under your weaknesses; showcase your strengths. Highlight all the reasons why you need to get better and this will shape your focus. *(LB)*

*Winds Against The Mind*

# Bipolar:
# RANDY'S STORY

Randy was a cute and adorable child growing up; everybody loved him. He was so full of energy and was always busy and very active. As parents, we noticed that he threw a lot more temper tantrums than the rest of his siblings, and he would get very destructive sometimes. We set firm limits with him, and complained about his frequent tantrums to his pediatrician. The pediatrician told us that we were doing everything right. He suggested that we continue to set limits with him when necessary and keep him very active, so that he could burn off some energy.

Randy played every sport we could fit into his schedule, and he was good at all of them. We enrolled him in a piano lesson, and quickly realized that he got easily frustrated. His attention span was a little too short for piano lesson because piano lessons require more concentration than most of the contact sports he played.

We also noticed rapid mood swings in Randy's interaction with the rest of his siblings. He picked quarrels with his siblings easily, became physically aggressive with them, and turned around a few minutes later to hug his siblings and say he was sorry. He did not bear grudges for a long time, but got very angry and frustrated very easily.

Randy brought a lot of notes home from school for getting into trouble, but it was nothing out of the ordinary. When we went to the parent-teacher conferences, the teachers always told us that he was a good kid at heart; he was just a little tougher than most little boys in his age group.

By the time Randy was in middle school, he got into more serious trouble at school. We became increasingly worried because we were hoping that he would outgrow some of this behavior. By the time he was in high school, he was into street drugs, smoking cigarettes and marijuana, going to clubs, sneaking out of the house at night, and getting into public fights. Randy was arrested several times by the police, and he ended up in the juvenile court system.

My husband and I did not know what to do with this child. We asked ourselves where we went wrong or what we had missed to have our child turn out this way. We tried to play by the rules and do everything right as much as possible with raising our children. Our other two children were nothing like Randy; we have never had any cause to worry about them. After some time, the stress started taking a toll on our marriage and the family.

We lived in a state of panic most of the time because life with Randy was always unpredictable. It became difficult to concentrate either at work or at home. How could we concentrate when we never knew who would be calling next about Randy? It might be anyone from a teacher to a police officer. Every time the phone rang, our hearts would start to beat very rapidly. This lifestyle was both disruptive and overwhelming for all of us.

Out of frustration, my husband and I started the "blame game"– we found ourselves "finger pointing" at each other, when the real issue was that we just didn't know what to do. What had happened to our adorable little boy?

Of additional concern, Randy was taking so much of our time that we found ourselves unconsciously neglecting the other two children in the house. This was never our intention; it just happened.

Randy was suspended from school several times for getting into fights. Finally, he was caught by a teacher for smoking marijuana on the school premises, which was against the school's policy. Randy was suspended from school, but the principal said he would give him another chance if he got professional help. Randy avoided every effort on our part to get professional help for him. He kept running the streets and finally got picked up again by the police. He was in the juvenile lock-up unit, and had to appear before the judge. The judge ordered a mandatory psychiatric hospitalization for him. We went to visit him in the hospital and met with the hospital staff. We were told he was going to be in treatment for a while. We were so relieved that he would at least be in a safe environment. We were always worried about the possibility of something bad happening to him on the street, especially the likelihood of getting himself killed in a fight.

My husband and I still continued to blame each other for Randy's problems. Both of us carried a lot of guilt, thinking that something was probably wrong with our parenting skills. There was always a constant tension in the house and a cloud of unhappiness.

When we attended a meeting at the hospital to discuss the plan of treatment for Randy, the psychiatrist explained to us that Randy was suffering from bipolar or mood disorder. He explained that it is a form of mental illness with mood swings where a person could be happy one moment and be sad one moment. He said people with mood disorder tend to take more risks during their manic phases, and some have the tendency to be violent and self-destructive. He also said that drug use is very common with teenagers suffering from this disorder.

The physician educated us extensively about bipolar disorder, and as he described typical symptoms of the illness, we felt as though he was describing Randy personally. The staff also gave us a lot of literature to read about mood disorder. My husband and I left the hospital feeling greatly relieved; after struggling with Randy for so long, finger pointing at each other, and dealing with our own issues of self-blame, it was truly a blessing to know what was wrong with our son. Now his problem had a name—bipolar or mood disorder.

Randy was started on some medications in the hospital, and he continued taking the medications at home. When Randy came home after being hospitalized, we noticed a difference. He was much more even tempered, and his behavior has improved. He did well when he stayed on his medications, but getting him to take the medication was a daily struggle for a while. He complained that the medication made him feel too sober and tired, but he is still taking it most of the time.

The bottom line is, most people suffering from mood disorder love the high or manic phase, and if they have a choice, they would rather keep the high. However with medication, they will stay more *euthymic* (more emotionally stable) instead of going up and down with their emotions. People need to understand the trade-off with being treated for bipolar disorder—people with mood disorder have to get used to having a euthymic mood, instead of going up and down with their emotions like a roller coaster. They have to give up the highs or the manic phase in order to have a stable life.

Randy, like most people with bipolar disorder, would get off his medications sometimes, and would go back to his old ways, consequently requiring medication stabilization and hospitalization all over again. We went through the struggle for about three more years, but we did not give up on him. We continued to emphasize that it was in his own best interest to stay on his medication. Finally, Randy came to terms with the fact that he has an illness, and needs to stay on his medication. He has been doing well; he attends college full-time and keeps up his grades. We are very proud of him.

We have our lives back as a family, now that we know what we are dealing with. We no longer blame each other for Randy's problems; we no longer blame ourselves. We realize that we are not horrible parents. After all, we are the parents of the other two children who are doing very well and are staying completely out of trouble.

Getting a diagnosis for the illness was a step in the right direction. Now we know we have a son with an illness, and we are trying our best to help him. Randy commutes to college from home. Having him at home gives us the chance to make sure he stays on his medications. He also goes to therapy and attends a support group. We have accepted the fact that Randy will always be a bipolar, and he will have good and bad days. We are grateful for the good days, and we love him unconditionally on the bad days. We are especially grateful that he is stable most of the time when he takes his medication. We have a lot to be thankful for as a family.

If Randy reminds you of your child, or our family story sounds like what you are going through, please do something. Get help. You don't have to live a miserable life. The situation can greatly improve with the right kind of help.

# Quotes of Encouragement...

As the wind blows harder and Randy's story sounds familiar to you, remember the following:

*"Any person who recognizes this greatest power... the power to choose... begins to realize that he is the one that is doing the choosing and that friends... cannot do the choosing for him, nor can his relatives. Consequently, he develops real self-confidence, based upon his own ability, upon his own actions and upon his own initiative."*

~ *J. Martin Rohe*

Peer pressure added to bipolar disorder could easily equal poor choices; choose wisely; remember you are writing your own script with your choices. If you are writing a script of shame, retrace your steps to the right track; it is never too late to write a script of joy and pride. *(LB)*

*"Close scrutiny will show that most...crisis situations are...opportunities to either advance or stay where you are."*

~ *Maxwell Maltz*

Bipolar disorder can turn your life into a turmoil and a continuous crisis; you can choose to live in turmoil and crisis, or turn your life around and make it productive; you can look for opportunities to grow, or become stagnant and be a victim for ever; you have the final "say" and the final "choice." *(LB)*

*"I have always believed and I still believe, that whatever good or bad fortune may come our way, we can always give it meaning and transform it into something of value."*

~ *Hermann Hesse*

Do not focus on your failures; focus on turning your failures into a success story. Divert your energy into helping other people in a similar situation to get up and not stay fallen; be able to say, "Look at me; I am still here. I made it; you can make it, too. I have bipolar, but bipolar does not have me." *(LB)*

# Bipolar or Mood Disorders:
# BASIC FACTS & UNDERSTANDING

Angela, Mr. Ladson, and Randy all suffered from *bipolar disorder*, a mental illness which affects our mood. We all experience happiness and sadness on and off in our lives; these feelings are normal if they are not extreme to the point of interfering with our ability to function normally on a day-to-day basis. People suffering from bipolar experience two extreme moods—they swing like a pendulum from an excited, expansive, euphoric, or elated mood to a very sad, depressed, or sometimes melancholic mood. People with bipolar disorder have described the elated mood as "feeling high like you are on drugs, except that there are no external drug influences producing the high; the high is produced by the chemicals in your brain."

During the elated mood known as the *hypomanic* or *manic phase*, they may be extremely happy, talkative, buoyant, and extremely sociable. They have endless energy levels and many grandiose ideas (heightened and false feelings of self-importance leading to a belief that they can do the impossible), and need little or no sleep. They may act out sexually. They cannot tolerate limit setting or somebody thwarting their plans when they are in this expansive mood. They may become very destructive and violent when others try to stop them or thwart their plans. They can be verbally abusive and emotionally aggressive toward others, or go into rage and pick fights with others for no reasonable cause. They may become the center of attraction or attention at a party; they have the tendency to violate the personal space of others, crack inappropriate jokes, use vulgar language and curse words, and become very loud and out-of-control in a social gathering.

In this state of mind, they might also make irrational decisions such as dropping out of school, quitting their jobs, or filing for a divorce. This out-of-control behavior characterizing the manic or the hypomanic phase can be very difficult on their significant others and immediate family members. They may go on uncontrollable spending sprees and make purchases without thinking, even when they know they cannot afford such purchases. They may go home to their spouses with expensive gifts they cannot pay for, and buy things they do not need on credit. For example, a typical bipolar bachelor may take a girlfriend on an extremely expensive vacation and use a credit card to pay for it, without having the resources to pay his credit card bill. Due to the poor judgment and impulsivity in the manic or hypomanic phase, these bipolar sufferers may give away expensive valuables and later regret their actions. They may even shoplift and embezzle money, believing they are invisible and are able to get away with anything. They may sign up for all possible overtime hours available at their jobs because they have endless energy levels. They are known for coming up with various grandiose ideas in this impulsive state. For instance, they may talk about starting a new business, changing their profession, or inventing something new. Some people with bipolar do follow through with their grandiose ideas, especially if the grandiose idea is something positive and achievable during the manic or hypomanic time frame. This is primarily because they have a lot of energy during that time frame.

Sexually inappropriate behavior is very common during the manic phase. Bipolar people may have increased sexual energy and become sexually demanding. They may show no sexual discretion, engaging in irresponsible and dangerous sexual acts, and have extramarital affairs. Sexual promiscuity may not be seen as a problem by a person suffering from bipolar, but rather as a form of enjoyment. Adolescents or teenagers with bipolar may be sexually promiscuous and be labeled as such by their peers. Such adolescents may also have problems with school, and use illicit drugs and alcohol. They may also engage in violent behavior.

The down side to the manic phase is this: there is a limit to what the body can take over a period of time. The body cannot cope with indefinite sleep deprivation and hyperactivity. If nothing is done to stop the non-stop physical activities, sleeplessness, and the acting out behavior, it could lead to physical exhaustion and death. An extremely manic person may require hospitalization for his or her own safety.

The hallmark of bipolar is the common switch from elation to depression, as opposed to a depressed person who constantly stays depressed. The switch from elation to depression could be gradual or sudden. A bipolar person can go from feeling that the world is a beautiful place to wanting to kill himself. The depressed phase of bipolar is typical of the feelings experienced by a person who is suffering from major depression. Bipolar people may experience hopelessness, worthlessness, *anhedonia* or lack of interest in pleasurable things, excessive fatigue or loss of energy, changes in appetite, which could go from no appetite at all to a voracious appetite, excessive sleep, poor concentration, and recurrent thoughts of death or suicidal ideation. They have the tendency to abuse drugs and alcohol. They may turn to illicit drugs to self-medicate, especially during the depressed phase of the illness.

For a better understanding of the management of bipolar disorder, it is important to make a distinction between the two different types of bipolar disorders, which are *Bipolar Type I* and *Bipolar Type II*. With *Bipolar Type I*, clients experience major depression with full-blown mania. The manic, expansive, or elated mood would eventually get out of control. Clients experiencing Bipolar Type I may require hospitalization to ensure their safety. They may go from laughter to rage, become extremely demanding, grandiose (false sense of importance), and psychotic or out-of-touch with reality. Judgment is extremely poor, and these symptoms may go on for up to a week or more.

With *Bipolar Type II*, clients may experience major depression with hypomania. Hypomania is a milder form of mania. People with Bipolar Type II still experience two extreme moods: the elated mood or the hypomanic state may be better controlled as compared to the full-blown mania in Type I. This is due to the fact that the hypomanic state is a less severe form of mania than a full-blown mania. Some of the manifested symptoms of hypomania may include grandiosity, buoyancy, over-confidence, euphoria, and poor judgment. The difference between the hypomania and the full-blown mania is that the symptoms of hypomania would not be severe enough to require hospitalization. The expansive or elated mood in the hypomanic state with Bipolar Type II may last for about four days.

The biological explanation of bipolar disorder, like some other major mental illnesses, links this particular form of mental illness to the dysregulation or abnormal regulation of some naturally occurring chemicals in the brain called neurotransmitters. When these chemicals occur in the right proportion in the brain, a person functions normally. When the levels of these chemicals are too high or too low, or when there is a problem with the transportation of these chemicals, a person may show signs and symptoms of bipolar disorder. The cells harboring or housing the neurotransmitters are called *neurons*; if there is a problem with the functioning of the neurons, it could also compound the problems and symptoms manifested in bipolar. Other biological factors are also involved.

Studies have shown that bipolar or mood disorder can be hereditary, and it can be passed down through the genes from one generation to the next generation. People with this disorder are likely to have a family history of relatives suffering from or who have suffered from this disorder. Twin studies comparing identical twins (twins who are mirror image of one another) with fraternal twins (twins that do not look alike) suggested a stronger hereditary factor and a higher genetic link in case of identical twins. Both of the identical twins may have bipolar, and only one of the fraternal twins may inherit bipolar.

There is no laboratory test to confirm the diagnosis of bipolar or mood disorder, so the diagnosis is made primarily on a personal history and the symptoms the person is exhibiting at that time. The person must have exhibited these symptoms for an extended period of time, and the time period necessary to make the symptoms meet the criteria for the diagnosis of bipolar must be determined by a licensed clinician in mental health or in a mental health related field. Such a clinician must have sufficient medical knowledge and training in the area of psychiatry, medicine, psychology, or nursing, or the clinician must be properly licensed to make such a diagnosis in that community. At times, the primary care provider, such as an internist, a family physician, or a nurse practitioner, may be the first to make the initial diagnosis. The client may then be referred later to a mental health specialist.

Treatment may include medication management, hospitalization if necessary, group and individual therapy, health teachings, and health maintenance. The type of medication to be used should be strictly determined by a certified, knowledgeable, and licensed clinician. Several factors are taken into consideration before deciding on what medication is to be prescribed for a client.

A bipolar person must be assessed for suicide during the depressed phase, and even in the manic phase. If a bipolar person has a suicidal plan, for example, if he or she plans to overdose on medication or have another self-destructive plan, this must be taken seriously. Help must be sought immediately. Bipolar people may also engage in extremely destructive behavior during the manic phase, such as racing a car at a dangerous speed which can result in their dying in a car crash. They must also be carefully watched during the extremely manic phase when they may go for days without food. They can be offered finger foods, or snacks when they are continuously active and are unable to slow down to eat. This is to keep them from starving to death.

Individual therapy is recommended in the treatment of bipolar disorder. It might be short or long-term therapy, depending on individual need. The therapist should help the client to identify irrational and impulsive decisions such as going on shopping sprees, and teach the client how to control such impulsive urges. The therapist can also help the client to identify other positive ways to look at life and to see light at the end of the tunnel during the depressed or down phase.

Group therapy is also recommended in the treatment of bipolar disorder. Being able to identify with other people dealing with the same illness can provide the clients the psychological relief that they are not alone with these struggles. They learn from one another and support one another in a group setting. There is openness, bonding, and a sense of community. People learn new social skills and more adaptive ways of dealing with their daily challenges. Most importantly, nobody is judging anyone else. There is unconditional acceptance of one another.

Family support groups for family members of people living with bipolar are also available in some communities. It is important for family members or significant others to learn how other families cope with this illness. These groups also provide an avenue to learn the best strategies for helping a person with bipolar disorder without becoming co-dependent (behavior that enables or encourage the bipolar person) or enmeshed (no boundaries or limit setting).

The financial implications of this disorder can also be very taxing on the rest of the family, especially in the area of impulsive spending sprees. Paying for the treatment of this disorder could also be difficult financially for the family. It cannot be overemphasized that bipolar disorder can be physically, emotionally, and financially draining on the family; it is responsible for a lot of family breakups.

ECT (electroconvulsive treatment) or shock treatment may be recommended as the last resort to treat the depressed phase of bipolar disorder, if the depression does not respond to medication or other treatments. ECT is relatively safe with few side effects. A psychiatrist will thoroughly explain and educate clients about ECT before recommending its use (see discussion on ECT under major depression, page 50.

In addition to other recommended treatment, living a healthy lifestyle, such as eating healthy food, exercising, meditating, relaxation, and stress management, is also helpful. Some of the treatment modalities are sometimes used in combination with one another. Appropriate treatment goals for each individual should be put together by a qualified clinician.

Bipolar or mood disorder affects people in many societies. It may be under diagnosed in certain cultures due to a lack of education regarding mental illness. It is probably better diagnosed and treated in the western world. Bipolar does not discriminate; it affects both male and female, young adults and older people. Having bipolar disorder is not totally horrible for those who suffer from it; some people suffering from bipolar have made great breakthroughs and achieved great successes. They can be higher achievers if they channel their energy properly toward positive use. Some tend to be very creative and are able to achieve higher levels of distinction and success in the manic phase, if they are not out of control. In addition, they tend to be more educated and also achieve a higher occupational status whenever the energy is properly channeled. They could be musicians, writers, artists, poets, producers, or company directors, just to mention some of the leading roles they play in our society. The ultimate key to the success of bipolar people is the ability to put their energy to positive use when they have excessive energy, strive to have a more euthymic or stable mood by also managing the depressed phase with medication and therapy, and stop the denial of the illness by seeking a professional help.

PART IV

# COMMON PROBLEMS RELATED TO MEMORY: ALZHEIMER'S DISEASE

## Alzheimer's Disease:
# MR. BOLTON'S STORY

Initially, I could not place what was wrong with my husband; he seemed a little more confused than usual. I thought he might be having a transient stroke because of his history of high cholesterol and hypertension. I scheduled an appointment for him to see our family physician, but every medical test came back normal. He became increasingly confused and forgetful. He would leave the house to go to the grocery store, and then would call me to say that he could not find his way to the grocery store he had been going to for years.

He loved to do things around the house, especially minor repairs. His favorite store was the hardware store, and he always looked for a reason to go to the hardware store at least once a week over the course of our forty-eight years of marriage. He would leave the house and not be able to find his way to the hardware store; he would have to ask for directions over and over again, which was very frustrating for him.

Around the house, he would misplace his glasses, his wallet, and other small items, and would have absolutely no memory of where he had put them. He would schedule appointments for people to come and work on the house, but when they showed up at the door, he would have no recollection of ever talking to them or asking them to come and do repairs for him. He would forget telephone numbers that he had dialed for years. When friends and family members called, he would not recognize who they were, or he would confuse them with someone else.

I was getting more and more worried and scared because it was becoming increasingly dangerous to leave him by himself. I took him back to the doctor and explained how his symptoms had progressively worsened since our last visit. At this point the doctor suspected dementia, in the form of Alzheimer's. He gave my husband some questionnaires to answer and repeated some tests. At the end of the visit, the doctor broke the sad news to me that my husband had Alzheimer's disease.

# Winds Against The Mind

I was not very well informed about Alzheimer's at that point in time. I knew it involved a form of memory loss, but I never imagined it would happen to my own husband who was always so quick to remember even the smallest of details.

The doctor explained that it is a degenerative brain disease, which causes the brain to lose the vital brain mass responsible for our ability to function. He pointed out that my husband was going to get worse because there is no cure for Alzheimer's yet. I was so devastated to hear this news. I couldn't imagine him being worse than he already was.

My husband was very energetic, hardworking, and full of life. He loved his family and took very good care of me and the children. We had worked together as a team for many years, but I was more dependent on him. The first question I asked myself was, "Where do I go from here?" It was very difficult for me to accept this diagnosis. I was in denial and quickly concluded in my mind that the doctor's diagnosis must be wrong, so I decided to get a second opinion from another doctor. Lo and behold, a second doctor confirmed Alzheimer's disease, despite my efforts to downplay the symptoms with the second doctor, in hopes of getting another diagnosis.

After working through the denial, I realized that I had to face the fact that my husband had Alzheimer's disease. This horrible illness has completely changed our lives forever, just at the time we were supposed to be enjoying the fruits of our hard labor in retirement. It was like a gradual death; you watch your loved one dying every day. I decided to keep him at home as long as I could. It was physically, emotionally, and financially draining. He got worse and worse every day because he became increasingly confused and forgetful. Initially, he was in and out of lucid or clear-minded moments, but the situation grew worse gradually. By lunchtime he could not remember what he had eaten for breakfast. Eventually he stopped asking for food even when he was hungry. I had to offer food to him, and if I put the food right in front of him, he would not know what to do with it unless I fed him. He was incontinent with urine and feces since he did not remember to ask to use the restroom. (He certainly did not go to the restroom of his own accord.) When I tried to change his wet or soiled clothes, he sometimes became combative. I think he must have felt that his privacy had been invaded because he was completely unaware of his incontinence. I had to bathe him and attend to all of his hygiene needs.

The most difficult part for me and the children was the fact that he did not recognize the children when they came to visit. Gradually, he completely lost memory of who I was. The grandchildren were especially hurt because they could not understand why Grandpa would not play with them. He used to play with the grandchildren a lot. He built a tree house for them in the back of our yard. We have a stream that runs through our backyard, and he used to play in it with the grandchildren; they reveled in playing in the mud with Grandpa. The grandchildren also enjoyed running errands with him to the grocery store and the hardware store. With his completely altered personality, they complained that Grandpa was not fun anymore, and we had to explain to them, at their level of understanding, what was wrong with Grandpa. Understandably to the grandchildren, at their level of comprehension, this change would hopefully be temporary, but each time they came back, Grandpa was still the same way, if not worse. Whenever they came over, our four-year-old grandson would ring the doorbell and immediately ask, "Is Grandpa better now so we can play?" That really broke my heart. I had to put dead bolt locks on the doors and install a security alarm because he wandered away from the house many times.

As much as I loved him, I felt stuck with him in these circumstances because I was always afraid to run short errands. I am thankful for the blessings of good friends — some of my friends would come and sit with him so that I could run errands.

For a period of time he had a good *remote (long-term)* memory, so if I showed him the pictures of the children when they were younger, especially in the toddler years and the elementary school days, he would smile. He would also sometimes make a passing comment about an interesting event that had happened during that time of the children's lives. When I played his favorite old music, he would get up and dance and even sing along. I always experienced mixed emotions, both joy and sadness, to watch him respond to anything. Eventually he lost the ability to remember any information, old or new.

After six years of taking care of him, I became exhausted and 'burned out.' I realized that I was not getting any younger myself, but it was not easy to let go. Early in our marriage my husband and I had made a promise to each other to be there for each other, no matter what. I hired a housecleaning service to come twice a week, and four of my friends volunteered one day every month to come and relieve me. My daughter would also come on some weekends to sit with him. While this was a viable solution temporarily, his health continued to deteriorate until I knew I needed help on a full-time basis.

Watching the daily downward decline was also very difficult; he was talking less and less, and when he did speak, his words did not make sense most of the time. Eventually he became mute with no communication at all, and he did not recognize me as his wife. I cannot begin to convey how painful this was for me. I could not afford to hire full-time help, as I had almost depleted all of our savings from taking care of him.

# Winds Against The Mind

I finally reached a turning point and had to make the decision to place him in a long-term care situation. Frankly, he needed more than I was able to give him. Although this was really the only choice I had, I experienced tremendous turmoil over it and felt as though a dagger through my chest might have been less painful. I never knew a day like this would come. Living with him and watching him decline with this illness was like a first death, but making the decision to put him in a nursing home was like a second death. I felt so guilty that I could not take care of him anymore, especially in light of our promise to take care of each other until the very end. Other people around me, such as my friends, community members, and my family, reminded me that if I were to die from exhaustion from taking care of him, he would have to go to a nursing home anyway.

With the support of my family and dear friends, I found a good nursing home near our house, so that I could go and see him every day. I reluctantly put him in the nursing home.

Finally, I have mentally accepted his new home. The staff is attentive to his needs, and I also go there to assist with his care, especially to feed him at meal times. I have also realized that although my husband and I are not living under the same roof, I can still be with him until the end.

I still cannot help but wonder about this illness called Alzheimer's disease; looking at my husband is like looking at an empty shell—the body is in one place, and the mind is locked up somewhere else. The memories of the good life we had together before his illness keep me going now, and sometimes I debate in my mind that maybe it was good for him that he was not aware of his own decline. He was a man with a lot of self-pride, very independent, and always preferred to serve others rather than be served.

During the early stages of his illness, I joined a support group for family members of people suffering from Alzheimer's, which was one of the wisest choices I made during this experience. I learned a lot from the group, and hearing the stories of others helped me to endure this hardship. I continue to monitor the medical news about this illness regularly, and I read a lot to gather information about what research is going into the studies of Alzheimer's. I pray that a day will come when there will be a cure for this devastating mental illness.

If this story sounds familiar, please get help. If you feel that you have reached the end of your rope in caring for a loved one with Alzheimer's, from physical or nervous exhaustion, or from depleting your financial resources, it may be time to find an assisted living situation for him or her. You can still be with your loved one until the end.

# Quotes of Encouragement...

As the wind blows harder and the story of Mr. Bolton sounds familiar to you, remember the following:

*"We must have strong minds, ready to accept facts as they are."*
                                            *~ Harry S. Truman*

If you have Alzheimer's, remember there is no cure yet, and the memory loss gets worse as the illness progresses. Face the difficult reality and be prepared for this unpleasant journey with Alzheimer's, put your house in order, make preparations for end-of-life issues, have a living will, durable power of attorney, and a personal will. If you so desire, make a documentary of good memories for your family which will give them a reminder of happy memories to hold on to as they gradually lose you to Alzheimer's. *(LB)*

*"The most important thing in life is not the triumph but the struggle. The essential thing is not to have conquered but to have fought well."*
                                            *~ Baron Pierre de Coubertin*

With Alzheimer's, there is no triumph until a cure is found, but do not be buried in your grief and forget to reflect on the good gifts that life has given you. Be thankful for the many blessings over the years before Alzheimer's, and do not see Alzheimer's as a dead end but as another difficult phase in the journey of life. Be able to say "I have fought well with the things I could control, and the things I cannot control I will leave alone." *(LB)*

*"How strange is the lot of us mortals! Each of us is here for a brief sojourn; for what purpose he knows not, though he senses it. But without deeper reflection one knows from daily life that one exists for other people."*
                                            *~ Albert Einstein*

As you struggle to take care of your loved one living with Alzheimer's, and you feel the tiredness and the exhaustion, remember that living for one another usually comes with a price called sacrifice, and sacrifice requires the willpower and strength to do things that are not convenient for us. *(LB)*

*Winds Against The Mind*

## Alzheimer's Disease:

# MRS. CAUDEL'S STORY

Mom was a librarian at a local university for thirty-five years. She was a very hardworking, friendly woman. She loved her work as a librarian and believed very much in reading. When we were little, she used to tell us children that reading is the root of all knowledge, and the only way we could be intelligent was to read. She read to us every night before we went to bed. When we were growing up, we read and wrote a report on at least one book a week. She made reading fun because she would always give us a treat for every book we read.

Our mother was active in our community, and she would organize a storytelling time for neighborhood children when she would read stories to them. This event was always well attended because she served homemade cookies and drinks! Did I mention Mom was an excellent cook? She was also very involved in our church, and she taught children in Sunday school. She read and told the stories so gracefully that if she could not teach on Sunday mornings, the children would cry and throw temper tantrums. We all knew that the children looked forward to going to Sunday School when she was there to teach.

But one Thanksgiving after we had grown up and left home, we came home for the holiday and our dad called a family meeting to share his concerns about our mom's health. He said Mom was becoming increasingly forgetful and confused and not remembering addresses and phone numbers. She was also misplacing things around the house, which was very unlike our efficient mother. We all laughed over it, and joked that maybe Mom was experiencing adjustment problems because she had only been retired for one year. She had been a very busy woman all her life, so maybe she needed to adjust to all the free time she had.

We had heard a lot about Alzheimer's disease, but had never been particularly concerned about this illness, though we were sorry for others who had it. It certainly had never occurred to us that we would learn about Alzheimer's firsthand through our mom. We were convinced that whatever was going on with Mom would all go away with time, but instead, the situation got worse. Dad told us that Mom was getting very tearful and frustrated because she kept getting lost on the way to familiar places. We also noticed that it took her a few minutes to identify who we were when we called the house, but she covered up very well. Mom would give excuses whenever she could not remember certain information. As time progressed, Mom began to confuse the days of the week and found it difficult to dial simple telephone numbers. She became frustrated and gradually removed herself from her community involvement.

Putting all the information together, we later deduced that some of these changes she must have noticed in herself were probably responsible for her decision to retire early. She could have worked for at least five more years before retiring, and as much as she enjoyed her career, her sudden announcement to retire had come as a surprise to all of us, but we hadn't questioned it. She had worked very hard all of her life, and only the two of them were left at home, Mom and Dad. The house was fully paid for, and they did not have a lot of expenses. They both had worked a little longer primarily to buy gifts for the grandchildren and to help us out with them if we needed any financial help. Everyone overlooked her sudden retirement.

After observing her steady decline for a year, the official diagnosis of Alzheimer's from her physician did not come as too much of a shock at this point, but it was still painful news to receive. Although Mom stopped volunteering in the children's church after she was finally diagnosed by her physician, the children still flooded around her every Sunday. It was very difficult for the children and her church members to accept her illness.

As I mentioned earlier, Mom was a good cook, and her favorite thing to do was to cook, especially for family and friends. With this illness affecting her brain, she would try to cook and would get confused about the ingredients and the process. She would get so frustrated and angry that she would throw pans around the kitchen out of frustration. She would leave pans on the stove and forget to turn the stove off. She came close to setting the house on fire on several occasions, but Dad always caught it just in time. She ran the tub one morning, and forgot to turn off the tap. Half of the house was flooded before Dad discovered it.

We suggested that Mom should be placed in a safer environment like an assisted living facility or a nursing home, but Dad refused. We watched him struggle daily to care for Mom, and it was very stressful for him. With our family setup, it would have been easier if it were Dad who had Alzheimer's, because Mom waited on him and really pampered him. We knew that if Mom could have communicated with us in a sound state of mind, she would have told Daddy to put her in a safer environment where she could be cared for instead of having him continue to care for her on his own.

Convincing Dad of this was another matter. He was also completely lost, and he was having an extremely difficult time taking care of Mom. He had to watch her very closely for safety, and somehow he was able to keep her from cooking.

In her confused mental state, she became anxious around the time for school dismissal every day—being a mother had occupied such an important part of her life that now she would worry that she hadn't picked us up from school. She did this for years, and Dad had to hide the car keys from her to keep her from trying to pick us up from school. Our devoted mother could not remember that we are all grown now and gone, and we all have children of our own. I cannot believe what Alzheimer's had done to our mother; her daily routine of picking us up when we were younger was still encoded in her long-term memory.

One evening, Mom and Dad were in the family room watching the television, and Dad accidentally went to sleep because he was exhausted. Mom sneaked into the kitchen and tried to prepare dinner. Dad was awakened by the fire alarm, only to discover that the entire kitchen was on fire. Dad called 911, the emergency service, and the fire crew came immediately to put out the fire. There was extensive damage to the kitchen and smoke damage to adjacent rooms. Dad and Mom had to move out of the house for about three months in order for the house to be renovated.

It was at this point that Dad agreed that Mom needed to be in a safer environment, and we all tried to be very supportive of Dad through this very difficult decision. As painful as it was for Dad to do this, we were relieved, because we had been worried that Mom might accidentally set the entire house on fire by trying to cook, while Dad was sleeping. We were afraid of the possibility that both of them could get killed in a fire accident.

Alzheimer's is a very difficult illness for family members to watch; it is like a death, but the body is still there, and the dead body is still moving. You don't know this new person anymore. It is truly a real-life scenario of a 'dead man walking. '

## Winds Against The Mind

We all visit Mom at the nursing home. At times she would remember us very briefly; she would say we looked familiar and she knew us for a long time. Other times she would have no idea who we were and would even ask us to get away from her. As time progressed, she completely forgot our names. If we visited her in the late afternoon, she would still worry about picking up the children and fixing the dinner. We cannot but wonder some times what happened to the mom that we used to know. What a terrible illness that would strip a person completely of her identity!

Watching Mom created an inner fear within all of us as her children. We are hoping we did not inherit the gene, and if we did, we hope there will be a cure for the illness before it takes over our lives. It was a very humbling experience to watch Mom endure this mental illness called Alzheimer's disease. Dad found it almost impossible to move on; we watched him gradually declining too, although he doesn't have Alzheimer's. We hope the day will come that nobody will have to live with this illness. If you have a loved one suffering from this illness, you are not alone. Do not hesitate to get help if taking care of your loved one is too difficult for you.

# Quotes of Encouragement...

As the wind blows harder, and Mrs. Caudel's story sounds familiar to you, remember the following:

*"Always think in terms of what the other person wants."*

~ *James Van Fleet*

As a caregiver, you may struggle with the guilt and the tough decision to place your loved one in a safer environment outside of the home, but ask yourself what your loved ones would want if they could make their own decisions. Would they rather see you die from physical and mental exhaustion? Or see you well and alive while they stay in an assisted living or nursing home? Make peace with yourself and know that it is okay to keep them safe outside of the home; you can only do your best in caring for your loved ones at home, but your best may not always be enough in caring for someone with Alzheimer's. *(LB)*

*"On the long analysis, then love is life. Love never faileth and life never faileth so long as there is love."*

~ *Henry Drummond*

As you helplessly watch your loved one gradually taken over by Alzheimer's, take a minute to cherish and reflect upon the love they have given to you; the love you have received from them, and the love they are currently receiving from you. Even if they are not aware of it, the life that may seem to be disappearing to you will be constantly watered by loving memories. *(LB)*

*"It is easy enough to be pleasant, when life flows by like a song; but the man worthwhile is the one who can smile, when everything goes dead wrong; for the test of the heart is trouble, and it always comes with years; and the smile that is worth the praises of the earth, is the smile that shines through tears."*

~ *Ella Wheeler Wilcox*

You cannot allow the sadness of having Alzheimer's to totally deprive you of the joy of living. Enjoy the moment that you have now. Even in your sadness, find joy. *(LB)*

## Alzheimer's Disease:
# MR. COVINGTON'S STORY

D ad was a janitor five days a week and a volunteer at the homeless shelter on weekends. He worked hard to put all of us through school. Our father always emphasized the value of education, and he encouraged us to aspire very high in life, and do whatever we chose to do very well. He could not afford to go to college when he finished high school, but Dad was undoubtedly a very intelligent man. He was so full of wisdom, and he was highly respected in the community.

After forty-two years of marriage, our mom died and Dad would not consider re-marrying. Our Aunt Marilyn, his younger sister who was divorced, decided to move in with Dad. Our aunt and our dad always got along well, and we were all relieved when she moved in with him. You see, Dad had struggled a great deal with our mother's death and had harbored a lot of anger over it. Mom died quite suddenly; she collapsed in the bathroom one day and died. Unfortunately, Dad was not in the house, and he blamed himself for not being at home when she collapsed.

Five years after Mom's death, Dad turned seventy. We decided to give him a big seventieth birthday party, inviting the entire community and the extended family. It was a very emotional occasion for Dad, especially because Mom was not there to grace the occasion with him. He was showered with a lot of gifts, and everybody spoke highly of his good work and his integrity. In his thank-you speech, he cracked a joke that he felt like he was getting married again, except that there was no bride. We noticed in his speech that he gave incorrect information, and he also struggled a few times to recall some details. We jokingly tried to help him to fill in the gaps, and nobody suspected any sort of serious problem. Dad also called some of the grandchildren by the wrong names and struggled to remember

93

some of the names and the faces of the guests. We blamed all of these little signals on the excitement of the day and did not think anything of it.

Shortly after the birthday party, our Aunt Marilyn started complaining about the bizarre behavior she was noticing about Dad. She complained that Dad was getting forgetful and confused. He would also wake up and knock at her door in the middle of the night, telling her to get up and go to work. She noticed that Dad was getting more aggravated and easily agitated. We suggested a visit to the doctor, and to our dismay, Dad was diagnosed as having Alzheimer's disease. Dad received the news very badly; he was very angry and went into seclusion for some time. He was a very independent man, and the thought of losing his independence was incomprehensible to him and very difficult to accept. You hear about Alzheimer's, but you don't know the seriousness of this illness until it hits close to home.

Gradually, Dad got worse—he would wander away, and people would find him and bring him back home. Luckily for us, it was a very small community. We reinforced the security in the house and installed an alarm system, but we did not put it on all of the windows. Dad was clever enough to know that the windows were not connected to the alarm, so he would climb out through the window in the middle of the night. Eventually we were forced to extend the alarm system to include all of the windows, too. My aunt tried to turn off the alarm in the daytime whenever she could watch him because neighbors were complaining about the alarm going off all the time. Dad became combative and agitated a few times, and he physically attacked my aunt. Thank heavens that she did not sustain any permanent injury.

One day around noon Dad went in the yard, took off all of his clothes, and started yelling "Help, help, help!!! Somebody help me!" The neighbors called my aunt, who was shocked to come outside and see Dad naked. She had left Dad on the couch taking a mid-day nap, while she went upstairs to do some housework. Dad got up from the nap and wandered into the yard while my aunt was upstairs, thinking he was still taking a nap.

My cousin, my aunt's youngest son, decided to move in to assist my aunt with caring for Dad. I also went over in the evenings and some weekends to relieve them as well. It was such a frustrating experience for all of us, but we did it with love. Taking care of him was worse than taking care of a child. We had to look out for little clues to figure out what his needs might be, because he reached a point when he could not tell us exactly what he wanted. Sometimes he would eat; sometimes he would not. He went to a specific bathroom in the house for a long time, and he sometimes forgot to go and had an accident.

A particular incident happened with Dad that really broke my heart; one day he started eating a bar of soap from the bathroom. By the time I found him, he had eaten half of the bar of soap. I tried to take it from him, and he got into a big struggle with me. He was very combative, telling me I had no business taking his dinner rolls from him. We ended up taking him to the hospital to have the soap flushed out of his system.

I was also trying to assist him with his hygiene one day, and I gave him a toothbrush with some toothpaste on it because he had indicated that he wanted a toothbrush. To my surprise, he started brushing his hair with the toothbrush and the toothpaste so his hair was full of toothpaste. Apparently, he had mistaken a toothbrush for a hairbrush. We started restricting guests from coming to the house to see him because he would suddenly take his clothes off, and by the time you knew it, he would be walking around the house naked. He was such a dignified man that it was difficult for us to watch him do some of the things he did. The whole situation was just unimaginable. When he could talk, he would tell us he was talking to his mom and dad, and he constantly talked about his childhood. He would also tell us at times that he was talking to our dead mom.

Another big challenge in the house was keeping the trash cans away from him. Being a janitor all of his life, Dad constantly went around the house changing the trash cans over and over again, even when there was no trash in them. We had to lock all the trash cans under the cabinet with a key. He believed he still had a job as a janitor. Dad's remote or long-term memory was intact for a while, and he would talk about paying the mortgage, electricity bill, and water bill. He would also ask us continuously for the car key so that he could take his paycheck to the bank to be deposited. After some years, we all became physically and emotionally exhausted from taking care of Dad, especially my aunt, who was almost as old as her brother.

We had a family meeting and decided that he needed to live in an environment safer than his home. It was a tough decision, but that was what was best for Dad and all of us. We had to put him in a nursing home, and we visited him there frequently; my aunt was there every day.

He became more combative as the illness advanced. On a few occasions he injured some of the nursing home staff who took care of him. Having cared for him at home for such a long time, we appreciated the selfless caregivers who took care of him in the nursing home. When I look at Dad, I see only a body, with the brain on a separate island on a vacation somewhere. This illness just does not make sense. We agreed for Dad to participate in an experimental study, taking a new drug, because we were glad to do anything we could to help advance research and to find a cure for this horrible illness. It hits too close to home for us, knowing that the gene could be inherited. We started doing our homework, researching the family history, and we discovered Alzheimer's had run in our Dad's family for a long time. We feel as a family that we are racing against time, hoping that they will find a cure in case we inherited the gene.

Dad finally died from Alzheimer's disease, and it was very difficult to let go. There was also a sense of relief that now he would rest in peace. Although he had long ago stopped being aware of what was going on in his life, for those of us who loved him and watched him struggle with Alzheimer's, his final years were heartbreaking.

# Quotes of Encouragement...

As the wind blows harder and Mr. Covington's story sounds familiar to you, remember the following:

*"Events will take their course; it is no good our being angry at them; he is happiest who wisely turns them to the best account."*

~ *Euripides*

When stared in the face by Alzheimer's, get angry but do not stay angry so that you will not die angry; enjoy the time you have to the fullest, try to fulfill the unfulfilled dreams that can still be fulfilled; remember that every moment counts. *(LB)*

*"You will find as you look back upon your life, that the moments that stand out, the moments when you have really lived, are the moments when you have done things in a spirit of love."*

~ *Henry Drummond*

When you sometimes feel like giving up on the care of your loved one with Alzheimer's, let the spirit of love renew your inner strength. This spirit of love is what radiates in you as gentleness and kindness, and it is the unconditional physical and mental sacrifice you make. This spirit of love is your unconditional presence until your loved one takes the last breath; this spirit of love is your relentless sacrifice to help your loved one live a comfortable life in an uncomfortable situation. *(LB)*

*"The best portion of a good man's life,*
*His little nameless, unremembered acts*
*Of kindness and of love."*

~ *William Wordsworth*

We tend to forget the professional caregivers in a nursing home or an assisted living facility who take care of our loved ones with Alzheimer's. We may not know their names; we may not be there to witness their acts of kindness toward our loved ones, but we must remember that they make a lot of daily sacrifices as they care for these people who are battling with Alzheimer's. They deserve to be appreciated; their job is more than a paycheck — it is a labor of love, and they must be encouraged always. *(LB)*

## Alzheimer's Disease:
# BASIC FACTS & UNDERSTANDING

M r. Bolton, Mrs. Caudel, and Mr. Covington all had *Alzheimer's disease*, which is one of the most dreaded and feared mental illnesses. It is characterized by a progressive decline of cognitive functioning and memory loss, and it totally robs its victims of their personalities. They lose their sparkle and seem not to be themselves. The physical body becomes an empty shell, and the mind is not there. Alzheimer's disease is often referred to as a thief of the human mind. The common age of onset for Alzheimer's is usually after the age of sixty-five, but it can occur at a much earlier age in some cases. People with early onset seem to have a strong genetic loading or a strong family history for the disease.

The early symptoms of Alzheimer's may be so subtle that they may go unnoticed by family members. People with Alzheimer's may try to compensate for the memory loss initially by hiding their memory deficits. Facing the reality of losing one's mind could be very frightening for anyone. People with Alzheimer's may stay in denial at first by putting up a charming persona or front to compensate for their memory deficiency. They may also *confabulate*, which is simply an unconscious mechanism of making up stories or answers in response to questions asked whenever they cannot remember the right answer to the question. Confabulation should not be regarded or seen as lying; it could be very hurtful for the people suffering from Alzheimer's if they are accused of telling lies when they confabulate. Confabulation is an effort on the part of the victim to protect their self-esteem.

During the early phase, people with Alzheimer's may not be conscious of what the problem is; they may feel extremely helpless, and they are usually frightened and depressed. They get very forgetful and start to misplace things around the house or in their environment. Gradually, they lose their short term or recent memory. With the progression of the disease, the ability to function gradually declines. They become more confused, and basic tasks such as housekeeping, driving, or cooking become more difficult. As a result, they may gradually withdraw from social activities.

Also with the progression of the disease comes the inability to attend to activities of daily living. Activities of daily living are simple and basic things that we do on daily basis such as toileting, grooming, dressing, and bathing. Such simple tasks become a major problem for them. Verbal communication is usually impaired and frustration may set in. They may become physically and verbally abusive out of frustration, or on the other hand, they may withdraw from their environment. They may also wander aimlessly and not know where they are coming from or going to. Restlessness is also common. Since Alzheimer's disease is a progressive degenerative disease, the progression goes from early to middle to final stages. These stages are usually characterized by their level of functioning at the different phases of the illness.

*Sun downing* may also be a challenge for caregivers. For example, at certain time of the day, usually at dinnertime, people with Alzheimer's may suddenly get restless and may become combative and agitated, insisting that they have to go home and prepare dinner for their family, when they actually live in an assisted living facility or a nursing home. If they live in the home with other family members, they may sneak into the kitchen and try to prepare dinner. Such a response is called *sun downing*. With sun downing, they are responding to the pre-coded routine, remote information in the brain programming them to do certain things at certain times of the day. They may talk about going to pick up the children from school or after-school care. They may also worry about taking the children to an after-school athletic event or practice. Since remote or long-term memory is the last to go, they will still remember the remote past for some time while letting go of recent memories quickly.

*Perseveration* is also common in people with Alzheimer's. Perseveration is simply an act of repeating a behavior or a phrase. For example, an elderly person suffering from Alzheimer's may continuously ask for his son, Jack, every five minutes, despite the fact that he has been told over and over again that Jack lives two hours away and will not be back to see him until the weekend.

People with Alzheimer's may also have *aphasia*, which is simply a loss of language. The loss of language is a gradual process, progressing from having difficulty with finding the right word to use to describe an object or a situation, to a gradual decrease in vocabulary, to babbling and finally to complete loss of words called *mutism*.

*Apraxia* is also common. This refers to a loss of purposeful movement with no underlying sensory or motor impairment. Common examples of apraxia include the inability to unlock a door, to drive, to walk, or to put on one's clothes.

Another common symptom is *agnosia*, which refers to the inability to recognize objects. For example, a person suffering from Alzheimer's disease may not recognize food as a substance to be eaten, clothes as something to be worn, or book as something to be read. If a telephone is ringing near them, they may not answer it because the ringing tone of the telephone may not mean anything to them. They cannot recognize the phone as a means of communication. The most difficult type of agnosia is their inability to recognize people, even their own children, grandchildren, spouse, and other family members. They may not even recognize themselves in the mirror. This is usually very devastating for family members.

Memory impairment is always a red flag in the initial diagnosis of Alzheimer's disease, especially if the memory impairment cannot be attributed to anything else. Once it is ruled out that nothing is wrong with the client medically, the clinician making the diagnosis will start narrowing down the diagnosis to Alzheimer's. The remote (old) memory stays intact for a while, and the recent (new) memory is lost very quickly. Again, this is primarily because the brain cannot encode or store new information. A person with Alzheimer's may not be able to tell you what she ate for breakfast, but may easily recount every food item on the table at the family's Thanksgiving dinner when she was ten years old. Eventually, both the remote and the recent memories disappear.

Communication with the victims of Alzheimer's may appear similar to that of a person with psychosis (losing touch with reality) or delusions (false belief held to be true by that person only, despite evidence to the contrary). For instance, they may claim to see things that are not visible to the people around them, and also to carry on a full dialogue with an imaginary person that is not visible to the people around them. Clinicians must be careful not to label the client as psychotic or delusional because the remote memory is the last to go with this illness. They may just be re-living their past experiences stored in their remote memory. For example, an Alzheimer's client in a clinical setting may continuously talk about a funeral and get really busy planning for this funeral. The staff may think she is delusional or psychotic, only to find out from a family member later that she was talking about her father's funeral that she planned thirty years ago. Since the remote memory is the last to go, clinicians must be sure of their facts before giving a diagnosis of a psychotic or delusional problem to these patients. If an Alzheimer's client is found to be actually psychotic or delusional, he or she could be treated with medication.

Another common symptom with Alzheimer is the *disturbance in executive function*. This simply refers to the impairment in a person's ability to make plans. For instance, planning a family vacation, organizing a picnic, planning a birthday party, and such common day-to-day planning become an extremely complex exercise for the brain of a person with Alzheimer's.

The final stage of the illness is characterized by the inability to recognize self in the mirror. They cannot recognize family members as well, and they may mumble or totally lack any verbal communication. Weight loss is common because they cannot remember how to eat, chew, or swallow at this stage of the illness. They may also forget how to walk, so mobility becomes a serious problem. Other complications of the disease include limb contracture (inability to completely stretch both arms and legs), bed sores or pressure ulcers, pneumonia, and finally death. The average lifespan from the onset of the disease to death is about ten years.

The cause of this terrible illness is still poorly understood. Some of the biological findings include the discovery of tangles and plaques in the brain tissues. These tangles and plaques affect the part of the brain that is responsible for our short-term memories and emotions. As the disease progresses, both the short-term and the long-term memories are finally lost.

There is also a strong genetic factor in the development of Alzheimer's disease. There have been a lot of studies into the hereditary predisposition. People with Alzheimer's usually have a strong family history. Twin studies of identical twins versus fraternal twins also show that genetically, both identical twins are likely to develop Alzheimer's, whereas one of the fraternal twins may develop the disease and the other may not. Identical twins are supposed to have the same genetic code and are usually mirror images of one another, whereas the fraternal twins are not a mirror image of one another.

*Dysregulation* or abnormal regulation of some naturally occurring chemicals in the brain called neurotransmitters have also been implicated in Alzheimer's disease. Too little concentration of certain neurotransmitters in the brain is believed to be partly responsible for Alzheimer's. Neurotransmitters are the chemical messengers that facilitate communication between the cells in the brain called neurons. Other biological factors are also involved.

It is easy to confuse Alzheimer's with other diseases that are very common in the elderly. Physicians and health care professionals must be able to rule out other diseases whose signs and symptoms may mimic those of Alzheimer's. Common examples may include infection, drug toxicity, drug overdose, and metabolic disorders such as diabetes. Infection such as urinary tract infections in the elderly can cause severe confusion, disorientation, and agitation, if left untreated. An elderly person with the diagnosis of diabetes whose blood sugar is uncontrolled may be confused and show symptoms of confusion that may mimic Alzheimer's.

Drug toxicity may also pose a problem because many elderly people are on several medications. Drug interaction or accidental overdose due to forgetfulness may cause some severe problems and confusion. For example, they could accidentally use a medication that was to be used once a day twice a day, due to forgetfulness. This could easily produce confusion and other signs and symptoms that could mimic Alzheimer's. Depression in an elderly person could also affect the memory and thus mimic Alzheimer's. A depressed elderly person may be confused, have memory loss, and show cognitive decline. It must be noted, however, that people diagnosed with Alzheimer's may suffer from depression, especially in the early stages of the diagnosis when they feel powerless. They face the reality that they have to live with this devastating illness until their death, and this thought could precipitate depression.

Precautionary measures must be taken to avoid possible misdiagnosis of Alzheimer's in elderly people. A clinician must do a very thorough history and physical, and must get a very good description of the recent symptoms.

A thorough laboratory assessment must be done, which may require some blood tests. Specific radiological studies or some special x-rays may be required. A mental status examination may also be required. It is used to evaluate the clients' level of orientation to the environment or to evaluate the clients' understanding of reality in their environment. Other tests such as a mini mental status examination must also be conducted. This is to further evaluate the level of orientation, mental deterioration, and the stage of the disease.

Diagnosis and management of Alzheimer's must be strictly handled by a licensed clinician with sufficient medical knowledge in the area of psychiatry, medicine, psychology, or nursing, or any other properly licensed clinician who is qualified to make such diagnosis in that community.

There are a lot of new medications in the market designed to slow down the progression of the disease. The appropriate medications for the client must be determined by a licensed clinician based on a comprehensive history of the client. A person with Alzheimer's should also be treated with medication for a possible underlying depression.

Safety concerns for people with Alzheimer include keeping them in a safe environment where they cannot wander away. This may require putting them in a locked unit in a long-term care unit or facility. The environment must also be clutter free, and the floor must be kept dry to prevent a fall. People diagnosed with Alzheimer's who are not kept in a safe environment may wander away and never be found. They may not be able to give any personal information which could help to locate their family members due to memory loss. A safety bracelet with personal information of the person that could help to locate family members or significant other must be worn always.

It is always very difficult for family members to put their loved ones in a nursing home or a long-term facility. Family members carry a lot of guilt and feel that they have failed their loved ones. Unfortunately, the caregivers can easily develop what is called the *caretaker's burn-out syndrome*. This is a situation in which the caregivers find themselves physically and emotionally drained from taking care of their loved one. Certified clinicians are usually available in the community to provide support and make this transition easier on the caregiver and the family members.

It is very important that family members of a person with Alzheimer's join a support group designed to help people like themselves. Sharing experiences, comparing notes, giving and receiving advice, and dealing with the loss are all very important in the management of this debilitating mental illness. Support groups provide emotional and psychological support and benefit family members and caregivers in working through this difficult process.

A person diagnosed with Alzheimer's disease can also join a support group of people diagnosed with Alzheimer's in the initial stage of the disease before the memory loss becomes advanced. The support groups could help the victim of this horrible illness deal with the stage of denial of not wanting to believe that this is really happening to them. At the initial stage, a person with Alzheimer's may harbor a lot of anger about the diagnosis. Going to a good support group could help the victim work through the angry stage, and finally reach a stage of acceptance. Working through all the emotions could help the victim deal with the diagnosis better. He would know what to expect as the illness progresses. This would enable him to tidy up his house in the area of making important long-term decisions that may affect him later when he is incapable of making such decisions.

Management of Alzheimer's disease could easily become a financial drain on the family. Families have been thrown into poverty in their efforts to care for their loved ones with Alzheimer's. This terrible illness does not discriminate; it affects people in most societies, and cuts across every ethnic and socioeconomic group. It affects male or female, and rich or poor equally. Due to lack of education or knowledge about this illness, it may be difficult for some people in some cultures to put a name to it, or to seek professional help. As a result, they may not be able to get the proper diagnosis. People with higher socioeconomic status or people who are wealthy may have the advantage of being able to provide a much higher level of care for their family members, especially in the well informed societies where information is readily available about Alzheimer's.

The common goal is to get help for the individual with Alzheimer's and the family members. This is important because family members are usually the initial caretakers. It is not wise to live alone or in isolation with this devastating illness, so reach out for help as soon as possible.

PART V

# COMMON PROBLEMS RELATED TO SUBSTANCE ABUSE AND ADDICTION

## Addiction:
# LARRY'S STORY

I wish I had accepted long time ago that I have one of the worst mental illnesses, called addiction. My outcome in life would have been different, and I would not be sitting in jail now. By the time I am eligible for parole, my life will be almost over.

I grew up watching my parents drink, and they would get into verbal arguments when they were drunk, which were usually followed by physical fights. Mom ended up in the hospital several times with physical injuries, but she always covered up for Dad, giving different excuses about her bruises to the hospital staff. Finally, they got a divorce.

When I was growing up, I despised the lifestyle of my parents. All the yelling, screaming, and arguments always played back in my mind. I told myself as a child that I would never live like that when I grow older. After Dad left, the situation got worse. Mom left us unattended, and came home drunk, frequently with different boyfriends. I was ten years old, and I had a brother who was eight and a sister who was six. We learned to fend for ourselves very quickly, but the neglect was so bad that we could not do a good enough job taking care of ourselves. We were still children who should be cared for. As much as we tried to hide our situation at home, the teachers picked up on it at school and started asking us a lot of questions about home. We did not have winter coats in freezing winter temperatures. We also wore summer outfits in the heart of winter. As little kids, we tried to do the best we could with our hygiene, but our hygiene was so compromised and obviously bad that anybody could easily figure out that something was not right at home.

The teachers called the Department of Human Services (also known as DHS) to investigate our family's home life. The Department of Human Services paid a surprise visit to the house and found very filthy living conditions with no food in the refrigerator. Our neighbors were interrogated by DHS, and the neighbors told them about how we come to their doors to beg for food, and how we were left home alone most of the time. This agency removed us from our home and placed us in temporary foster care, and an effort was made to locate our father. At that time, we had not seen our dad for over a year, and DHS discovered that our dad was in jail in a neighboring state.

Our grandmother, who was about sixty-three years old at that time, came forward to take custody of the three of us. Grandma had some medical problems, and she was declining in health, but she tried her very best to take care of us. Mom would show up at Grandma's house occasionally, always drunk. She would then disappear into thin air for weeks. I harbored much anger and resentment toward my parents, but unfortunately I took out my anger and frustration on my innocent grandma, who was struggling to take care of us in her old age. By the time I was fourteen, I was already a problem; I caused my grandma a great deal of stress, and I regularly lashed out at her.

I lied about my age to get a job, and I was working by the age of fourteen. I worked very hard and started drinking by the time I was fifteen. I was always drinking and staying out with the wrong groups of friends. I actually felt that I was having fun, while a soft, quiet voice inside of my head reminded me from time to time that I should not be going in that same direction that had destroyed my parents and my family. I was too angry to listen to my inner voice.

Knowing what I know now, I was drinking at that time to numb my emotional pain. By the time I was seventeen, I had moved out of my grandma's house. It was a good decision because I had stressed her out so much with my irresponsible behavior that her health declined even more.

I met a woman at the restaurant where I worked, and we used to go out to a bar and drink together almost every night. Before I knew what was happening, we had moved in together and were getting drunk regularly. We ended up getting married and having two children together. The marriage was utterly chaotic, doomed to fail from the beginning because we were both alcoholics. I saw the cycle repeating itself; this was exactly how my parents lived. My wife and I argued constantly because we were always drunk. There was rarely a sober moment around the house. My wife and I had the same codependent relationship as my parents—just one generation later.

I found myself beating my wife, and she covered for me with the law just as my mom had covered for my dad. She ended up in the hospital several times, and she lied about the cause of her injury in order to keep me out of jail. We eventually divorced. My ex-wife cleaned up her life after we divorced; she went to rehabilitation, became sober, and re-married. The court granted her the custody of our two boys. I was too drunk to pay her child support, and I could not be bothered about my children.

Life began and ended with the bottle every day. I went from one low-paying job to another menial job; somehow, someone always employed me. By the time I was twenty five, I was a serious addict and a dangerous alcoholic. I had several tickets for driving under the influence of alcohol. I was always detained in the jail for a short period of time and then released back into the community. The jail was so congested with criminals that people with issues like mine were not of serious concern to the law enforcement agency. Unfortunately looking back now, I know that repeat offenders like me should have been at the top of the priority list of the law enforcement agency. We are no doubt a serious threat to our society.

One fateful evening, I left one bar to go to another bar. I got into my truck in a completely drunken state. I had no business driving at all, but I did not have it together enough mentally to know right from wrong. I always played down my drinking. I was in total denial because of my addiction. I had been lying to myself for years about my addiction and had convinced myself that I could handle alcohol; the only thing that mattered to me in life was the bottle. My life was to work and drink. On the way to another bar, I blacked out, and the next thing I remembered was the sound of an ambulance and several police cars. Apparently I ran into a pregnant woman in a head-on collision; I went completely out of my lane and did not know it.

Instantly, I woke up from my dream state. I was terrified; the woman was covered with blood, and I saw the emergency and fire truck personnel trying to get her out of her car. I was taken to jail, and for the first time in my life, I knew how to pray. I spent all my time in jail praying that the woman would not die because I was so terrified by what I saw at the scene of the accident.

The woman was rushed to a nearby hospital, where she died the next day; she was five months pregnant. Taking her life was bad enough but finding out that she was five months pregnant made me hate myself. I was so depressed I wish I would die. I had taken two precious lives because of a senseless addiction.

I went on trial, and the prosecutor and the family were extremely bitter, which I expected them to be. The lady had two other children both under the age of five, and their pictures were brought to court. The jury had absolutely no mercy on me, because I was a repeat offender. I got the maximum sentence for every count against me, which meant serving a total of thirty-five years with no option of parole.

## Winds Against The Mind

The reality dawned on me that I would have to be in jail for thirty-five years as a consequence of making wrong choices and for remaining an addict until I had taken two innocent lives. I have never been able to forgive myself until today. The picture of the lady's two children kept haunting me; I could not stop thinking about how I deprived two innocent children of being raised and loved by their mom, and how I also deprived her husband from having a wife.

Sooner or later her children will know the story of their mom — that she was killed by a drunk driver, and that I was the drunk driver. Her children will also find out that they were denied a chance of having another baby brother or sister because of me. I could not believe that I ruined two precious lives in a mere instant and destroyed the joy of an innocent family. I read a letter of apology to her family during the trial, but my sorrow will definitely not bring her back. I hope others reading my story will learn from my experience, and not wait until they kill somebody. I was in total denial until this tragic accident, believing that I could always handle a few more bottles.

When something completely takes over your life and your mind, and you are completely powerless and controlled by it, face the reality that you are dealing with an addiction. Get help and stop telling yourself that you are in control, because you are not. The truth is that you are totally out of control. Whatever your addiction is, get help for it. If it is alcohol, please do something about it, and don't wait until another person gets killed. Please do something before it is too late.

# Quotes of Encouragement...

As the wind blows harder and Larry's story sounds familiar to you, remember the following:

*"The lecture you deliver may be wise and true,*
*But I'd rather get my lessons by observing what you do,*
*I may not understand the high advice you like to give,*
*But there is no misunderstanding how you act and how you live."*

~ *Edgar A. Guest*

As parents, the greatest textbook you can write for your children is the behavior you model to them; you cannot act irresponsibly and teach responsibility to your children; you set your children up for failure when you model bad behavior; children are likely to do what they learn by observation rather than what they are told to do; you cannot be an addict and expect to raise a sober child. *(LB)*

*"Man must cease attributing his problems to his environment, and learn again to exercise his will— his personal responsibility."*

~ *Albert Schweitzer*

As a child, you cannot choose your parents and you cannot choose your birth environment. What you can choose is what you want to make out of your life and what you want to make out of your birth environment. You have the willpower to succeed and the willpower to fail. No matter what unfortunate circumstances you were born into, activate your willpower to succeed. Do not be a victim; there is always a room to grow for a willing heart. "Will" and "power" yourself to make the wrongs in your life right and to turn your misfortunes into fortunes. *(LB)*

*"How shall I habit break?*
*As you did that habit make,*
*As you gathered you must lose;*
*As you yielded now refuse.*
*Thread by thread the strands we twist*
*Till they bind us neck and wrist,*
*Thread by thread the patient hand*
*Must untwine 'ere free we stand."*

~ *John Boyle O'Reilly*

Addiction is a self-imprisonment of the mind and the body. You have to be determined to get yourself out of this jail and to exercise your option of parole; otherwise you are doomed with a life sentence. Accept your failures, set a goal to succeed, and never give up. Get up whenever you fall; do not stay down. Refuse to quit; you fail only when you quit. *(LB)*

*Winds Against The Mind*

## Addiction:

# MR. SHAW'S STORY

**E**very time I looked at my wife, I told myself that she deserved a much better man than I was. My wife is a stunningly beautiful, articulate, brilliant woman, who is also extremely kind. I don't know what else is there to look for in a woman that she does not have. Unfortunately, I had an addiction, and I could not understand why I was doing what I was doing. I wanted to stop, but I could not make myself stop. I was addicted to sex. The feeling was like a rush, an intense and powerful feeling of wanting to have sex all the time. I wouldn't stop until I had satisfied this selfish desire. I am ashamed of so many things I have done, and for years I also lived with the day-to-day fear that one day the rest of the world would know the truth about me and my addiction.

Being privately employed and running my own business did not help my dilemma. I had a successful business, and made a lot of money. I primarily ran my private office like a motel for years, and I got away with it. I had affairs with several women who worked for me, both single and married. My longest affair, with a former secretary, lasted for twelve years; we were having sex at least two to three times a day in the office for twelve years. I used to schedule several business trips so that I could feed my addiction; some were frivolous trips, others were important. I always looked forward to the nights with different prostitutes. I had affairs with the wives of friends and close associates who trusted me. I was eager to have sex with anybody who would feed into my addiction, with little discretion. I found myself in our bedroom one day with the housekeeper that my wife employed to clean the house. I always felt ashamed and disgusted with myself and my infidelities, but I could not make myself stop. I have cried several times and have told my wife to feel free to file for a divorce, because I always knew she definitely deserved a better man than I could ever be with this addiction, but she did not leave. I did not want to divorce her, because I could never leave her to marry another woman, but I knew I deserved to be divorced by her.

# Winds Against The Mind

My problem did not stem from a desire to marry another woman; there was no doubt in my mind that I loved my wife very much. The problem was, for some reason, I just could not make myself stop cheating on her. Still, my wife continually refused to leave the marriage, despite the fact that she had caught me cheating on her several times. After some time, I convinced myself that she had accepted me, even though I had been unfaithful, so I gave myself the very selfish and self-centered permission to continue to cheat on her.

Beauty was not an issue for me because I would have sex with any woman who was willing to feed my addiction. Most of the women I slept with did not even compare to my wife's beauty. The only line I never crossed to feed my addiction was the line dividing me from my children, but anybody else was fair game. We have three beautiful girls, and I could tell that my wife kept an eye on my interaction with the girls; she did not trust me at all with the children.

My wife would not allow other children to spend the night in our house unless I was out of town. If I suddenly cancelled my trip, she would immediately cancel a previous arrangement to allow other kids to spend the night with our girls. Our daughters' feelings were hurt many times because their mom would suddenly cancel their plans to have their friends over; they would even come and complain to me about their mom's decisions. Unfortunately, I could not tell the girls that I was the problem, not their mom.

I was disgusted with myself one day when I realized that I was making passes at one of my daughter's teenage friends. Fortunately, the young girl did not pick up on my passes. I remember a time when I was scheduled to be out of town for one week, and unfortunately the trip was cut short and I was back at home three days later. My wife was expecting me to be gone for a week, so she had planned for her friend's younger sister to come and visit. My wife could not turn around and ask her to leave when I returned, but I know she was worried. The young woman was very attractive, and from the moment I set my eyes on her, I was obsessing with how to seduce her. I could not take my mind off her, and I was constantly trying to figure out how I could have sex with her. Somehow, my personal charm and money always gave me an edge to trap vulnerable women very easily. My wife, who was all too familiar with my 'social habits', tried very hard to keep an eye on the young woman.

All week long my wife encouraged her to be out of the house whenever she had to go somewhere. Before the end of the week, however, I found a window of opportunity that allowed me to be alone for a few hours with the young woman. I had already been working on her with my usual charm. She fell into my trap, and I found myself in bed with her in no time. We were not caught by my wife, and

I enjoyed another of my 'secret' victories. The affairs I enjoyed most were those involving the dangerous risks that I took in my matrimonial home and got away with. My wife suspected something with the young lady, but she could not prove it. She never allowed the young lady to come back and visit again.

The only thing I think about apart from food and keeping my successful business going is sex. One time I gave my wife a sexually transmitted disease, and she would no longer have anything to do with me unless I was wearing a condom for protection. I would schedule unnecessary trips to previous destinations where I had been, just to have a repeat experience with some specific prostitutes that I had previous encounters with. I was a frequent flyer visitor to an adult club outside of our community. I always made sure I did not go to any adult club close to where we lived for fear of being identified. I also wore lots of disguises to the places I went. I was a big collector of pornographic magazines, and I ran up huge telephone bills calling sex lines.

There were several times that I hated myself for what I was doing, even to the point of not wanting to live. Sadly these feeling that controlled me were so compelling that it felt like my existence was tied to this addiction. My wife would discover the most degrading things in my suitcase when I returned from a trip. I always made sure that most of my bills from the trip were sent to the office, so that I could spare my wife a few more eyesores. Some people in the community were aware of my sexual misbehavior, but nobody seemed to talk about it because I was a philanthropist in the community. I gave a lot of money and sponsored a lot of community projects.

On one of my trips, I was in a room with a prostitute who was on the run from a law enforcement agency, and I was not aware of it. Unfortunately for me, there was a drug bust by the police, and I was terrified. I was arrested and later released because I was not in possession of any drugs. My addiction was to sex, not drugs, but I was always willing to pay for the women to buy the drugs. I found it easier to manipulate these women to do whatever I wanted them to do when they were high on drugs. I also had another fake identity card that I carried with me whenever I was in a place where I should not be. The fake identity saved me from being recognized several times.

All along I carried a lot of guilt and shame. I was never a cold-hearted addict, and although deep inside me I had an unparalleled love for my wife, I simply could not make myself stop this irresponsible sexual behavior. Loving my wife so much but still cheating on her was what puzzled me about this horrible addiction; it was a serious bondage. I continued to keep the good family man image in the community and lived a phony double life.

I came back from a trip one day and heard a knock on the door, I was asked to sign for a letter. I opened it and I was shocked. My wife had just filed for divorce. Apparently she had planned the divorce a long time ago; she was just waiting to do it in her own time. She wanted our youngest child to be in college before asking me for a divorce. I was so shocked that I almost fainted. I had asked her to leave me several times in the past because I was convinced she deserved somebody much better than I could ever be, but she stayed married to me all these years. I thought she had decided to stay married to me, regardless of my dark baggage of sexual addiction. Lo and behold, I was totally wrong. She told me that she decided to keep the family together while the children were younger because of her own sad childhood. Her father walked away from her mom and the children when she was seven years old, and she never got over the pain of being left at an early age by her father.

My wife said she made a promise to herself that she would never divide our family. She had determined the only reason she would divorce me while the children were younger was if any of our daughters ever complained to her that I had attempted to abuse or molest them sexually. She would be ready to fight me publicly at that point. Fortunately for me, I never crossed that line in all of my insanity; I never attempted to molest my children.

My wife made the divorce very simple; she asked for the divorce on the grounds of irreconcilable differences. She even protected me by not exposing all of my deviant behavior in the divorce papers she filed. She said the divorce record is a public document, and she did not want any future public embarrassment for the children. Throughout our marriage, I was not a particularly doting father, and this was perfectly okay with my wife; she did not trust me with the children anyway. She was always glad to limit my involvement with the children throughout the marriage. She explained to the children that their dad had to work very hard to be able to take care of the family, which was why I was not so involved with them. She said she gave up her career in order to compensate for their dad's busy schedule. The children were okay with the arrangement, and I was a good financial provider anyway. It all worked out well.

All of a sudden, I found myself begging my wife not to leave me, but her mind was made up. She threatened to expose me to the world with all the overwhelming evidence she had collected over the years if I tried to fight the divorce. She confronted me with the fact that I was a sexual addict who was in total denial, and that I needed to go get help. She clearly stated that she was not willing to be part of this arrangement anymore, because I caused her too much pain and suffering that would take a lifetime for her to heal from.

**119**

# Winds Against The Mind

After the divorce, it dawned on me that I would not be able to get away with my addiction without everybody knowing the truth about me. I had been hiding for so long under the perfect family-man umbrella, and now that the cover was removed, the truth about me would soon be known on the streets if I didn't do something. I frantically started searching for help; I didn't even know until my wife left me that there was help for sexual addiction. I thought it was something you just had to endure.

Finally I am in a long-term, out-patient treatment program. I am also in a support group which has really been helpful. I was shocked to find out that there are many other people out there who are battling the same addiction. When I listened to other people's stories, I realized that a lot more people suffer from this illness than we actually realize. It's been a long journey to recovery. I am traveling the pathway one day at a time. I feel sad every time I think about the years of pain and hurt I caused my wife. She is re-married now, and looks very happy in her new relationship. Every time I see her, I always feel very envious of her current husband. I wish I could retrace my steps and make decisions that would have stopped my addiction from ruining my marriage to such a wonderful woman.

She finally told the children about my sexual addiction and about what she had endured for years. She showed the children some evidence she had collected over the years to justify her decision to leave. The children were shocked; they could not understand how their mom was able to deal with this situation for so long, and to hide it from them in order to protect them from hurt and pain. The children forgave me, and we have good father-daughter relationships. I am the one who needs to forgive myself. I lost the most precious thing to me in life, which is my family, and it all happened because of this senseless and selfish addiction.

If your story sounds like mine, please do something. Sexual addiction is a terrible addiction, and it is always downplayed by society. As a result, a lot of people don't take personal responsibility for it or make any attempt to get help. It is especially condoned as acceptable behavior for virile men; most societies indirectly rubberstamp their approval for men to run around with other women. Sexual addiction is not only a problem with men; a lot of women, both young and old, also deal with this problem. Don't allow sexual addiction to destroy you; it is not worth the risk. Get help because it is better late than never.

# Quotes of Encouragement...

As the wind blows harder and Mr. Shaw's story sounds familiar to you, remember the following:

*"When you do the wrong thing, knowing it is wrong, you do so because you haven't developed the habit of effectively controlling or neutralizing strong inner urges that tempt you, because you have established the wrong habits and don't know how to eliminate them effectively."*

*~ W. Clement Stone*

Addiction is like a firmly established bad habit; there is a strong element of selfishness to addiction because feeding the addiction produces some satisfaction, and this makes it very difficult to give up this bad habit; you continuously give in to the urge because of the selfish reward; to break the chain, you have to step aside, confront the problem, look within yourself, and be willing to change; utilize every resource available to you to break this bad habit; otherwise the bad habit will eventually break you into pieces. *(LB)*

*"We may think there is willpower involved, but more likely... change is due to want power. Wanting the new addiction more than the old one. Wanting the new me in preference to the... person I am now."*

*~ George Sheehan*

An inner drive, a willing heart, a strong desire to change, and self-determination are some of the ingredients for "want power." It is not going to be an easy journey, but you have to be sick and tired of being that dog that constantly goes back to its vomit. *(LB)*

*"If I had to select one quality, one personal characteristic that I regard as being most highly correlated with success... I would pick the trait of persistence. Determination: the will to endure to the end, to get knocked down seventy times and get up off the floor saying, 'here goes number seventy one!'"*

*~ Richard M. DeVos*

Addiction is not easy to beat; you are at war fighting for your life, and you have to win or your life may be at stake; it is not going to be a smooth ride, it is a step-by-step process; no matter what you face, do not quit. *(LB)*

Addiction:

# TONY'S STORY

**W**e live in an affluent suburb of a very big city; we are a wealthy
family living in an upper class community. We sent our son to an
exclusive private school, and we were able to give him a lot more
than we had when we were growing up. We knew about drugs and
saw drug related killings on the news all the time. We lived in a fool's paradise,
actually believing that drugs and violence were restricted to the other side of town
where the poor people lived. We thought we did not have to worry about drugs, and
we believed our community should be drug-free since it was crime-free.

Tony was our only child, and we tried to do everything right in raising him.
He always did very well in school, so we thought we were doing a great job as
parents. He was involved in many youth activities; he was the president of two
youth clubs and was a speaker against drugs and alcohol. We had no reason to
suspect that Tony could be involved in drugs and alcohol. We had a huge wine
cellar in the house, and none of the wine bottles were missing.

Tony wanted to be a lawyer, and as his parents, we were excited about this
goal. He was very outspoken and a good public speaker. Our house has three levels,
and Tony's room was on the third floor. We were on the middle floor. Tony was a
typical teenager with a lot of friends, and at age fifteen he asked to move to the
basement of the house in an effort to establish some independence. He told us that
the primary reason he wanted to move to the basement was to keep from
disturbing us, because his friends were always in and out of the house. We thought
this was very considerate of him, and we readily agreed to his request. Most of his

friends were children from the neighborhood, in a comparable station in life with Tony's; we just automatically assumed that they were all good kids. We walked around in ignorance and could not see beyond our own little world. Tony had his own fair share of disagreements with us as parents, just like most typical teenagers, but these were nothing out of the ordinary.

On this fateful day, around three o'clock in the morning, we heard a knock at the door. It was very strange. We had never before had anyone knocking on the door in the middle of the night. We could not imagine who it might be. We assumed that Tony was home, and if he was not home, he had a key.

My husband got to the door, looked through the side window, and saw a police officer. He opened the door in panic, and asked the police officer what was wrong. "I am so sorry," the police officer said. "For what?" my husband questioned. The officer continued and said, "We received a call from a rave that a boy was unconscious; we responded with an ambulance and did everything we could. We gave him CPR [cardio pulmonary resuscitation] and rushed him to the hospital emergency room, but it was too late. I am very sorry to tell you that the boy died, and he was identified as your son." (A rave is an all night party frequently attended by a very large number of youth).

My husband told the police officer that there must be some mistake because our son did not go to raves. Besides, his car was outside, so we thought he was home. The officer told my husband to check the house and make sure that our son was at home. My husband and I rushed down to the basement to check if Tony was in his room, and to our surprise, Tony was not in the house.

We got dressed and went to the hospital to identify the body, even though we were still convinced in our minds that it could not be Tony. We were shocked when we got to the hospital. It was like a bad dream when we discovered the body was Tony's, and he was dead, as cold as ice. We both felt like dying at the spot; we held each other and simultaneously wondered how we had missed such a serious problem. The autopsy later revealed that he died of a drug overdose.

After Tony was buried, we went through a phase of severe depression and not wanting to live. Every day became a struggle. Our lives were like a shattered dream. We were not alone—the incident shook the entire community, and everyone was in shock. Tony was a nice, polite young man, and his death was mourned by many people.

One day when I was mourning the loss of my son, I made a decision to do something before another child wound up dead. Our Tony used to come in and out of the house with a lot of other teenagers. I was convinced that there must be more teenagers at risk. I searched Tony's room for any possible clues that I could find, and I was surprised by what I discovered in his room. I found pills, needles, syringes, and street drugs. I was totally shocked because Tony was exceptionally skilled at hiding everything from us. It took an extensive search and almost tearing his room apart to discover some of the dangerous drugs that Tony had in the house. He had things hidden inside his mattress and pillows. He disguised drugs in obscure places and corners around his room. He would hide cocaine inside his cologne box, and hide needles and syringes inside his shaving kit. You really had to be searching for these items to discover where they were in Tony's room.

We also realized that a lot of the wine bottles in the house had been replaced with water. My husband and I rarely drank alcohol. We used wine only for formal entertainment or on holidays. We were both from families of alcoholics, and we decided to stay away from alcohol to prevent us from falling into the same trap as our parents. We had no clue that Tony had been drinking the wine and filling the bottles with water.

We also wondered how Tony got the money to support his drug habit since he had no job. Our money was never missing in the house, so we knew he hadn't stolen money from us, which we know now some children do in his condition. We gave Tony a weekly allowance which we thought was very reasonable and comparable to other neighborhood kids. Tony would ask for money to buy new clothes and other items such as electronics. He said he was trying to keep up with the fashion whenever he asked for money for new clothes. We did not see the need to deprive him of the money because he was doing so well in school. We were very generous to him as parents, and we never questioned him about what he did with the money or asked for receipts. We realized that we might have indirectly supplied the money to support Tony's habit. Looking back now, we probably gave him too much money without even realizing we were doing it.

I decided to interview other teenagers in his school and also in the neighborhood. I was sick at my stomach with the information that came out of these children. Apparently, using drugs and alcohol and going to raves were extremely common among the youth in the neighborhood and also at Tony's school. Tony had been drinking and using drugs since age thirteen without our knowledge. I learned that he even owed friends money which he had borrowed to support his habits.

As we processed this information, my husband and I reflected on our memories of Tony with a new perspective. We remembered that Tony wore a lot of cologne, and he was sometimes too happy around the house. At the time we thought this was part of teenage life, and we never thought much about it. Whenever Tony was home to eat a meal with us, Tony acted like a normal kid, and occasionally he would even watch a movie with us. We thought we had the ideal, nearly perfect family. Needless to say, we were shocked to learn that Tony had been sneaking out of the house to go to raves for more than two years.

He also asked to spend a lot of nights over at his friends'. Whenever he was out of the house, we would call Tony to check on him. He was always where he said he would be. Little did we know that a lot of drug activities were going on inside our basement and also at the homes of Tony's friends. Our son's friends confessed that Tony had been in need of more and more drugs lately, and they believed his death was purely an accidental overdose. His friends also confessed that they were also involved with drugs and alcohol. Some of them stopped after Tony's death, and some of them could not stop, even with Tony's death.

One of the mistakes we thought we made as parents was not being observant and not checking when his friends were over to find out what was happening in Tony's apartment. He asked for privacy with his friends when they were in the house and we respected his request. One of Tony's closest friends approached me to confess that he was scared that he would be the next victim. He said his parents still did not suspect his frequent use of drugs and alcohol, and he was scared to tell his parents.

I put together an early education awareness program, especially for unsuspecting parents like us. I also sponsored a public forum and open discussion forum in the community about drug and alcohol issues. Some other parents joined me to set up centers with telephone numbers to call for help. While I knew that whatever I did could not bring Tony back, I did know, however, that my efforts could help to prevent further tragedy in our community. It was a rude awakening for everybody.

Addiction is self-destructive and is a silent killer. My husband and I never thought it could touch us personally. We saw it as something that happens to other people, but now we are the "other people." The truth is, there is no exception to the rule, and there is no safe neighborhood. Addiction is a serious problem cutting across every socioeconomic class, killing our youths and adults alike. It is a national battle that must be taken seriously and fought seriously. It cannot be taken lightly or ignored; it is a national destroyer of precious lives, worse than an epidemic.

Now we are left with only our memories of Tony; he is gone forever. We feel good about the fact that we have made a difference in the lives of other people's children. Some of the children in our neighborhood ended up in rehabilitation and got their lives back on track. Tony became the sacrificial lamb, and we set up a memorial for him. Our advice to parents is to keep an eye on their children. You cannot put the same standard of trust in a child that is expected of an adult because children may not always make the right choices. Do something immediately if you have any suspicion that your child may be on drugs or alcohol. Do not let the story of your child become another story like Tony's.

# Quotes of Encouragement...

As the wind blows harder and Tony's story sounds familiar to you, remember the following:

*"Man becomes a slave to his constantly repeated acts ... what he at first chooses, at last compels."*

~ *Orison Swett Marden*

Addiction may start as having fun or an innocent choice, only to become an insatiable desire that could be so demanding, so controlling, and so compelling that the addict feels as if his survival depends on the substance or drug of addiction, just like the air he breaths in; when something completely takes over your life, take a self inventory and confront it; addiction does not discriminate; you can never be too young or too old to be an addict, so the earlier you get help the better; do something before it is too late. *(LB)*

*"If fifty million people say a foolish thing, it is still a foolish thing."*

~ *Bertrand Russell*

The same goes for foolish choices, if fifty million people do a foolish thing, it is still a foolish thing. Just because a lot of people make wrong choices, a wrong choice will not turn into a right choice; it takes courage to stand alone. Beware of peer pressure and do not follow the crowd blindly; do not allow peer pressure to introduce you to addiction; once you become an addict, your peers will not come to your rescue — you are on you own. *(LB)*

*"No man, for any considerable period, can wear one face to himself, and another to the multitude, without finally getting bewildered as to which may be the true."*

~ *Nathaniel Hawthorne*

You can only hide an addiction for a season, not for a lifetime; sooner or later it will catch up with you. People will soon know the truth about you, and you will be forced to face the reality and the consequences of your actions; if you think you are deceiving others, you are very wrong. You are actually deceiving yourself; the unfortunate truth is, your self-deceit can cost you your life if you do not step up and do something about the addiction. *(LB)*

## Addiction & Substance Abuse:
# BASIC FACTS & UNDERSTANDING

L arry, Mr. Shaw, and Tony all battled with different types of addiction. *Addiction* or addictive behavior is a behavior that completely takes over a person's life, making the person totally powerless, helpless, and unable to let go of that behavior. The behavior usually produces an adverse effect on the major areas of the person's life. A person who continuously engages in such a behavior that completely takes over his or her life is referred to as an addict. The behavior may affect the addict's physical, psychological, occupational, social, and financial well being. Although the addict is fully aware that this behavior is counterproductive, dysfunctional, disruptive, and destructive to his life, the addict constantly goes back to engage in the behavior. An addict feels completely trapped and unable to escape the behavior. He or she sometimes uses denial to minimize the addictive behavior, claiming that it is not that much of a problem and they can stop whenever they like. An addict could be a male or female, young or old, rich or poor, and could be of any ethnic group or race.

Addiction is a major problem in most societies. Illicit drugs and alcohol seem to get a lot of attention, and they are prevalent in the Western culture. Other types of addiction that seem to be overlooked include sex addiction, game addiction, food addiction, gambling addiction, and pornographic addiction. These are just a few of the types of addictions that people deal with from day to day.

For more public education, understanding, and awareness, some of the commonly abused drugs will be discussed. The side effects and the consequences of the use on the body of the user will also be highlighted. Hopefully, more understanding of the short and long-term devastating effects may serve as a rude awakening for some readers, especially young people. Part of the goal is to discourage people, especially the youth, from using any substance that could be addictive, or could destroy their bodies and their brains.

# Commonly Abused Drugs

**Central Nervous System Stimulants (common examples are: Cocaine and crack, amphetamines, nicotine and caffeine)** – Some of the commonly abused drugs of addiction are the *central nervous system stimulants*. The central nervous system is the area of the brain that controls our mood, thoughts, memory, emotions, language, sleep cycles, and basic drives, such as hunger, sex, and aggression. Stimulants act on the nervous system by speeding up all the normal functions of the body. Some stimulants are short-acting (exerting their effect in a very short period of time) and some are long-acting (exerting their effect over a longer period of time). Illegal use of central nervous system stimulants can be life-threatening, especially with overdose. For example, some people may have a mild, undetected, non-life-threatening heart condition and function well in life. If they ingest excessive stimulants, it may produce the effect of a sudden assault on the heart by hyper-stimulating the functions of the heart. They may collapse and suddenly die from a heart condition that was ordinarily benign or non-life-threatening. A scenario such as this would be very unfortunate, because this heart condition may not have killed them if they were not abusing stimulants. A person with a normal functioning heart could die just as suddenly from the excessive use of stimulants because of the hyper-stimulating effect on the heart and the other parts of the body.

**Cocaine and Crack** – *Cocaine* and *crack* are short-acting stimulants. They speed up everything in the body. Cocaine is made from the leaves of the coca bush, and crack is made from cocaine. Both cocaine and crack are readily available for illegal purchases in many communities. Crack is much cheaper to make and to purchase than cocaine. A few years ago, cocaine was used as a recreational drug of the affluent. Crack and cocaine can be smoked, sniffed, or used intravenously (needle injection through the vein). Crack and cocaine are highly addictive, and users get hooked on them very easily. The period of high varies from three minutes to thirty minutes, depending on the method of ingestion. Users go from the state of high to a state of deep depression. They usually need more drugs to attain another high. This may lead to binges (using crack or cocaine continuously over and over again) to maintain the high, and to keep them from going into or staying in the depressed state. The continuous binging may sometimes lead to overdose.

The state of high usually produces *euphoria* (heightened happiness), *hyper-alertness* (constantly on guard), *grandiosity* (heightened and unrealistic sense of importance), and improved self-esteem. Users may also lack inhibition, which is usually manifested by lack of ability to discriminate between right and wrong. For instance, they may have sex with four to five strangers in one night without any awareness of such behavior. They may not care about the consequences of such an irresponsible behavior, even when they are aware of it. The continuous use of crack or cocaine comes with medical consequences to the body. Users may develop sore throat, nasal passage deterioration (damage to the passage in the nose), upper gastrointestinal problems (problems in the upper part of the digestive system or stomach), heart attack (sudden failure of the heart), stroke, seizure, chest pain, tachycardia (rapid beating of the heart), as well as exposing themselves to HIV (human immunodeficiency virus) and hepatitis (inflammation or swelling of the liver). Hepatitis and HIV may be contracted from needle-sharing among addicts.

**Amphetamines** – *Amphetamines* are long-acting stimulants. They speed up everything in the body as well. Amphetamines are used in the treatment of some medical conditions. Unfortunately, they have been widely abused and used illegally. Overdose or excessive use can be lethal or life-threatening. People abuse amphetamines to stay awake for a longer period of time. For instance, an executive who is trying to meet a deadline to finish a project for his company may use amphetamines to stay awake to complete the project. Amphetamines were used for a long time in the movie industry to keep actors and actresses awake for a long period in order to finish shooting a movie. It was done unintentionally at that time. That generation was ignorant of the long-term consequences of the effects of the drugs on the body. We know a lot more about different drugs and their effects now than we knew several years ago. Unfortunately, some actors and actresses in that generation got hooked on amphetamines and had to deal with drug addiction later in life. Some students also use amphetamines to stay awake to study for examinations; this is a very dangerous practice. Abuse or excessive use of amphetamines can cause *delirium* (a state of confusion) and *psychosis* (losing touch with reality). The psychosis could mimic a more serious mental illness like schizophrenia. Users may become suspicious, paranoid, hyper-talkative, hypersexual and have auditory hallucination (hearing people that are not there), and visual hallucination (seeing people that are not there). After the high effect of using stimulants, users go through a stage called *crashing*. They may sleep for days, and they may feel physically and emotionally tired or exhausted. They are fatigued,

131

drowsy, severely depressed, and apathetic (they look pitiful). The tendency for users to commit suicide at this point is very high. They must be carefully watched. Some users could end up committing suicide during the depressed phase.

**Caffeine and Nicotine** – *Caffeine* has a stimulating effect and can be very addictive. A lot of people have to have their coffee before they can start their day, and some people just gulp coffee all day long, refilling their cups every few minutes. Essentially, there is nothing wrong with moderate consumption of coffee. Some people need that initial boost to start their day. However we must always recognize that excess of anything is bad. When the consumption or intake is not controlled, it becomes a drug and becomes addictive. The use of caffeine is not restricted to drinking coffee or caffeinated drinks only. The abuse of caffeine extends to the use of caffeine pills as well as mixing caffeine with other stimulants or suppressants to increase the desired affect. Mixing caffeine with other stimulants increases hyper stimulation. Likewise, mixing caffeine with depressants such as alcohol produces masking effect, by appearing to reduce the intoxication level of the alcohol. Some of the side effects from abuse of caffeine include: nervousness, increased heart rate, agitation, insomnia, headache and stomach ache.

*Nicotine* has stimulating effects and it is equally addictive. It can be smoked or chewed. Nicotine chewing and smoking predisposes a person to cancer of the mouth and lungs, respectively. Some of the common side effects include jitteriness, irritability, agitation, and headache. Nicotine is not treated aggressively as an addictive substance because it is socially acceptable. People cannot pull out a bag of cocaine and smoke it in the public. On the other hand, people can pull out their cigarettes and smoke them in public. For a long time, the public understanding and education about the dangers of cigarette smoking were poor. The truth about the health risks was also hidden from the public by the cigarette industries for years. Two or three decades ago, cigarette smoking was socially acceptable. The truth about lung cancer is now exposing the dangers of cigarette smoking.

Turning on the news and seeing people that we love, respect, and adore die from lung cancer is also a rude awakening that lung cancer has no respect for any person. The wise thing to do is to cut down the risk of having lung cancer by not smoking or exposing ourselves to secondary smoking. Secondary smoking entails being in the presence of somebody who smokes all the time, and inhaling the smoke or fumes without personally smoking a cigarette. It is very common to have a spouse, child or close associate who smokes all the time. The smart thing to do is not to stay around somebody who smokes all the time. Fortunately, many public figures who suffered or are suffering from lung cancer are also doing an excellent job of increasing the public awareness about the dangers of cigarette smoking. They are publicly discouraging cigarette smoking, especially among youth.

**Opiates (common examples are: Opium, Heroin, Morphine, Codeine, Percocet, Demoral, Dilaudid, Talwin, Methadone)** – *Opioid* abuse is witnessing a significant increase, especially in countries where its availability and use are not controlled. Opiates are very addictive. They are used as medications, and a lot of medication in the opiates class are sedatives and strong pain killers. Opiates are classified as narcotics and used for medical purpose to control pain. Common examples of opiates are heroin, morphine, codeine, percocet (oxycodone hydrochloride), demerol (meperidine), dilaudid (hydromophone hydrochloride), and talwin (pentazocine). Some of these drugs are sold illegally on the street, making them readily available to addicts. Some of the side effects from overdose or intoxication include drowsiness, slurred speech, decreased blood pressure, decreased respiration, or possible respiratory arrest. Others include impaired judgment, convulsions, shock, coma, and death.

*Heroin* is a synthetic form of opium. Greater emphasis is placed on heroin as an opiate because it is very popular with young addicts. Heroin is very potent and is readily available on the street. Needle-sharing with heroin users increases the chances of contracting HIV (human immuno deficiency virus) among the users. Overdose of heroin can be fatal and life-threatening. Overdose on heroin can produce changes such as drowsiness, stupor (a state of unresponsiveness except to strong stimuli), reduced pulse rate, reduced blood pressure, decreased respiration (decreased breathing rate), constricted pupil (decrease in the size of the pupil in the eye), and impaired judgment (poor decision-making).

**Marijuana** – *Marijuana (cannabis sativa)* has both euphoric (heightened happiness), and sedative (state of drowsiness) effects. The active ingredient in marijuana is found in the leaves and flowers of Indian hemp plant. The use of marijuana is very common in the United States. It is used socially the same way some people use alcohol. Marijuana is primarily smoked and people have different names for it. Some call it "hash," "roach," "joint," or "refer." Smoking marijuana can cause confusion, increased heart rate, redness of the eye, euphoria (heightened happiness), heightened sensitivity (hyper-stimulation and sensitivity of the body, for example: jumping when touched), paranoia (feeling that people are trying to hurt them or are coming after them), anxiety, or relaxation.

There has been a lot of controversy over the use of marijuana in the United States. Some groups are fighting to legalize the use. It is used medically in the form of pain pill for cancer patients. Marijuana reduces the nausea side effect and pain from receiving chemotherapy. It also serves as an appetite stimulant for some people with HIV/AIDS who may be wasting away. However, the advantage versus the disadvantage of legalizing marijuana must be carefully considered because marijuana is easily abused. Marijuana is also addictive.

**Hallucinogens (common examples are: Lysergic Acid Diethylamide-LSD, Mescaline-Peyote, Psilocybin, Phencyclidine Piperidine-PCP)** – *Hallucinogens* put the user in a psychotic state by altering the user's state of awareness or mental status on a short-term basis. Hallucinogens have been used for religious purposes in different societies for centuries. Some are synthesized like LSD (lysergic acid diethylamide). Some hallucinogens are naturally occurring like the mushroom (psilocybin) and peyote cactus (mescaline).

Hallucinogens produces a state of euphoria (heightened happiness), illusion (for example, confusing a bottle for a gun), grandiosity (feeling of self-importance, for instance, falsely believing oneself to be a president of a country), confusion, and loss of boundaries. Intoxication from the use of hallucinogens can cause high blood pressure, rapid heart rate, muscle weakness, and fever. The user's experience, which the user looks forward to by using LSD or hallucinogens, is referred to as a "trip." When a user experiences a bad reaction to hallucinogens, it is referred to as a "bad trip."

*P*hencyclidine Piperidine (PCP) produces an altered state of mind in the user in a short period of time. It produces a hallucinogenic effect. It can be sniffed, smoked, ingested orally, or used intravenously (injected into the vein). PCP is primarily licensed for use as an immobilizing, anesthetic agent for animals. PCP is called different names such as "angel dust" or "peace pill" or a "horse tranquilizer." PCP produces changes in behavior, clouded judgment (poor decision making), belligerence, and anxiety in the user. Intoxication from PCP use can cause kidney failure, respiratory arrest (user can stop breathing suddenly), hypertension (high blood pressure), seizures, muscle spasms (muscle contraction), and muscle rigidity (muscle stiffness). Other side effects include blank stare (empty stare into space), nystagmus (an abnormal eye movement), decreased sensation to touch or pain, violence, and sometimes death.

**Methylphethamine** – *Methylphethamine*, usually referred to as "meth" or "tina" or "crank," is another addictive drug that has become a nightmare of the drug enforcement agency in the United States. Addicts may report feeling euphoric, happy, energetic, hyper-alert, hyper-sexual, grandiose, unable to sleep, and overly confident. Meth addiction and abuse is a financial drain on the healthcare industry. Severe burn injuries result from explosions caused during the manufacturing of meth. The major ingredient is pseudoephedrine, which was relatively easy to get over the counter until recently. Pharmacies no longer readily dispense pseudoephedrine as an over-the-counter drug; anyone who obtains this drug is required to sign a log book. Only a limited quantity may be purchased. Other ingredients that are used to manufacture meth such as iodine are also more controlled. It is very unfortunate that the recipe used for making such a dangerous drug is so readily available in the community and even on the internet. It is especially important for parents to check the internet sites that their children are logging into.

The manufacture of meth has gotten out of control in the United States. The use of meth started in the rural areas or the suburbs, but it has now found its way to the mainstream. The use of meth cuts across every socioeconomic group. Suppliers or dealers of meth are setting up laboratories all over the country to make large quantities for sale and consumption. Addicts are making meth in their kitchens with their children watching. Users and their children are showing up at the hospitals with burn injuries from explosions during the preparation of this dangerous drug. Law enforcement agents are constantly striving to search out the laboratories where meth is being prepared and closing them down. Apart from the danger of burn injury from explosions, intoxication on meth can cause paranoia, hallucination, severe weight loss called the "crank diet," stroke, liver damage, dental erosion, disfigurement and skin infection from intravenous use of needles.

**Steroids** – *Steroids* refer to the group of drugs classified as anabolic, androgenic, and corticosteroids. Corticosteroids are used in the treatment of inflammation that is not caused by infection. The sex hormone estrogen and progesterone are used in the making of oral contraceptives. (Contraceptives are medications used to prevent unwanted pregnancies.) The steroid that is getting all the attention is called the anabolic steroid.

**Anabolic steroids** – *Anabolic steroids* are the synthetic derivative of the male hormone testosterone. Anabolic steroids increase the body's ability to maximize the use of nitrogen ingested in protein by increasing protein synthesis. Increased protein synthesis helps the body to build body muscle mass and also prevents the breakdown of body muscle. The effect of the muscle growth and increase in strength is called the anabolic or tissue building effect. Anabolic steroids also promote the development of male sex characteristics, such as voice deepening, and increased body and facial hair. This is referred to as androgenic or masculinizing effect of the anabolic steroids.

The abuse of steroid by athletes is making news all over the world. Athletes take steroids because it is believed that anabolic steroids increase the strength and the ability of an athlete to train longer and harder. It is also believed to increase lean muscle mass. Anabolic steroids can be taken orally as pills or powder, or can be injected into the muscle with a needle. A lot of athletes who share needles or inject steroids are exposed to the serious danger of contracting hepatitis or the HIV/AIDS virus. Anabolic steroids can also be used topically on the skin. For use in abusive circumstances, its popular form of administering is orally or intramuscularly with the needle. These steroids which are to be injected are either oil or water-based. The oil-based last longer than the water-based, and they are released very slowly into the body for a long period of time.

Anabolic steroids are mostly abused by athletes who rely on strength, size, and endurance for their sport. Athletes who are involved in weight training and body building also fall into the class of those who would likely abuse steroids. Football players, wrestlers, baseball players, track and field athletes, swimmers, and body builders are among the athletes who are likely to use steroids.

The use of anabolic steroids is popular among adolescent boys who are involved in sports in high school. Some adolescent boys are also taking steroids to enhance their looks. It is unfortunate that adolescent girls are also abusing steroids to maintain thinness. Steroids make them lose body fat and gain lean muscle. Some normal adults who are also trying to have the "ideal" body look are also abusing steroids.

Athletes have different styles or schedules for their steroid use. Some may take it in cycles of weeks or months instead of taking it continuously. This schedule is called "cycling." Some users combine different types of steroids simultaneously to maximize the steroid effect. This schedule is called "stacking." Some users gradually increase the dose over a period of time, usually weeks to months. This schedule is called "pyramiding."

The adverse effects of steroid abuse outweigh the benefits. Steroid use causes a lot of medical and psychological problems. Adolescents who take steroids in the early or middle puberty may have stunted growth or short height. They may never mature fully. This is because anabolic steroid can affect bone growth, causing the bone plates in the bone to mature too quickly or fuse too quickly. This is called premature closure of the epiphyses. Steroid use can also cause skin and hair changes. It could also cause baldness and feminization in males, resulting in formation of breasts. Other male-related problems also include impotence, inability to maintain an erection, enlarged prostate, shrinkage of the testicles, and decreased sexual drive.

Steroid abuse can also cause masculinization in females by producing excess facial and body hair (called hirsutism), acne, baldness, enlarged clitoris, menstrual irregularity, breast atrophy (hardening), infertility resulting from uterine atrophy, and increased sexual drive. Other possible side effects include headaches, high blood pressure, kidney damage, liver problems, and cardiovascular or heart problems such as heart attack, strokes, and blood clots. Steroids usually harden the arteries. Arteries carry blood throughout the body. Urinary and bowel problems, such as diarrhea, may occur. Urinary problems could be manifested by pain and problems with urination, which is very common.

Abusers may experience sleep problems, joint and body aches, plus an increased risk of ligament and tendon injuries. Others include jaundice (or yellowing of the skin), nausea and vomiting, dizziness, and trembling. Steroids can also cause water and salt retention, making the skin appear puffy and swollen. Steroid abuse also decreases the body's immune response or immune system, a condition known as immunodeficiency. The body's immune system is usually suppressed, and the body stops producing its own steroids, relying on the artificially induced steroid into the body. It decreases the body's ability to fight infection.

Emotional side effects of steroid use include depression, thoughts of suicide, wild mood swings (going quickly from very happy to very sad), manic or out of control behavior, anger, hostility, and homicidal acts (wanting to kill others). Others include paranoia (extreme feelings of mistrust of others), and fear.

Hallucinations, especially visual and auditory (seeing or hearing things that are not there), may also be present. Anxiety and panic attacks are also common. Extreme or severe aggression that may result in violence such as fighting or other destructive behaviors can also be observed. This extreme aggressive, out of control behavior is referred to as "steroid rage." An overwhelming feeling of wanting to die, called suicidal feelings, may lead to suicidal attempts and death.

The health problems resulting from steroid abuse may not appear until several years after the steroid is taken. Some of the side effects from steroid abuse may be reversible if the use is discontinued. Some of the damage could be permanent and irreversible. Steroids can be detected by a simple urine drug screen in a physician's or healthcare provider's office. It is very unfortunate that a lot of fake steroids are sold through the black market. Users put themselves at risk of injecting or swallowing poisonous or dangerous substances that are not steroids. These could have dangerous or deadly consequences.

**Party Drugs or Date Rape Drugs** – *Party Drugs* or *Date Rape Drugs* are common drugs used among youth mostly in the Western world, especially in the teenage years. They are used most commonly by teenagers and young adults in high schools and colleges. These drugs are getting a lot of attention because they are widely accepted by this age group and are causing a lot of havoc in young people's social lives, particularly in larger social gatherings.

**Raves** are all night parties attended by a very large number of youth. At these parties, one may find party drugs and hypnotic music. Some common party drugs include ecstasy (3,4, methylenedioxymethamphetamine), ketamine, and GHB (gammahydroxybutyrate), and the date rape drug called rohypnol (flunitrazepam). *Ecstasy* is very commonly used, and different derivatives of ecstasy are also called "Adam," "love," "Eve," among several different names. The drugs produce euphoria (heightened happiness), increase self-esteem and self-confidence, cause users to lose their inhibitions (loss of control over one's instincts), and produce hyper-sexuality as well as enhancing sociability (feeling of belonging or acceptance by others). Intoxication from the drugs can cause acute renal failure (sudden shut-down of the kidney), psychosis (losing one's mind and the ability to distinguish between what is real and what is unreal), severe anxiety, memory impairment, hostility, hyperthermia (sudden rise in body temperature), severe depression, and death.

Winds Against The Mind

*Rohypnol* (flunitrazepam) is a very popular date rape drug because it produces the effect of quick relaxation on the voluntary muscles of the body. It reduces inhibition while inducing forgetfulness, causing a prolonged state of amnesia or memory loss, in relation to recent events. When date rape drugs are used with alcohol, they act more quickly and their effects last longer. Many young women have been the innocent victims of date rape drugs. They were sexually assaulted without their consent. A person cannot consent to an act that she is not aware of. Parents should educate their children about the danger of the date rape drugs.

**Inhalants –** *Inhalants* are now getting very popular in the Western world. They are called different names such as "dusting," "huffing," "bagging," or "wagging," depending on the product and the method of use. The drugs produce a state of euphoria (heightened happiness) for approximately ten to fifteen seconds, and users may experience the feelings of high for a few minutes. It is very commonly used in the age range of nine to seventeen years, and the use cuts across every social and economic class. Child users have found inhalants to be a cheap and easy way to get high and become addicted. What's more, they falsely believe that they are not using drugs; therefore such usage cannot hurt them. Unfortunately, inhalants can kill, even with the very first attempt. The sad reality about inhalants is that they are very readily available. Common household products such as paint thinners, spray paints, hair spray, household paint, wax removers, nail polish remover, whipped cream dispensers, glue, cigarette lighter fluid, shoe polish, cooking spray, colored markers, gasoline, correction fluid, rubbing alcohol, scotch guards, and several other common household products are all readily available products that can be used as inhalers. When the substance is put in a plastic or paper bag and breathed in, it is called "bagging." When the substance is breathed directly from the can or through a cloth soaked in the solvent, it is called "huffing."

Another popular inhalant is Dust-Off, a common compressed air used to clean or blow dust from computers. The children inhale the Dust-Off, using a method called "dusting," when they inhale the Dust-Off as it is sprayed. Dust-Off contains a propellant called difluoroethane, which is heavier than oxygen. It displaces oxygen from the lungs and replaces it with heavier air, causing reduced oxygen to the brain and the heart. Dust-Off can cause instant death.

Several other inhalants work in a similar way by reducing oxygen flow to the brain and the heart, and subsequently causing death or severe brain or organ damage to the body. Users may slip into unconsciousness. They usually have a sudden airway obstruction, resulting from swelling produced in the lungs from the products inhaled. Some may throw up or vomit from using the inhaled substance and aspirate the vomited substance and die. The products could also cause irregular heart beat which again could lead to sudden death. The state of euphoria may also propel the user to engage in life-threatening behavior or unintended trauma, such as driving recklessly at high speeds and ending up in a car accident. Other dangerous behavior could include jumping off a cliff, drowning, or accidentally setting one's self on fire. Users carry out such destructive behavior because they cannot make sensible decisions in this dangerous state of euphoria. Some inhalants may catch fire accidentally when being used because they are highly flammable. Inhalants can cause light headedness, drowsiness, agitation, and lack of inhibition (inability to control one's instincts). Other possible complications include liver damage, permanent cognitive decline or confusion, heart damage, bone disease, breathing problems, central nervous system damage, and eye damage. The danger of inhalants as mentioned earlier is the easy accessibility and affordability.

Every household uses these different products that can be easily inhaled. Since the products are relatively inexpensive, and can be purchased legally by anyone at any age, it makes it very difficult to control the addiction. Unless the user is caught or the people around the user are very attentive or observant, there is no track mark or physical evidence to implicate the user. Equally neither needles nor syringes are needed to shoot up the drug, and so there is no evidence of broken veins on the user. This type of drug use is extremely easy for users to conceal. Unfortunately, it is easily concealed from concerned parents, whose children may be using inhalants. It could be easier to catch a child who is smoking marijuana, drinking alcohol, or using other street drugs than to catch a child using inhalants. It is a very serious problem, and parents or parental figures of children who are abusing inhalants must be overly vigilant to detect this addiction on time before it is too late.

**The Choking Game** – The *choking game* is another form of dangerous addiction among youth. Some temporarily cut off oxygen to their brains for a few seconds by tying a rope around their necks. This produces a very short state of high or euphoria. Youth who engage in this act are very ignorant about the serious danger of the choking game. They sincerely and honestly consider it as a game. Sadly, it is a fast way to die. Since nothing is sold or purchased in the choking game, there is a rationalization among youth that it is not an addiction. Unfortunately, it is so dangerous that a child may never have a chance to try it a second time. He or she could die the very first time it is tried. Some youth have been found hung on trees and on other unusual places, trying to play this choking game.

Parents need to be very vigilant with their children and also to educate them about the dangers of these few seconds of high that could cost them their lives. Children can be innocently introduced to dangerous addictions such as this choking game or inhalant use simply from spending the night with a friend. This is why it is so important to discuss the dangers of this addiction with your children openly. The society at large should also increase the public education about the dangers of these drugs and dangerous games such as the choking game in the community forums and schools.

**Central Nervous System Depressants (common examples are: Barbiturates, Benzodiazepines, Alcohol)** – Some *Central Nervous System Depressants* are medications that are used to treat anxiety problems in the medical profession. Some of these central nervous system depressants are widely abused medications. The most common ones are the benzodiazepines, barbiturates and other sedative hypnotics such as valium, xanax, klonopins, librium and serax. These medications produce a relaxing or calming effect on the body. They are usually referred to as downers. Addicts prefer to use them with alcohol because it makes the mellow effect lasts longer.

Despite the fact that the central nervous system depressants are prescription drugs, they are readily available for sale illegally on the street. People who are addicted to this group of medications usually doctor shop. Doctor shopping is going from one doctor's office to another and fabricating lies and stories to get a prescription for these medications. Some of these medications were prescribed by physicians for decades to treat anxiety before it was realized much later that they were very addictive. Addicts could die from accidental overdose of these medications. Some public figures in the entertainment industry were known to have died from the accidental overdose of these medications.

*Alcohol and addiction to alcohol (alcoholism)* is usually downplayed as a major addiction problem because drinking alcohol is socially acceptable. Alcohol is used readily, and it is easily available in many societies. Alcohol addicts sometime mix other addictive drugs together with alcohol to intensify or to prolong the effect of the drugs, or to extend the effects of both the drugs and the alcohol. Such behavior shows the extent to which the addicts will go to get the desired effect they want from the drug of addiction.

There are so many psychological and emotional changes that come with excessive use of alcohol on its own or combining alcohol with some other drugs. Some of these changes may be life-threatening if the side effects are not aggressively treated. These include decreased respiration (decreased breathing), changes in speech (slurred or hyper-verbal), drowsiness, constricted pupils, euphoria or dysphoria (heightened state of happiness), impaired judgment, and a short attention span. Others include palpitations or sweating, tremors or shakes, lack of coordination, muscle rigidity, elevated vital signs (manifested by elevated temperature, blood pressure, and respiration), seizure, blank stare, restlessness, impulsive behavior, agitation, hostility towards others, as well as the user's making unreasonable demands on others or even assaulting them. Auditory and visual hallucinations (hearing voices or seeing things that are not there) and paranoid behavior (mistrust of others or feelings that others are trying to hurt them) may also be present. Bizarre behavior such as chanting or barking like a dog, grandiosity (false sense of self-importance), an unusually aggressive sexual drive or lack of sexual interest, cardiac arrest (the heart may suddenly stop), and stroke may also occur. Users may also go into a coma (a state of unconsciousness), and die.

Alcohol withdrawal may be life threatening and requires medical emergency attention. The withdrawal symptoms usually develop within a few hours after the last drink. The withdrawal symptoms may peak in one to two days and gradually disappear or progress to delirium (a state of confusion), which is considered a medical emergency. Some of the early signs of alcohol withdrawal include nausea and vomiting, anxiety, insomnia (inability to sleep), hyper-excitement or jerky movement, (becoming easily startled), inability to eat (anorexia), and nightmares.

Other more severe symptoms of alcohol delirium include complete disorientation, severe changes in vital signs such as high temperature, high blood pressure, and rapid heart rate, and diaphoresis (excessive sweating, sometimes making the addict look like someone who has just had a bucket of water poured on him). More symptoms include paranoia, extreme agitation, tactile hallucination (feeling that bugs are crawling all over him), visual hallucination or seeing things that are not there (they usually see spider or snake), and illusions (wrongful perception of an object such as seeing a bottle and believing that it is a gun). Addicts may also fluctuate in their level of consciousness by going from consciousness to unconsciousness and vice versa.

Alcohol addiction comes with sad medical consequences such as developing cirrhosis of the liver (a medical condition that can stop the liver from functioning), Wernicke's encephalopathy, and Korsakoff's syndrome (alcohol induced amnesia or forgetfulness). A person experiencing Wernicke's encephalopathy can have ataxia, (falling or inability to walk or stand or maintain a wide-based gait), clouded consciousness (conscious but not fully aware of his environment), and ophthalmoplegia (weakness of the muscle controlling the eye movement). The onset of these symptoms is rapid and can be life-threatening. It can cause brain damage. The treatment involves aggressive medical intervention and the addition of some essential vitamins that were depleted from the body as a result of the alcohol abuse. Korsakoff's syndrome is chronic, and the victims may experience recent memory loss or memory impairment. They use confabulation (fabrication of answers to questions to fill in the details they cannot remember) to compensate for the memory loss. Alcoholics develop Korsakoff's syndrome from improper diet and malnutrition. Severe alcoholics may quit eating and just consume alcohol only. They usually lack some essential vitamins that are required by the body.

It is believed that alcohol addiction is more prevalent in men than women, especially in the western world. However, the incidence among women is increasing, especially with more women working outside of homes. Alcohol and drug problems are responsible for several deaths. A lot of violent crimes, senseless killings, and motor vehicle fatalities are caused by people under the influence of drugs and alcohol.

# Factors Affecting Drug Use

The question arises as to why some people abuse drugs and alcohol. Obviously there is no one contributory factor but many factors. Genetic factors, environmental factors, socioeconomic factors, cultural influence, mental illness, and the effect the drug has on the user are some of the contributing factors. Others include availability of the drug, development of tolerance, and physical dependence. Knowing some of the contributory factors may promote awareness and possible prevention in some situations.

143

**Genetic Factors** – Genetic factors are highly influential in alcohol and drug addiction. From adoptive studies, if a child was born to an alcoholic parent and the child was adopted at the time of birth by a non-alcoholic parent, the child still carries a far greater risk of developing alcohol problems compared to a child born to non-alcoholic parent, who was adopted at the time of birth by a non-alcoholic parent. Some naturally occurring chemicals in the brain have been implicated for this behavior. The child may inherit the same distribution of this naturally existing chemical that is supposed to be responsible for drug and alcohol addiction from his or her biological or natural parent. As a result, the child is already genetically predisposed or genetically coded to develop drug or alcohol addiction. In other words, there is a strong biochemical factor that may already predetermine the fate of the child from the time of his birth to become an alcoholic when he or she is older. Genetic factors should not be used as an excuse for personal responsibility. A person with a strong genetic history should try to prevent the onset of alcoholism by avoiding alcohol in the first place. Remember, 'prevention is better than a cure.'

**Environmental Factors** – Environmental factors also play an important role in the development of drug and alcohol addiction. Children tend to pick up the habit of a significant other or their role model. If a child is raised in an environment where there is a lot of drinking and drug use, the child may grow up to copy this behavior.

**Easy access to drugs and alcohol** – Availability or easy access to the drugs and alcohol may also affect use. For instance, people in the healthcare industry such as doctors, nurses, pharmacists, who may already have a tendency to be addicted to prescription drugs, may quickly pick up the habit because of availability and frequent exposure to the prescription drugs. Also, someone who works as a bartender and has the natural tendency or inclination to become an alcoholic may very easily become one because of the availability and frequent exposure to alcohol as a bartender. The lack of restriction on the sale of prescription drugs and the sale of alcohol to minors may influence addiction problems early in life among youth in some countries. Easy availability and access allows underage children to start drinking early and quickly develop tolerance to drugs and alcohol at a younger age. Even in the parts of the world where there is an age-limit rule and restrictions for alcohol purchase, people still find a way around the rules. The case gets compounded when there are no rules or restrictions.

**Socioeconomic Factors** – Socioeconomic factors also influence the addiction to drugs and alcohol. Socioeconomic factors influence accountability because the law enforcement authorities are more likely to catch poor people with addiction problems than wealthy people with addiction problems. Addicts could be doctors, lawyers, housewives, engineers, teachers, students, law enforcement agents, politicians, actors, actresses, janitors, or construction workers—all the way down to the stereotyped core addict who lives on the street, selling drugs to support his or her habit. Nobody is excluded from developing drug or alcohol problem. The only difference is that people with higher socio-economic status are less likely to be held accountable because their money can hide them for a long time. Likewise, they are less likely to be labeled as addicts because of their station in life as compared to people in the lower socioeconomic group.

Also, people with higher socioeconomic status may be able to afford the substance more than poorer people. They may not have to steal to support the habit because they have a better financial cushion. Unfortunately, sooner or later, addiction catches up with the addict, irrespective of their station in life or socioeconomic class.

**Cultural Factors –** Cultural factors also affect drugs and alcohol addiction. Some cultures and religions prohibit the use of drug and alcohol, especially among children, adolescents, and sometimes women. Such cultures may socially sanction the use or abuse of drugs or alcohol if the user is not legally allowed to use it. The social sanctioning may result in the people getting punished for using alcohol. Alcohol and drug use may be less prevalent in such an environment. There is also a general belief that people who live a more stressful life, which is believed to be more of the lifestyle in the western world, are more likely to abuse drugs and alcohol. It is believed that the pressure to optimize their productivity and to be able to do more work and activities than their bodies would naturally allow them to do may be the reason for turning to drugs and alcohol.

**Onset of the action of the drug –** If the drug is readily available and quick to exert its action on the body to produce the desired effect, it may be frequently abused. For example, illicit drugs that are readily available and quick to produce mind altering effects may be more popular than those that exert their effects much longer. Alcohol is very commonly abused because it is fast acting in its mind-altering property as well. It produces a feeling of elation or happiness and also easily available. Similarly, some prescription drugs are likely to be more commonly abused for the same reason.

**Mental Illness –** Mental illness is responsible for a lot of alcohol and drug abuse.

It is unfortunate that a lot of people who abuse drugs and alcohol use them out of ignorance to self-medicate and to treat underlying mental illness. They may not be able to name the mental illness that they are experiencing, but they realize that they always feel better when they drink alcohol or use illicit drugs. Again, more public education is needed in the understanding of mental illnesses, especially in the adolescent years. A lot of children in high school use drugs and alcohol to treat emotional and mental problems, especially major depression and mood swings (or bipolar disorder).

For those young adults who do not mask the symptoms of mental illness with drugs and alcohol, early signs and symptoms of most mental illnesses will start to become evident in the adolescent years. It will be early enough to get the attention of parents and caregivers because the true picture of the illness would not be clouded by the drugs and alcohol. More public education is needed to increase early detection and to promote increased awareness of mental illnesses in this population. Increased awareness can help to increase the early intervention. Detecting and treating the problem early may forestall, and thus prevent, the future probability that these young adults will become adult addicts, struggling with addiction for the rest of their lives.

The problem of drug and alcohol addiction cuts across every age group; a lot of adults and older people use alcohol to self-medicate as well. For instance, *depression* is a very common mental illness that is always downplayed. A depressed person who is experiencing sadness most of the time may unknowingly or unconsciously turn to alcohol and drugs to treat the depression. If such a person lacks proper public education about depression, anything that relieves the depression will be considered as life-saver. For instance, a depressed person who is using alcohol to treat the depression could say, "I feel happy and I don't feel down in the dumps when I drink."

Another common mental illness that is treated by many people with drugs and alcohol is *anxiety*. A person who drinks a lot to relieve anxiety may say, "A couple of beers will calm me down when I am anxious."

*Psychosis* (marked inability to differentiate what is real from what is unreal or losing touch with reality) is also commonly treated with drugs and alcohol. People who are experiencing early psychosis with a sudden overwhelming feeling of not being able to control their thoughts may turn to drugs or alcohol to self-medicate. The drugs and alcohol temporarily cloud their judgment or numb them, and make them forget that they are not in control of their thoughts. Such a person may say, "I feel out of this world, like I am on another planet when I am on cocaine."

The majority of the homeless people living on the street and in the homeless shelters who are addicted to drugs and alcohol actually have mental problems. It is very unfortunate that the healthy ones in the society who are fortunate enough to have their minds functioning right are very quick to judge this class of people. Derogatory comments are made about them, and they are treated as outcasts. The focus should be on helping this population to seek help and to get better. Blaming them for their mental illness and ostracizing or abandoning them will not keep them off the streets. With proper assessment, a distinction could be made between mental illness that resulted from substance abuse and mental illness that previously existed before the person turned to drugs and alcohol. Lack of knowledge and understanding on the part of the victims about mental illness is primarily responsible for the self-medication with drugs and alcohol.

**Emotional Factors and Physical Addiction** – Emotional pain also contributes to drug and alcohol addiction. Many people have had horrible experiences in life, and these experiences shape their outlook and reaction to life. Horrible childhood experiences are usually very painful, and many people carry emotional scars from their childhood. Such people may initially turn to drugs and alcohol to feel happy and help numb their pain. They try to forget about their emotional hurts and scars by drinking or using drugs. By the time they realize what is happening, they have become addicts. Unfortunately, if a pain is emotional, it will still be there when the effects of the drugs and alcohol wear off. Until the underlying problem is dealt with, the victims will be in psychological and emotional bondage to the pain. Sadly, they will also be in bondage to the drugs and the alcohol as well. For instance, a prostitute who is abusing drugs and alcohol may have an emotional scar from a childhood history of physical and sexual molestation. She may be using the drugs and alcohol to treat her childhood pain and unpleasant memories. Until she gets to the root of the problem and gets some psychological help, the pain will never go away.

To make things even worse, many people who are addicted to drugs and alcohol may develop a tolerance for and physical dependence on the drugs and alcohol. A lot of people are aware that they have drug and alcohol problems, and sincerely make several personal attempts to quit. However, the symptoms of withdrawal are usually very unpleasant and uncomfortable. These may sometimes be life-threatening. As a result, an addict would continue to use drugs and alcohol to avoid the horrible symptoms of withdrawal. It may sometimes take professional help and a lot of will power on the part of the addict to change this habit or behavior.

# Diagnosis and Treatment

Alcohol and drug problems are public health problems. The negative effects of alcohol and drug addiction are always very expensive in any economy.

*Codependency* is very common among people battling with addictions and their significant others. Usually, the closest people to the addict such as spouse and family members may be protective of the addict. Other people who are very close and very involved with the addict apart from their relatives may also find themselves in a codependent relationship with the addict. Codependence is simply a situation in which people who are supposed to confront and discourage the addictive behavior of an addict enable the behavior instead of discouraging it. The codependent person or enabler may feel overly responsible for the addict's behavior. He or she may feel guilty and spend a lot of their time thinking about the addict and how to save or rescue the addict. The enabler may try to control the addiction, but usually has no success in doing so. He may excuse the behavior of the addict and cover up the addiction. He may try to break off the addict's connection with his or her drug supply, but usually to no avail or with no success. He may threaten to leave the addict and continuously bargain with the addict, but he can never leave nor follow through with his threats. A codependent person may avoid and also keep the addict from attending social and family events in order to avoid public embarrassment caused by the addict. He may try to control the finances of the family, with the hope of preventing the addict from buying the addictive substance. He may try to cover up by taking over the addict's work and responsibilities. A codependent person may co-exist with the addict in an emotionally charged environment. The addict's mood may influence the mood of the people around them. There may be a lot of verbal and physical abuse, or both, around the house or in the environment. A codependent relationship does not help the addict or the enabler. It is a dysfunctional and destructive relationship.

## Winds Against The Mind

Diagnosis and treatment of addiction is usually a big challenge. There are too many denial and codependency issues with alcohol and drug problems. Many people are unwilling to seek help. Most addicts try very hard to hide their addiction from the rest of the world. Some family members and significant others may try to keep the problem within the family because of the stigma attached to drug and alcohol addiction. We must remember that nobody wakes up in the morning one day and says, "I want to be an addict for the rest of my life." Unfortunately, diagnosis of alcohol and drug addiction cannot be made primarily in a laboratory. There are no diagnostic tools invented yet that are available to predict that a person would become a drug and alcohol addict. There is scientific-based research that could project the probability or possibility, but they are not conclusive. Making the diagnosis is primarily based on the comprehensive history of the addict. In addition to the history, every clue and intuition that may point to the direction of possible diagnosis of drug and alcohol addiction must be carefully followed.

Dealing with addiction is always difficult for the addicts as well as for the people around them. Usually the addicts are aware of the problem, but unfortunately, as mentioned earlier, they sometimes stay in denial. They may also feel powerless and try to rationalize or justify the reasons for the behavior. A common denial phrase or language of an addict is, "I can handle it," or, "It's not as bad as you think." Addicts minimize the problem and hide it for as long as possible. The first people to notice the problem of addicts are usually those who are close to them, such as their spouses, children, parents, significant others, boyfriend or girlfriend, coaches, teachers, associates, and friends. It may be very tough on the addict and the person who confronts her, but it is in the best interest of the addict if she is confronted about the addiction.

Confrontation does not need to be negatively or emotionally charged. The purpose of the confrontation should not be to create a drama or a scene. The goal of the confrontation is to help the addict face the truth about his or her addiction. After confrontation, the next step is to encourage the addict to seek help. If an addict does not know how to go about seeking help, the person who confronted the addict should try to get help for him or her.

It must be mentioned that some people have been able to quit their addiction willingly on their own, although such people may not be in the majority. Usually, such people have come to a point of disgust with their addiction and gotten sick and tired of living such a lifestyle. Such people are the few fortunate ones with

149

very strong willpower. The majority of addicts, on the other hand, need prompting and professional help to fight their addiction.

The treatment of addiction is multifaceted and may be broken into multiple stages. Many certified clinicians and treatment centers specialize in the treatment of addiction. Dealing with addiction is a tough challenge for a lot of clinicians. The first goal is to look for a non-judgmental clinician who has not already concluded that a client's case is a hopeless case before even taking it on.

A certified clinician would usually start with taking a very comprehensive and thorough history of the client. In addition, a thorough medical and psychiatric evaluation is usually done, taking into serious consideration the underlying emotional problems. At times, addicts are reluctant to seek professional help because of confidentiality issues. They do not want their business or stories on the streets. They do not want the entire world to know about their addiction problems. It must be noted that certified clinicians know the importance of confidentiality. Clinicians always sign a confidentiality statement with their clients. However, if the treatment facility is in an open-treatment center, it may be difficult to keep the knowledge of the client's treatment away from the public. If the addict is a known name or public figure, keeping the treatment confidential may be difficult in such an environment.

Treatment of addiction could be in an inpatient or an outpatient setting. Some people may need an initial short-term inpatient stabilization period where they work through the withdrawal from the drugs or alcohol under strict supervision. They may later transfer or transition to an outpatient setting. People with a long history of struggle with addiction may need a long-term residential program. The long-term program could last anywhere from three months to two years, depending on the facility or the individual. The long-term residential treatment may be the only way out for people with a high rate of recidivism or relapse.

Employee assistance programs are also becoming popular. Employers provide therapeutic services for their employees by way of medical and mental rehabilitation. Instead of firing a talented employee with an addiction problem, employers are trying to play a part in the solution. It cannot be overemphasized that addiction cuts across every socioeconomic group. Many professionals such as doctors, nurses, lawyers, teachers, engineers, accountants, and several other elites are dealing with addiction issues. Addiction is not written on the forehead of the addict. Stereotyping addicts as only those who are homeless under the bridge or a prostitute on the street will make clinicians overlook many people out there in need of help. There is no perfect description of an addict; it is time for everybody to stop the stereotyping.

One of the major goals of therapy is to help an addict identify a positive way to cope with stress, and also to identify some underlying factors that may be responsible for the addiction. Dealing with the underlying problems is usually very helpful towards recovery.

Another major focus of the therapy is relapse prevention. Addicts see relapse as a sign of weakness and failure. As a result, a lot of addicts give up after several relapses. Some addicts may consider suicide, or even commit suicide. The goal of therapy is to let the addict know that every sober period, no matter how short-lived is a step in the right direction. Addicts have to keep working hard at beating the addiction until they finally get it right. When there is life, there is hope. An addict must compare her survival to that of a person competing in a running race—a failure is a runner who falls during a race and stays fallen. A winner is a runner who understands that after every fall, he has to rise up and keep going to the finish line to complete the race. Sooner or later the runner will get it right and will be able to run without falling, and hopefully make it to the finish line. There is always hope for recovery only if the addict does not give up.

Treating underlying psychiatric or mental illness such as depression, anxiety, post traumatic stress syndrome, schizophrenia, bipolar, and other major psychiatric or mental illness is an important part of the recovery process. There are several medications used in addition to therapy in the treatment of addiction. The appropriate medication must be prescribed by a certified clinician only, after a thorough and a comprehensive assessment of the client has been completed. Several factors are taken into consideration before a medication is prescribed; this is because clinicians are usually cautious when dealing with addiction problems. They do not want to accidentally move the client from one addiction to another addiction.

Initial detoxification and crisis management may be needed at the beginning of the recovery process. The detoxification process serves to get the drug of addiction out of the addict's system or his body. The process is primarily determined by the substance the client is addicted to or the substance that was used. For instance, initial detoxification and crisis management for somebody addicted to alcohol will be different from that of a person addicted to cocaine.

Family therapy and marital therapy may also be needed with the help of a certified clinician. Addiction introduces very negative dynamics into the family. There may be a lot of physical and emotional abuse and neglect of the spouse and the children of the addict. Sexual problems are always common in marriages when one or both parties are addicted to drugs or alcohol. The spouse with the addiction problem may be sexually inappropriate. For example, he or she could be very demanding, and aggressive when high, or have no sexual desire when low or depressed. If the addiction issue is sexual addiction, it may be difficult for the spouse of a sex addict to meet the insatiable demands of the addicted spouse. The spouse of a sex addict may also be exposed to the risk of contracting sexually transmitted diseases because of multiple partner exposure from the addicted spouse. When under the influence of drugs or alcohol, addicts may sexually molest or abuse their children or other people's children. This introduces a more serious dynamic into the problem, which may require the involvement of the law enforcement authorities. An addict may be emotionally labile (going from very angry to very sorry, and going from very quiet to very loud) because of the influence of the drug of addiction.

Support group participation is also an important part of the treatment of addiction. There are several self-help groups available. They all serve the common purpose of helping an addict to stay sober. There are several advantages in joining a support group. Addicts are able to identify with other addicts, and come to realize that they are not the only persons on this planet or in this world dealing with the particular addiction and struggling to be free from the addiction daily.

Some support groups help to provide role models and sponsors who serve as around-the-clock support for new members of the group. It is always good to know that there are people out there who have won the battle with addiction. Addicts learn new functional ways of doing things and work on replacing the old dysfunctional ways that did not work for them. Members of the support group learn to deal with their underlying emotional factors and possible psychological or mental problems that are contributing to the addiction problems. Common examples are fear, guilt, anxiety, anger, and depression. They learn to stay motivated and to work in positive physical and spiritual growth, and to aim at living a peaceful and enjoyable life, free from addiction. They also learn how to take personal responsibility for their behavior as well as how to treat and respect others. They learn that other people are not to be treated as objects to be used to satisfy their addiction. They are encouraged to love and respect their bodies by eating well, meditating, and exercising.

Support groups provide an environment where members are not constantly judged and criticized for their struggles with addiction. There is unconditional acceptance in a support group because everybody is dealing with the same issue or the same kind of problem, and is trying to stay in recovery.

There are many support groups available in the United States for the treatment of addiction, but Alcoholics Anonymous, also known as AA, is the founding father of most of the support groups. AA is based on a twelve-step program, which could basically be applied to or used in other addiction programs. The three major concepts that Alcoholics Anonymous emphasizes are:

- Individuals with an addictive disorder are powerless over their addiction, and their lives are unmanageable.
- Although individuals with an addictive disorder are not responsible for their disease, they are responsible for their recovery.
- Individuals can no longer blame people, places, and things for their addiction. They must face the problems and their feelings.

The twelve-step program has been both criticized and greatly praised. The ultimate goal is for an addict to find out which program works for him or her and to stay with it.

Support groups are sometimes called maintenance therapy, and they primarily keep several addicts out of trouble. These meetings are available literarily for any type of addiction in the United States. Other societies that may need such groups can copy the established model from Alcoholics Anonymous. Some other common support groups are Al-Anon (family members of alcoholics), NA (Narcotics Anonymous), Al-a-Teen (support groups for adults and teenagers dealing with addiction issues), Cocaine Anonymous, Pornography Anonymous, Pills Anonymous, Sex Addicts Anonymous, and several other groups addressing different addiction issues.

The importance of support groups for the family members of an addict cannot be overemphasized. Addiction is not only frustrating for the addict; it is equally frustrating for the family members, the significant others, and society at large. People who are close to the addict, especially the family members, can learn how to cope from a good support group. They will be able to help the addict without becoming enmeshed or codependent. Support groups for family members can also provide an appropriate avenue for family members or people close to the addict to vent their frustrations. Family members can also learn how to set limits, and to deal with the constant manipulation that is common with addicts. People who are very close to the addict sometimes experience deeper emotional pain than the addict himself.

A very controversial program that is available in some countries in the Western world is called the needle exchange program. Addicts can return the needles they have used in injecting intravenous drugs in exchange for sterile or new needles. The goal is to decrease needle sharing and spread of blood transmitted diseases, especially the HIV/AIDS. The societies that allow needle exchange programs operate on the hope that addicts will possibly clean up their acts one day. If this happens, they will have a second chance at a sober life.

The needle exchange program has been criticized in some countries as an enabling program that would encourage the addicts to continue their dysfunctional lifestyle. The advantages versus the disadvantages of such programs should be carefully weighed before establishing such support programs.

The ultimate goal in dealing with addiction is not to give up because there are a lot of success stories out there. It is hoped that the majority of the people struggling with addiction problems will eventually be successful in overcoming the bondage of addiction. Every step of progress made, irrespective of any relapse, is a giant step in the right direction. With more scientific research, better public education, the already available success programs, and more promising future programs, we can hope that the battle against addiction will be permanently won one day.

# Addiction Problems among Youth and What Parents Can Do to Help

A strong foundation has been laid for this discussion by providing extensive information about the different types of drugs, their special names, and the horrible consequences of using these drugs. Many parents are totally unaware of what drugs are out there and the everyday dangers that their children are constantly exposed to. It is almost a norm for most teenagers to experiment with drugs and alcohol. Although it is hard to point to one root cause for the widespread use of drugs and alcohol in our young people, parents can nevertheless examine some of the reasons why young people try drugs and alcohol. First, they need to be aware of their children's environment and pay special attention to what is going on around their children.

It is very important for parents to spend meaningful time with their children especially in the younger years. It would build their children's self-esteem and self-confidence, and prepare them for the teenage years. There is a lot of pressure on youth to belong and to be accepted by their peers. A child with a very poor self-esteem is more likely to follow the crowd down a wrong pathway just to gain approval of his peers. It is important to let a child know that it is okay to be different in some situations, and it takes courage to stand alone.

Parents should know the type of people that their children are keeping company with and get to know their children's friends. If possible, they should get to know the parents of their children's friends, and acquire some knowledge of their background. If your child is a close friend with a child from a dysfunctional home where there is no parental guidance or control, your child will be endangered by this lack of supervision. It must be noted that dysfunctional home has nothing to do with socioeconomic status of the family. A family could be poor or wealthy and be dysfunctional. Many adolescents are more easily influenced by their peers than even by their parents or any other person. They might listen to their peers before they listen to their parents. Youthful years are a vulnerable period when children are trying to establish their own identities as young adults and to assert their independence. Unfortunately, they may not always be ready to make that transition into adulthood. If a child spends the night outside of the house with a friend, it is important for the parents to have a direct phone number of the friend's parents. It is also wise for a parent to call and check, to be sure that the child is actually honest about his destination. It is common among youth to tell their parents that they are going to a particular place but end up somewhere else that could be dangerous.

Parents should not be afraid to investigate further into their child's private life if they suspect the use of drug or alcohol. It is safer to catch the problem early and intervene quickly. Early intervention could prevent the future possibility of the child committing suicide, developing emotional problems, becoming an adult addict or going to jail.

If a parent's fear is confirmed with further investigation that a child is experimenting with drug and alcohol, such parents may want to go through the child's belongings every now and then without being disrespectful to their child. It is best if this is done in such a way that the child would not know or suspect that it was done. If an addicted teenager finds out that her parents are going through her personal belongings, she may invent more sophisticated hideouts to keep drugs and alcohol away from her parents. Going through the child's purse, handbags, schoolbags, drawers, wardrobe, toiletries, or even searching under the pillows and mattresses may not be a bad idea in this situation. The goal is to be alert and not take chances just in case the child is still actively using drugs and alcohol. The intention is not to police the child or to invade her privacy, but to make sure that the child is not moving towards a dangerous pathway. It is better to be safe than to be sorry. The decision to search the child's belongings should be at the parent's discretion. A parent who is not comfortable with searching his or her child's belongings should not do it.

It is also important for children to be able to account for their money, especially if they are employed in a part-time or summer job and are earning some money. Excessive spending may be the first clue to alert a parent that the child may be spending money on drugs and alcohol. If a child cannot account for the majority of his or her money most of the time, the parent should take the initiative to investigate the child's spending. Parent should always make sure that no money or valuables are missing around the house. This could also be the first clue to a child's alcohol and drug problems.

Early education about alcohol and drugs is another key to preventing our youth from getting involved in alcohol and drugs. Parents need to spend a lot of time talking to their children about drugs and alcohol during the early years of life. The earlier they hear about it, the better prepared they are going to be able to deal with it. Children should be taught at their level of understanding. For instance, parents should try to educate their little ones about the importance of respecting their bodies. As soon as a child develops the moral concepts of right from wrong, he or she will start to make decisions based on what they learn. Children must be taught early not to put anything that can destroy their bodies into their mouths. When they acquire more understanding as they grow older, the dangers of drugs and alcohol should be discussed with them. For instance, a child must be educated as early as possible about the dangers of "huffing", "dusting" or "bagging" because most of the products used to feed this dangerous addiction are readily available around the house. Remember, a child could be innocently introduced to "huffing", "dusting" or "bagging" from spending a night with a friend. As mentioned earlier, many children are of the opinion that the products used in "huffing", "dusting" or "bagging" are not drugs because they are household products. Unfortunately, this is not true. A child who has no education about the danger of these addictions may consider "huffing", "dusting" or "bagging" a fun prank or play, and end up becoming an addict or dead.

Parents should also encourage continuous early education about drugs and alcohol problems in the school system and the community. A one-time or sporadic drug and alcohol education class in the middle or high school is not enough to keep children out of trouble. There should be a movement to have schools incorporate drugs and alcohol education and prevention into the school curriculum. Continuous education and reinforcement about the dangers of drugs and alcohol may help to reduce youth involvement with drugs and alcohol. We hope that we can have fewer or zero future addicts with such teachings. It is very unfortunate that many youth innocently get involved with drugs and alcohol with the intention of having fun, getting accepted by their peers, and belonging to the group. They may not know the extent of the lifelong struggles that would follow this decision, especially the possible danger of premature death. Prevention would be cheaper for taxpayers than a cure. The cost of drug and alcohol rehabilitation is outrageous. There is no doubt that continuous early education and possible preventive measures are a lot cheaper than trying to cure the problem after it has occurred.

Parents need to model good behavior for their children. Children learn more from what they see than what they are told. Alcoholic parents may not be respected by their children if they try to tell their children to stay away from alcohol. Parents also need to talk with people who are in constant interaction with their children, such as the teachers, sport coaches, camp leaders, counselors, and friends. Those who interact closely with a child may be the first to pick on the signs of drug and alcohol problems with that child, even faster than the parents.

Parents should encourage their children to get involved in organized activities such as sports, community service, and productive recreational clubs. Children who are involved in contact sports like basketball, soccer, track and field, and other interactive sports usually have a good outlet to expend their energy. Adolescents have a lot of energy to burn off because of the physiological changes going on in their body at this phase of their development.

It is also important that parents make sure that their children are not using drugs to enhance their athletic abilities. It must be emphasized to children that the primary purpose of sports is for physical fitness, and if they excel in the sport, it is okay. Many parents put too much pressure on their children by trying to make them into "star athletes." Some parents try to live their own dreams through their children. They become desperate to make their children become that athlete that they could not become. Such fanatical behavior and excessive pressure could indirectly push a child to go to any extent to excel in order to please the parent. Parents should take a self-inventory and be mindful of the degree of pressure they are putting on their children who are involved in sports.

Clubs such as the YMCA, Boys and Girls Club, YWCA, community service clubs, volunteer clubs, and school service clubs give children a sense of responsibility and usefulness. Young people feel that they are doing something good and beneficial for their community, and this is a healthy feeling. For those who are raised in Christian homes, a lot of churches have organized, structured church youth groups that offer opportunities for spiritual growth, service projects, mission trips to help those who are less fortunate, and social outlets. Getting involved in such groups and in other church activities can be very beneficial. Children who are seriously and sincerely involved in good religious and non-religious clubs may be able to stay out of trouble. They learn the moral code of right and wrong. Embracing such values early in life could influence the future decision making of a child in the vulnerable youthful years. It is equally important that parents instill good values in their children at home. The common saying, "Charity begins at home," may still ring true.

Parents must also be educated about drugs and alcohol addiction. Many parents may have a general idea about such problems, but are ignorant about the extent of the problem. Some parents do not know how much the world has changed around them. Parents must try to understand the street language and the drug language among youths. They may want to casually listen to their children's conversations with their peers occasionally for possible clues of suspected drug activity. Parents must be willing to discuss drug and alcohol openly without holding back, especially if their own children are dealing with drug problems. Many parents cover up for their children. They usually avoid coming out and talking openly about their children's struggles because they feel a sense of shame and failure as parents. This is understandable. People can be very unkind and judgmental, thinking that drug addiction can never happen to them. Sometimes when children die from a drug overdose, their parents may say that their child committed suicide as a result of major depression, or come up with different stories to cover up the true cause of their child's death. When parents who have experienced this difficulty with their children begin to speak up boldly, such openness will increase the awareness of this problem. When more parents realize that drug overdoses could happen to their children, they will get involved in finding solutions to this horrible problem. With increased openness and awareness, the rest of the society will begin to wake up to the reality that this is a serious problem that needs a very serious intervention.

Parents need to find out how much their children know about drugs. They need to find out what their children think about drugs, and how they plan to handle a situation that puts them under a lot of pressure to use drugs and alcohol. Rehearsing and talking about a possible scenario may psychologically or mentally prepare a child to deal with a real life situation in the future, if the situation ever arises.

It is important for parents not to treat a child or a youth like an adult. Parents sometimes forget how they betrayed the trust of their own parents when they were younger. It is okay to trust our youth, but at the same time, we must be very vigilant and remember that youth will always be youth. Parents must always remember that teenage years are very vulnerable years in the life of a child. This is a period when decisions made by a child may not always be the best or wisest decisions. Many parents run a hectic daily schedule and live stressful lives. As a result they are willing to allow their children to drive as soon as possible, without properly monitoring their movements. It is wise for parents to make sure that their teenagers are ready for the responsibility that comes with the independence of driving and the ability to go to anywhere they want. A lot of problems occur when teenagers have this great independence of having or driving a car. It is wise for parents to check on their children's movements because teenagers may not always make good decisions about where they go. Some parents will take the time to check the mileage on the car's odometer before the teen drives the car to an event, and then recheck the mileage upon the teen's return if they suspect that their child may be going to dangerous places.

Parents can also take some simple precautions to assess their children for drug and alcohol problems. For example, meeting your son or daughter at the door when he or she comes back late in the night allows the parent to make a simple assessment immediately. The brief assessment could provide the first clue to the parents that their children are using drugs and alcohol. Parents could assess their children's mental alertness or check for the smell of alcohol or signs of drug usage when they meet them at the door. Youth are constantly trying to be ahead of their parents. They could rinse their mouth with mouthwash to mask the smell of alcohol before coming home. However, a parent may still be able to tell if a child is drunk. The parents may not detect the problem early if the child is not met at the door. The child could come in late at night, sleep off the drug and alcohol hangover, and clean up his or her acts before the parents could suspect anything the following morning.

As mentioned earlier, many parents do not spend time with their children anymore; this is creating a big vacuum in some families. Gone are those days when one parent stayed at home with the children. We must, however, not forget that there are some homes where both parents have to work because the family needs both incomes. The need to keep up with inflation may also require that both parents work. With the increased rate of divorce, more homes with single parents are also springing up. At the same time, there are some two parent homes where one parent could stay home. Sadly, the need to acquire more material things takes priority over spending quality time with the children in some of these homes. In the homes where both parents have to work out of necessity, work should not be used as an excuse to abandon parental responsibilities. There are many parents who both work, but at the same time make a determination to set guidelines for their children and follow through with them. There are many single parents as well who have raised successful and functional children. Sometimes good parenting is a matter of setting priorities and backing them with strong determination, dedication, and love.

The technological advances have made a lot of parents buy more sophisticated electronic equipment and gaming systems for their children, especially in the adolescent years. Unfortunately, many children are busy competing to see who has the best gaming system. Mixed-up priorities can lead some parents to try unconsciously to buy their children's love by excessively spending money on them. Instead of giving their children the most valuable gift of spending constructive time with them, some parents spend money on their children—buying for them expensive clothes, shoes, gifts, toys, and electronic gadgets. Some parents work two jobs to be able to buy the newest electronic gadgets and expensive gifts for their children every time a new model or style comes out. This has become a rat race among some parents.

We cannot put all the blame on the electronic industries or other manufacturers for feeding on the insatiable appetite of the consumers. After all, they have products to sell. We have to blame the consumers partially for not prioritizing. Some parents buy all these gifts primarily out of a guilty conscience for neglecting their most important responsibility, which is "parenting". The present generation is gradually losing the family closeness. Some parents even use the television and electronic games to babysit their children, instead of engaging them in meaningful conversation and interacting with them. They would rather have them watch the television or play electronic games because it is more convenient. It must be mentioned that some of the electronic gadgets and gaming systems are educational, however, they must not be used to replace parental responsibility. Family members living under the same roof rarely interact in some households; everybody stays in different parts of the house doing different things like a group of strangers sharing the same address. Spending constructive time with children will help to develop their character.

Parents should work on bringing back the old family closeness, typical of most families not too long ago. Family closeness could help to fill the void some of our youth are trying to fill with drugs and alcohol. Many youth join a gang and call their gang members their family members. This is very unfortunate. Sadly, if gang members are providing the support that should be provided for the child at home, then the child will think of the gang as his family, even if it is a dysfunctional and a dangerous family.

Parents should also encourage public and private funding into the study and research of addiction problems. It is hoped that with time, a lot more will be known about the addictive gene, and the involvement of the brain in addiction. There are lots of studies out there already, but more is still needed. Maybe the day will come that "craving," which is the biggest trap in addiction, will be treated with a pill or a vaccine, just as high blood pressure can be easily controlled by medication. This may be the future solution for those who cannot beat their addictions very easily with willpower and rehabilitation. After all, many things are possible with science; new information is unveiled every day. Maybe, science will one day help us to identify and to control the "craving" gene.

The final conclusion is that parents can never take too many precautions when it comes to their children, especially in the areas of addiction issues. The truth of the matter is that prevention is always better than a cure, and parents must always strive toward the welfare of their children.

## PART VI
# COMMON PROBLEMS RELATED TO THOUGHTS: SCHIZOPHRENIA

## Schizophrenia:
# BRYAN'S STORY

It was around three o'clock in the morning, I thought I heard movement in my room, but I dismissed it. A few minutes later, I heard another movement and reached for the lamp next to my bed. I was shocked to see our middle son, Bryan, standing next to our bed with a sharp knife. I screamed at the top of my lungs, and my husband woke up. Bryan was laughing inappropriately, and he said, "I have finally learned that both of you have been poisoning my food and calling me crazy; you have both been giving me the poisonous pills to make me crazy. I'm going to kill both of you! Don't move — it's payback time." I didn't know what to do. I covered my head with a blanket, saying my last prayer. The next I heard was a sound of a struggle in the room. I quickly removed my covers to see what was happening. My husband and my son were in a big struggle; my husband was trying to take the knife from him, and he was trying to stab my husband. I reached for the phone, and the phone was dead. Our son had cut off the main telephone line to the house. Unfortunately, there was no wireless phone at that time.

I ran out of the house to the next door neighbor's and frantically knocked on their door asking them to call 911, the emergency police and ambulance service. I went back in the house to try to help my husband. He had overpowered our son, but our son was still fighting back. The knife had been thrown across the room, and my husband and son were both struggling to get to the knife. My husband's arm was bleeding, and there was blood all over the floor. I quickly ran to pick up the knife. Our son was screaming all sorts of obscenities and cursing, but my husband refused to let go of him. The police finally came, and although it took them fifteen minutes to respond, it felt like fifteen hours.

**165**

The police completely overpowered Bryan and took him away in handcuffs. Watching Bryan was very heartbreaking for me as a mother; Bryan continued to scream all sorts of obscenities, threatening that when he comes back, he would make sure that both of us died. Bryan was frantically trying to explain to the police, in his delusional and confused state of mind, that my husband and I were trying to kill him by gradually poisoning his food, drinks, and medications, so that we could collect a life insurance policy on him. My husband was taken in the ambulance to the nearest hospital where he was treated for his stab wound and was later released to come home.

We are a typical middle-income family with high hopes and aspirations for our children, and we never once imagined that our child could be struck with an illness like this. Bryan's illness began when he was in college. He was a great child growing up; very athletic, straight-A student, and graduated top of his high school class. In college, Bryan wanted to do something that would allow him to work with airplanes, which always fascinated him as a child. His college was a seven-hour drive away from home, and he went there to study aerospace engineering. As parents, we were excited and hopeful about his future. We told everybody how proud we were of Bryan, and how well he was doing. The illness struck the very first semester of college. Initially, he was calling us and was complaining about how people were talking about him and were ganging up against him.

As parents, we told him to ignore the people talking about him, that such experiences are part of growing up. He would call at very odd times of the night, complaining of not sleeping. He complained that some people in his dormitory were talking by his window and his door at night, and they were determined to make his life miserable because they did not like him. We suggested to him that he should look into changing his dormitory. We were very worried as parents, but we thought it was all part of the stress of going away from home for the first time. We were hoping that he would adjust and do well by the end of the first year.

One fateful day, we received a call from his college for us to come immediately. We were told on the phone that Bryan had had a nervous breakdown. He had taken off his clothes, and he was screaming obscenities in front of the dormitory, threatening to jump off the third floor. He was overpowered by the security officers, taken to the emergency room, and transferred to a mental hospital. My husband and I were totally clueless about the seriousness of some mental illnesses. We knew that people have mental breakdowns, but it was not something that we particularly knew much about. You always think it could never happen to you; unconsciously, you walk around thinking that it is something that happens to other people until it touches you personally. When we arrived at his school, we were shocked when we saw Bryan for the first time. He looked like a totally different person. He was spaced out; his affect or facial expression was flat (expressionless look), and he was unusually slow from the effects of the medications he was being given. All of a sudden, we could not communicate with our son anymore because he was saying a lot of things that did not make sense to us. He told us that his life was in danger because some people were monitoring him and were trying to kill him. He was looking around, talking in whispering tones, and was extremely suspicious of others.

We met privately with the doctor, and he sadly told us that Bryan was suffering from a mental illness called schizophrenia, the paranoid type, and this was why he believed people were after him. The psychiatrist further explained to us that this illness is not totally curable, but Bryan could be stabilized to function optimally as best as he could function with medication management and therapy. The psychiatrist explained schizophrenia to us in detail, and told us that this was basically a malfunction of Bryan's brain, and that Bryan would experience things that would be real to him, but not real to anybody else.

As parents, we were not willing to believe that this could be happening to our son. For us, the most difficult part of dealing with this illness was the acceptance part. We were not convinced that the psychiatrist knew what he was talking about. My husband and I came to the conclusion that Bryan, just like a typical young college student, had probably experimented with street drugs and had these complications from the effects of the drugs. We both knew deep inside us that Bryan was not likely to use street drugs, but we had our own explanation for this problem, other than what the psychiatrist was telling us. We asked the psychiatrist if Bryan tested positive for any street or illicit drugs, and he said there was no trace of any illicit or street drugs in his system.

We were still convinced that the drug was probably out of his system at the time of admission, and that was why he did not test positive; and we were bent on getting a second opinion. We checked into a local hotel, and Bryan was kept in the hospital for about two weeks and was later released to us. We took him home with us and sought a second opinion with a local psychiatrist when we got home. The local psychiatrist reached the same diagnosis of schizophrenia, the paranoid type, and that was why Bryan believed that other people were out to get him or hurt him. We eventually accepted the diagnosis, but we could not stop wondering how this could happen to our son. That was the most difficult part, why us? What had we done wrong to deserve this?

Bryan became a totally different person with little or no interest in life, and he was very suspicious of the rest of the family. For more than five years we struggled to keep Bryan at home. He was seen regularly by a local psychiatrist, and he has been on medications and therapy. Even so, Bryan would accuse us of poisoning his food, and he refused to eat at home sometimes. He would refuse to take his medications sometimes; he complained that the medications made him feel tired and sleepy a lot. He would also accuse us of trying to poison him at times when we offered him his medication. However, he agreed to take the medications because he did not want to be hospitalized. We always told him that we would have no choice than to put him in the hospital if he did not take his medication. We made him understand that this was not a threat; it was the only way we could keep him from constantly relapsing. It was a continuous battle because he did not believe that anything was wrong with him. He had a few relapses that required hospitalization despite all of our efforts to keep him out of the hospital, and he hated the hospitalization experience very much.

Bryan spent most of his days in front of the television, and he sometimes talked to himself in front of the T.V., claiming that the people on the T.V. were talking to him or talking about him. We tried to re-enroll him in college part-time, but he could not handle the pressure. He would come home and would tell us that some people were watching him in the classroom and reading his mind. We acquired a lot of information about schizophrenia and tried very hard to keep the family together. Despite all of our efforts, Bryan's illness changed the family dynamics. Our older son Travis refused to come home from college on most of the holidays. He said watching his younger brother with this illness was too difficult for him to handle. Travis and Bryan were very close siblings growing up; they had done everything together. They were not only brothers—they were also like best friends. Travis got very angry and bitter about this illness called schizophrenia every time he was around his brother Bryan. He even promised never to have any children, because he read in the books that schizophrenia is hereditary.

Bryan's illness has been very devastating for all of us. Schizophrenia is physically, financially, and emotionally draining on the family. My husband and I managed to survive with the help of therapy and our support group, and we managed to keep Bryan at home until this last incident. It was very scary, because he could have killed both of us. You raise your child with lots of love and hope, especially a child like Bryan who was so full of life and very purpose-driven. Like many other parents, we looked forward to a very bright future for him—graduation, marriage, and a good life. Unfortunately, this is what fate handed to us. For more than five years now, we have had to worry about Bryan performing his daily hygiene. The Bryan we used to know was a very tidy and organized child. With this illness, we can never tell from day-to-day if he would trust us enough to take his medications or to eat at home. Now we have to keep him permanently locked up in the state mental institution after our last brush with death. It dawned on us that it may not be very safe to live with Bryan with this illness, which really hurts. We go to visit Bryan on weekends, and he is more stable on medication. We take him outside the hospital on passes to shop and eat, if the voices in his head will allow him to eat.

Bryan has a better insight into his problems now, but he still cannot trust anybody because of his paranoia and suspicion of others. We know clearly that he hears voices and sees things that are not there. Sometimes Bryan is able to identify that the voices are not real, and knows that what he sees is not real. Other times he falsely believes that what he hears are real people talking to him, and what he sees are real people as well. We don't know if Bryan will ever come back home to live again; it really hurts to leave him at the hospital every weekend when we visit. We have to face the reality of keeping Bryan in a safe environment and also to consider our safety as well. We have not given up hope on Bryan for when there is life, there is hope. Who knows? There may be a cure for schizophrenia in Bryan's lifetime.

Bryan's illness has taught us the humility of the serenity prayer—to accept what we cannot change, to change what we can, and the wisdom to know the difference. If Bryan's story sounds familiar to you, please get help. Every schizophrenic is not locked up in a mental hospital. There are so many schizophrenics functioning in the world, holding down jobs and living in the community with the appropriate help. Please do not hesitate to do something before it is too late to help someone you know who could be suffering from this illness. We will always love Bryan unconditionally, but at the same time, we wish he never had schizophrenia.

# Quotes of Encouragement...

As the wind blows harder and Bryan's story sounds familiar to you, remember the following:

*"In the final analysis, the question of why bad things happen to good people transmutes itself into some very different questions, no longer asking why something happened, but asking how we will respond, what we intend to do now that it has happened."*

~ Harold S. Kushner

No parents deserve to watch their child suffer from schizophrenia. The truth is, it is not your fault, neither is it the fault of your child. Now that you are faced with this illness, don't go down in self-pity or try to figure out why it happened to your child. Instead, go after every available resource that can help you and your child function effectively with this illness; set a goal to maximize the quality of life for your child and your family. This is the winner's attitude in the midst of despair. *(LB)*

*"Man's mind is his essence; he is where his thoughts are."*

~ Nahman of Bratzlav

A man's actions are a reflection of his thoughts. If your thoughts have not deceived you for many years of your life, it could be incomprehensible to you to believe that your thoughts can suddenly turn against you. This, in essence, reflects the daily struggle and conflicts of schizophrenics; even when their actions hurt your feelings, remember they are victims of their own minds, Give them a helping hand, no matter how difficult it is for you; don't forget that their thoughts have misguided and misled them. Unfortunately they don't even know it. *(LB)*

*"What we do not understand, we cannot control."*

~ Charles Reich

Schizophrenics with an active illness lack the ability to comprehend or to understand their own minds and situations. They cannot control their actions and their reasoning, so be supportive and helpful. Set aside your personal feelings, try to forgive them for their actions, and remember it could have been you, because schizophrenia does not discriminate. *(LB)*

# Winds Against The Mind

## Schizophrenia:

# MRS. BUTCHER'S STORY

Whence I was in college, I took a class in abnormal psychology, which was probably the closest book knowledge I had about unusual behavior in people. I knew that people do have mental illnesses, but being raised in a wealthy and affluent family, I actually thought mental illness was mostly poverty induced. I did not think I had to worry too much about it since it was mainly a problem of poor people, I always said to myself. My thinking was very naïve and ignorant, but I actually did not know better.

I met my wife one summer at a picnic organized by a well-respected family in our community, and it was love at first sight. I proposed to her after one year of dating, and we got married the following year. I worked with my parents, running the family business, and my wife stayed at home to raise our three children. At age forty-five, she had a minor surgery to have her appendix removed due to an infection. I first noticed some very strange behavior after this surgery, but the doctor dismissed it as a possible effect of anesthesia. She later fully recovered, and everything was back to normal. About six months after the surgery, I noticed an increase in her drinking and stranger behavior. I was worried and insisted she get professional help before her drinking got out of hand. We both tried to be very cautious about alcohol, because alcoholism runs in both of our families.

The appointment for my wife to see a therapist was set for when I returned from a five-day business trip. My teenage son who stayed at home called me twice on the trip to say that his mom was behaving strangely. I was very angry with her and concluded that she must have been drinking a lot more since I was away. I tried to talk to her a few times, but she would come to the phone and laugh hysterically, and say things that did not make sense. I was very irritated and upset by her reactions. After four days, I cut my trip short and came home to one of the biggest surprises of my life.

First of all, my wife was not at home when I arrived. As I walked into the house, I noticed something strange: one of the rooms in the house was completely furnished like a baby's room. This made no sense to me. We have three boys, two in college and the youngest in high school. Obviously boys don't get pregnant, so what was going on? Why did we have a baby's room in the house? My wife could not be pregnant because she had had a total hysterectomy (had her womb removed) five years earlier. Questions flew through my mind. I finally concluded that maybe one of the boys had gotten a girl pregnant, but my wife should have at least told me first, out of courtesy, before preparing a room for a grandbaby in the house. At this stage of my life I really could not imagine living in a house with a baby. If this were the case, I would rather support my son, the baby, and the mother in a separate apartment.

In the middle of my mental debate, my wife came in. She had bags of groceries and bags of baby items. I noticed that she had a strange look about her. "What in the world is going on?" I asked with an expression of shock on my face. "I have only been gone for four days. What happened?" My wife turned around and told me that she had been impregnated by some supernatural beings and that we were going to have a baby. It was the most bizarre thing I had ever heard in my life, especially since she had a hysterectomy five years earlier. I reminded her that she had hysterectomy few years back and her womb was removed; therefore she could not have a baby. She laughed at me hysterically, telling me that she had another womb supernaturally implanted in her. She went on to talk about some people living in the house with us who have magical and supernatural powers, and she even said they can make both of us disappear if we want to disappear. She said these people gave her their power, and impregnated her by using their magical powers, and the child she was going to have would change the world, clean out bad people, and rule the world. She was so excited to tell me that the baby was due anytime, and she planned to involve me in the delivery.

I knew immediately that something was seriously wrong with her. Everything she said just did not make any sense. I called our family doctor to explain the situation; he told me to bring her to his office, but she refused to go. The doctor later agreed to come to the house.

After spending few hours observing her, our doctor told me that if there were no medical problems causing these types of symptoms, she might be experiencing an adult onset of schizophrenia. The doctor said it was very unusual for people to develop schizophrenia at my wife's age, but it does happen. He also went on to say that the people she was seeing and communicating with were very real to her. To my surprise, she was very cooperative with the doctor. She treated his visit more like a social visit than a patient-doctor visit, but she agreed to do whatever he asked her to do. She allowed the doctor to take her blood for a check-up and cooperated with a general medical examination. She believed that the doctor was checking on the baby she was going to have.

The doctor called back the next day and told us that every test he did on her came back clear and normal. There was no indication of a medical problem. At dinnertime, she set the table for seven, and there were only three of us in the house. She insisted that four other people were sitting at the table with us. She was dishing out food into four other plates, and she carried out a full conversation with these invisible people at the dinner table. Our teenage son was so disgusted with what was going on, he left the dinner table and went to his room. I was totally paralyzed with shock. I tried to convince her to go to the hospital with me, but she insisted that she had to have the baby at home, and she did not want to be tricked into having the baby in the hospital. I called our primary care physician again, who suggested that I should call a psychiatric hospital and have her evaluated for mental illness and then have her admitted to the hospital for further evaluation.

We called a psychiatric hospital and tried to commit my wife, and we explained what was going on with her on the phone. We were asked several questions, and one of which was if she was destructive or endangering her life or other people's lives, and we said 'no.' To my surprise, we were told that if she was not a danger to herself or other people, such as trying to kill others or herself or being physically aggressive to others, there would not be any basis to want to hospitalize her. They told us that they did not have enough grounds to commit her forcefully or admit her to the hospital. They suggested that we try the outpatient care of a psychiatrist, but my wife continuously refused to go. Unfortunately, we could not find a psychiatrist who would come to our home to see her. I was frustrated and had to turn to my family for help. No one could convince my wife that something was wrong with her. She was in this state of euphoria, totally excited about the baby she was going to have. She bluntly refused to seek or get help.

Her symptoms continued to escalate gradually. She was pacing the house, talking to herself, but was claiming to be talking to the aliens living in the house. She was getting more and more restless, staying up all night arranging the baby's room, and laughing inappropriately. I found myself crying for the first time in my adult life; this was not the woman I married twenty-three years ago. I felt a sense of shame about the situation, and I was hoping that no one would find out except my immediate family. Our family name was a household name in our community, and I was worried about how this situation was going to be perceived if it got out to the public. I was convinced that I would definitely not be able to take the embarrassment. Life was at a standstill at my house; everything totally revolved around trying to bring my wife to reasoning. Our youngest teenage son, who was watching all of what was happening, got very frustrated with his mother, because he could not understand what was happening to her. My wife was trying to convince even our son to believe some of her strange beliefs.

By the fourth day, her symptoms had gotten worse. She approached our son in the kitchen on his way to school and asked him if he could give one of her guests in the house a ride to the store. Our son, who was obviously a typical teenager and was extremely frustrated with the situation, turned around, lashed out at my wife, and drove out of the house in anger. When he came back from school, my wife accused him of intentionally trying to drive over one of her guests and then physically attacked him. She got into a fight with him and was completely out of control. It was so strange to those of us outside her world that the people she was seeing were so real to her, and she actually believed that my son tried to drive into one of them with the intention of killing him.

After she attacked our son, we had a valid reason to commit her, so we called the police, and she was finally taken to the hospital. The whole scenario lasted about four to five days, but it felt like ten years of horror. I could not believe that this was really happening in my home. It was like a bad dream. I was relieved that she was finally admitted, and she would at least be getting treatment. I love my wife very much. She is my life, and I could not take watching her with this illness. It was too painful for me. I was hoping that the diagnosis would be different, but unfortunately, every test ruled out any medical or organic problem for her behavior, and the final diagnosis for her at the psychiatric hospital was adult onset of schizophrenia.

We later found out that my wife's great-grandmother on her father's side who lived in Europe also had a similar illness in her mid forties, and ended up being confined to a mental institution for the rest of her life. Fortunately for us, my wife's story did not end up like her great-grandmother's story. She was stabilized on medication and hospitalized for a few weeks. The voices went away, and she did not see the aliens anymore. I noticed a drastic decrease in her energy level. We had to have a sitter stay with her and help her around the house. She went from being a very active, energetic, always on-the-go woman, to a very slow person. I later found out that her low energy level and some of the side effects she was experiencing might be due to the side effects of her medications. She had one relapse since the first incident, and this was when she quit taking her medications, believing she was healed. Fortunately, she has been very compliant with taking her medications ever since, and we are able to have as close to a normal life as possible. Our youngest son recently went to college, leaving only the two of us in the house.

Just when we felt that another phase of our lives was beginning, with the children gone and a lot more free time, an illness like this struck and changed everything. I looked forward to our taking many wonderful vacations together when the children were gone, but since the illness, she feels safer in the home environment instead of outside the home. She is not the same energetic, fun-loving woman I married, but we still have each other. We have enjoyed a few wonderful vacations together; I just wish we could take some more. What really baffles me is how I managed to live into my forties without an in-depth knowledge of an illness like this until it was happening close to me. I now know everything I need to know about schizophrenia. When you have to live with it, you will know about it. I have since learned to educate myself about other mental illnesses since this experience. The children are very supportive and understanding, and they love their mom unconditionally.

If this story sounds familiar, please go and get help. Every case is not a hopeless case. Our family life is by no means a horrible life, although it could be better. I look forward to a day in human history when there will be a cure for schizophrenia, I hope, during my wife's lifetime.

# Quotes of Encouragement...

As the wind blows harder and Mrs. Butcher's story sounds familiar to you, remember the following:

*"Surely there is grandeur in knowing that in the realm of thought, at least, you are without a chain, that you have the right to explore all heights and all depths, that there are no walls nor fences, nor prohibited places, nor sacred corners in all the vast expanse of thought..."*

*~ Robert G. Ingersoll*

The above quote is the perfect description of the mind or the thought of a schizophrenic; they live in this imaginary world that has no boundaries and no limitations; this world is real to them just as your world is real to you. Before you judge them, remember that this is not a choice that they made. This illness chose them; they did not choose the illness. *(LB)*

*"I am thought, I can see what the eyes cannot see, I can hear what the ears cannot hear, and I can feel what the heart cannot feel."*

*~ Peter Nivio Zarlenga*

The world of a schizophrenic is ruled by his malfunctioned thoughts or malfunctioned mind. He can truly see what you cannot see, hear what you cannot hear, and feel what you cannot feel. Before you judge him, remember that you live in a world that everybody can see, but he lives in the world that is visible only to his eyes. Your reality is not his reality, so help him as much as possible to see the difference between the real world and the imaginary world he lives in. *(LB)*

*"What is going on in the inside shows on the outside."*

*~ Earl Nightingale*

The truth as it is perceived inside of a schizophrenic governs his external actions that are observable by the people around him. When he talks or acts strangely, remember his constant inner struggles before you get frustrated with him. Some schizophrenics act out or give many external cues that are ignored until something dangerous happens, so be alert to the external cues. These are usually the only connection to what is going on inside of them. *(LB)*

177

*Winds Against The Mind*

## Schizophrenia:
# MR. CRUTCHER'S STORY

My aunt called and told my sister and me to come home immediately because our mom was in a critical condition. We asked her for the hospital information where Mom was, but she insisted that we had to come home first, and she would be waiting for us at the house to take us to the hospital. Since my aunt rarely calls us, this was a very frightening phone call. We were extremely nervous with all sorts of thoughts flying through our minds. Our aunt refused to give us any detailed information about what was wrong. She insisted that we had to come home immediately. We took the very next flight home in a state of panic.

Upon our arrival at home, we noticed that there was a tape around our house, and a sign that read, "Crime Scene. Keep Off." My aunt was already waiting for us at the entrance gate of the house. She said to us tearfully that our mom was dead, and she was killed by our dad. She hugged us both and told us that she was very sorry. My sister and I felt like she was speaking another language, and we both broke down and cried bitterly. The whole time I kept thinking that it must be a bad dream, because the dad we know and love would never kill our mother. We finally went to the morgue (mortuary) to see our mother's body. It was a very depressing sight to see her innocent body lying there, badly stabbed.

Growing up, we knew something was not right with our dad at times, because he had to be hospitalized on and off. Mom would tell us that Dad had an illness that affected his mind, and he needed his medication adjusted, which was why he had to go to the hospital. The explanation was good enough for us at that time, and we were always happy to see Dad come back home. We did not know that Dad had schizophrenia. He was so loving and caring whenever he was home. He was such a doting and giving father to us. He spent a lot of time with us and was a happy father.

His family was his universe. Dad worked very hard at his job whenever he was not in the hospital. He worked as the assistant manager of a big grocery store in our community. He worked at this store all his life, and our parents actually met when they both were working at this same grocery store. Mom had since moved on to other jobs. Mom was aware of Dad's illness from the time they met, but she loved him unconditionally. Dad was such a wonderful person when he was not ill that you could not help but love him. Life was great for us when we were growing up, and we did not feel different from other kids. We did not lack material things, or miss out on childhood fun. Our grandparents, knowing Dad's health limitations, spent a lot of time with us. They were extremely supportive. Dad was stable most of the time, and we had a wonderful childhood with him that was full of good memories.

After graduating from high school one year apart, my sister and I decided to venture out and explore the world apart from our little town where we grew up. We both moved to a bigger city. My sister decided to pursue a music career because she had an incredible voice, and I decided to go to college and major in political science, with the hope of going to law school one day. Our move was very traumatic for our dad, and he became more and more paranoid (feeling suspicious of others) after we left. His paranoia was centered on our mom. Dad constantly accused Mom of having an extramarital affair, and even had her followed by a private investigator. He started telling other members of the family that Mom was having an affair.

Everybody knew about his illness and about how he would become paranoid whenever he was very ill, but it had not really been a big problem. He was always fine in the past when his medication was adjusted. Everybody in the family tried to convince Dad that his accusations were wrong, and that they were all false beliefs coming from his mind. Mom constantly reassured Dad of her unconditional love for him and continually told him that she would never cheat on him. She took him to his psychiatrist to have his medication readjusted several times, but there was no improvement. He was eventually hospitalized. Mom was very supportive of Dad as usual, and she went to the hospital to see him each day of the hospitalization.

Shortly after his return from his last hospitalization, he claimed that Mom had spent the entire time that he was away in the hospital with another man in the house, and insisted that he saw a lot of evidence around the house to prove that another man stayed there. Mom was very concerned, but never thought of anything too serious about his accusations, because he had had paranoid beliefs in the past. He was able to let go of the beliefs when he felt better. Dad continued to express serious anger about his false beliefs, but he was never violent about it. He had never been a violent man all of his life, even in his most confused state of mind. Mom laughed over his accusations most of the time, while she continued to reassure him that she would never be unfaithful to him.

On the fateful night of Mom's death, Dad stabbed her to death, claiming that she brought her boyfriend to the bedroom, and Mom and her boyfriend were making love next to him on the same bed. Dad actually believed he killed two people, his wife and her boyfriend. Dad was apparently seeing somebody else that was not there in his state of confusion or delusion, but nobody else could see what was so real and believable to him. It was all in his mind. Obviously the imagination part of his brain just malfunctioned and went wild. It really hurts that an illness will make somebody commit such a grievous and horrible crime based on false beliefs. We later found out that Dad had stopped taking his medications for a long time because the imaginary voices told him not to take them, and that Mom was trying to kill him and marry someone else. Mom never found out because he had been very compliant about taking his medications for most of their lives together. He was very well informed about his illness, although he relapsed at times. Not taking his medications was the major primary cause of this bizarre behavior. He had done well over the years on medication. We were full of anger and resentment, and it hurt very much to lose our mother.

My sister and I decided to visit Dad at the mental institution; we demanded an explanation for his actions. To our surprise, Dad showed no remorse. He emphatically said that he would kill 'both of them' over and over again for disrespecting him on his matrimonial bed. We asked what he meant when he said that he had killed two people, and we emphatically told him there was no other person. Dad maintained that he killed our mom and her boyfriend for humiliating him, and he saw them with his two eyes making love next to him on the bed. He was so grounded in his belief, which was the most frightening part of this illness. A side of you really hates the man you know as your father, but a little voice in your mind tells you to only hate the illness, not your dad. What a terrible illness, that would make somebody behave like this, to foolishly take another person's life and be completely unaware that there was no basis for such a horrible murder! How do you live with or reconcile these facts? How do you forgive such a man who himself was a victim of a terrible illness, who himself has no control of his own mind? We felt such an unbearable pain.

Currently, my sister and I have no trace of mental illness, but knowing what happened to our dad frightened us, and we hope we will never develop this illness. You might be wondering how we face the world and tell our story, or how we explain that our mom had to die a painful death because our dad has schizophrenia. If we ever have children, how will we tell them about their grandparents? We suddenly felt like orphans, because Mom is dead, and Dad is locked up forever. It was a big struggle for us to go back to see our dad.

The next time we saw him, he was medically stable and rational. He was not psychotic or out of touch with reality anymore; the voices were not as bad as before, and all of his hallucination was gone. It finally dawned on him that he had killed his wife whom he loved very much and had left his children with no mother. He was extremely sorry for his actions, and he talked about killing himself so that he could go and join our mom. The hospital staff told us that they had to watch him closely because he was preoccupied with death, and he had tried to kill himself twice since his realization that he had killed his wife when he was psychotic. He confessed that he had stopped taking his medication a long time ago, but our mom had never found out, because he hid it very well from her.

My sister and I have been a good support for each other, especially since we share the same apartment. Sometimes we wonder how we have managed to survive from day-to-day, walking around with so much emotional pain. We were also in therapy and a support group. Our grandparents have been a great source of strength for us, and our extended family members are also wonderful, providing great support. We volunteered to participate in a research study at a local hospital for family members of schizophrenics in our search for a cure. We hope that one day no human being will ever have to suffer from such a cruel illness that takes over your life, controls your mind, and makes you commit a terrible crime, leaving you totally clueless of how wrong you were.

Dad was constantly watched for suicide at the hospital, because he talked about killing himself all the time. We found a place in our hearts to forgive him, reminding ourselves of the good memories of him as a wonderful father and that he was a victim of a terrible illness that controlled his mind. We went to the hospital to see him whenever we could. Our visits were always very difficult for him, and we noticed that he never forgave himself. He also had a few relapses in the hospital, but these were properly managed since this was a controlled environment. His visual hallucinations, whenever he had them, were primarily seeing our dead mom, despite contrary evidence presented to him that his wife was dead. After about two years in a mental institution, Dad went home on a weekend pass with our grandparents one weekend, and ended up successfully killing himself. Dad's suicide re-opened a new chapter, and now we are real orphans. It was very painful, but we know our grandparents could not have been able to prevent his suicide.

Please do not allow our story to frighten you. We are sharing this story with the world to help somebody out there suffering from the same illness. If you also have a loved one with this illness, let this story increase your awareness. Don't take too much for granted with schizophrenia; please get help as soon as possible.

Do not dismiss what a schizophrenic says or sees because it is not real to you. Please remember it is real to the victim of this illness. Most importantly, make sure they are properly managed with medication. After all, this same father of ours kept his jobs for years, had a close-to-normal life, but everything changed when he decided he did not need his medications anymore. It is not a hopeless situation; there is help out there, and a lot of schizophrenics contribute constructively to society when they are properly managed with medication and therapy. Please get help before it is too late. We should all work together and report any dangerous clues or signs by people with schizophrenia with the hope to get help for them. With increase awareness, we can all work together to prevent more tragedies.

# Quotes of Encouragement...

As the wind blows harder and Mr. Crutcher's story sounds familiar to you, remember the following:

*"I know but one freedom, and that is the freedom of the mind."*
~ Antoine de Saint-Exupery

Some of us enjoy the total freedom of our mind; we are in total control of our actions and the choices that we make; a schizophrenic, on the other hand, cannot enjoy the same freedom. He is totally in bondage or slavery to his own mind. His mind has chosen to go to war against him, and the victim of this war is the schizophrenic. *(LB)*

*"One might as well try to ride two horses moving in different directions, as to try to maintain in equal force two opposing or contradictory sets of desire."*
~ Robert Collier

The splitting of the mind of a schizophrenic is like riding two horses in two different directions. While he struggles to be part of the life that is real to all of us, his delusional mind also escapes to the life that is very real only to him; he constantly struggles to maintain in equal force two opposing or contradictory sets of desire; the desire to be here and to be there; unfortunately, the mind might eventually escape to the delusional world, a very private world that could be very scary and make a schizophrenic do things that are unimaginable or incomprehensible to the normal mind. *(LB)*

*"Invariably it is true— as is the inner so always inevitably will be the outer."*
~ Ralph Waldo Trine

Just as you believe what your mind tells you and you base your actions on your beliefs, a schizophrenic also believes and reacts based on what his mind presents to him; remember to put yourself in his shoes, for he is trying to be just like you in believing and trusting his own mind, but he is totally unaware that his beliefs are all false, and his mind has totally malfunctioned. *(LB)*

*Winds Against The Mind*

### Schizophrenia:
# BASIC FACTS & UNDERSTANDING

Bryan, Mrs. Butcher, and Mr. Crutcher all suffered from schizophrenia. Their minds that they trusted for years turned against them and started to deceive them, but they did not know it. *Schizophrenia* is a malfunction of the mind or the brain. People suffering from this illness usually have a completely altered sense of outer and inner reality, and they usually respond to the altered reality as if it is real or true. The inability to perceive reality accurately is manifested by the disturbance in their thinking, emotions, speech (or language), physical ability, and social behavior. The illness could be described as the total breakdown in the networking or the communication system of the brain. Unfortunately, victims may be ignorant of the fact that they are living in an altered reality.

Some of the common signs and symptoms of this illness include delusions, hallucinations, disturbed motor ability (such as problems with walking normally, holding eating utensils, or writing), and speech disturbance.

*Delusions* are falsely held beliefs that cannot be corrected by normal reasoning or by presenting the schizophrenic with facts. There are different types of delusional thinking; some common ones are delusions of persecution, delusion of grandeur, delusion of control, and somatic delusion.

A schizophrenic may have a groundless belief that somebody is poisoning his food and is trying to kill him, despite the fact that there is no rational evidence to support this belief. This is called *delusion of persecution.* It is also referred to as a paranoid belief or paranoid feelings. For example, a victim of this illness may believe that somebody has been sent to kill him, and this potential killer is watching him round the clock, looking for a perfect opportunity to attack him. He may live in fear and try to carry a weapon for protection. He may also believe that his medication is being poisoned.

*Delusion of grandeur* is displayed when the schizophrenic believes that he is somebody who is highly influential, perhaps an important person or a very powerful, famous figure. He could believe that he is Jesus Christ, Elvis Presley, or the President of the United States of America. He may insist on being addressed as Mr. President, or Mr. Elvis Presley. With *somatic delusion,* the false belief is about the body, or the body function. He may belief that he has HIV/AIDS, cancer, or a form of deadly disease, despite every medical proof to the contrary. *Delusion of jealousy* may make schizophrenics believe, falsely, that their spouses are cheating on them. They may be convinced that their wives or husbands are having extramarital affairs, despite the fact that there is no evidence to support the accusations. With *delusion of control,* schizophrenics may believe that their bodies or minds are controlled by another person or an object that is external to them, such as a computer. For instance, they may believe that they are being controlled by the secret service or the CIA. A schizophrenic who is convinced that she is being controlled could say, "There is a computer chip inside my head that tells me what to do" or "there is a ghost that controls my mind with electrical waves." She truly believes and is convinced in her own mind that she has absolutely no control over her thoughts and actions. She believes that she is strictly taking orders from somebody or something else external to her.

It can be very difficult at times to communicate with or initiate a dialogue with a schizophrenic. It can be easily noticed in a conversation that her brain is not making any connection with the outside world. The person may be busy trying to filter out the voices in her head to the extent that she may not even hear a word of what you say to her during a conversation.

Apart from their delusional thought content, the thought process of those suffering from this illness could also be very unique to them. Some of the terminologies used to describe their thought process include circumstantiality, perseveration, flight of ideas, tangentiality, thought blocking, thought broadcasting, thought insertion, ideas of reference, and looseness of association. *Circumstantiality* is a thought process in which the schizophrenics take an extra unnecessary tedious route before answering a simple question. They may go into countless details and irrelevant explanations to get to their point or to reach their goal. For instance, if you ask a schizophrenic what he ate for breakfast, he might first talk about all the food in the refrigerator, all the groceries available in the house, the process of breaking an egg, beating the egg, adding salt to it, and frying the egg. He could then go on to talk about putting the bread in the toaster and adding some butter. Finally, he could now tell you that he had a fried egg and toasted bread for breakfast.

*Perseveration* is a thought process in which a schizophrenic repeats the same word, phrase, or idea again and again in response to a different question. For instance, if you ask him for his name, he could respond by saying "I want a burger," "I want a burger," "I want a burger," and keep going on and on. Perseveration could also be a motor response. For instance, a schizophrenic may want to brush his teeth every five minutes. Perseveration may also involve the inability to shift the focus of a conversation away from a particular topic. For instance, he may want to talk about basketball all the time, and nothing else.

*Flight of ideas* is a thought process in which a schizophrenic jumps rapidly from topic to topic. His thought process is racing at this time, and his mouth is trying to keep up with his thought process or his brain. The topics may be illogical, or there may be understandable links between the topics, but the talking or the speech is usually very rapid. The theme of the topic may be grandiose and full of fantasy, but usually, the listener cannot put in a word or interrupt the talking. The listener may be forced to just listen, because it is usually not a two-way dialogue. It must be noted that people with other types of mental illnesses apart from schizophrenia may also have flight of ideas. A good example is a person with bipolar disorder, who may also have flight of ideas when he is in the manic (heightened happiness) phase of his illness.

*Tangentiality* is a thought process in which a schizophrenic goes off topic in response to a question, or will completely talk past the point of the question asked. Her response may be totally obscure or irrelevant to the question asked. She may finally come around to answer the question, or she may never even answer the question. For instance, if you ask a schizophrenic about the well being of her child who has just been discharged from the hospital after a prolonged illness, she may answer by talking about the child's last birthday party, the child's ballet or dance performance, or the child's soccer tournament. She may finally address the issue of the hospitalization after going round in circles and tell you that the child is recovering well, or she may never even address your question.

A schizophrenic experiencing *thought blocking* may have a sudden obstruction or interruption in the spontaneous flow of their thought or speech, and this obstruction is perceived by the schizophrenic as an absence or deprivation of thought. For instance, a schizophrenic may suddenly stop in the middle of a conversation and say that his mind went blank.

A schizophrenic may believe that thoughts actually escape from his head, and that these thoughts could be heard by others. He may also believe that other people can read his thoughts, just like reading a magazine. He may not see the need to respond to your questions because he is convinced that you can hear and read his thoughts on your own. It may not make any sense to him to say out loud what he is thinking because he believes that you have already heard and know what he is thinking anyway. Why repeat himself? This delusional thinking process is called *thought broadcasting.*

*Thought insertion* is another common thought process that may be experienced by a schizophrenic. A schizophrenic experiencing thought insertion may believe that other people have the ability to insert their thoughts in his mind, and consequently his thoughts are not his own thoughts. For instance, a schizophrenic could say, "They are making me think of killing my wife, but I really love my wife; I don't want to think like that."

*Ideas of reference* is seen when a schizophrenic interprets outside events as having direct personal reference to him; for instance, watching the television and believing that the television discussion is about him. It may be impossible to convince him that the television discussion is not about him.

*Looseness of association* is a thought process in which the person shifts from one subject or idea to another without any relationship or logical meaning or connection between the ideas discussed. The individual is unaware of the lack of connection in his or her thoughts and communication processes. For instance, a schizophrenic could say, "I am very hungry, all animals live in the zoo, I don't want to go to a shoe store, there is a river near my house..." and keep going without any awareness of the disconnection between the ideas expressed.

A schizophrenic may also experience hallucinations. *Hallucinations* are sensory perceptions a person believes to be real, despite the fact that there is no outside or external stimulus that exists to justify this belief. Hallucinations could affect all the senses: sight, hearing, smelling, taste, feelings, and touch.

A schizophrenic who is actively experiencing *auditory hallucination* hears voices or sounds that are not there. For instance, he may say "I hear my grandfather telling me to kill myself," although it is a known fact to everybody around him that his grandfather died five years ago. *Visual hallucinations* make a schizophrenic see things that are not there. For instance, he may say, "I see the image of the devil on the wall," or "I see my wife sleeping with another man in my bedroom every night." Despite all evidence to the contrary, he still believes what he sees. Unfortunately, what he sees is real to him, but not real to the people around them. He may argue and struggle very hard to convince others to believe what he sees. He does not know that the deceitful visual images are all produced by his malfunctioning mind.

Sometimes, a schizophrenic may smell something that does not exist or is not there. This is referred to as *olfactory (smell) hallucination*. For instance, he may insist that the whole house smells like a fish, when there is no fish or any type of seafood in the house. A schizophrenic may also experience what is called *gustatory (taste) hallucination*. He may claim that he tastes something that is not in his mouth. For instance, he may say "I taste rotten meat in my mouth all the time," despite the fact that he is a vegetarian who does not even eat meat. *Tactile hallucination* occurs when a schizophrenic feels something on his skin, or has a body sensation of something that does not exist. For instance, he may say "Insects are crawling all over me," despite the fact that there are no insects anywhere near him.

A very fearful type of hallucination is called *command hallucination*. It is fearful because the voices can ask a schizophrenic to do violent things such as hurting or killing themselves or others. Command hallucination must be taken seriously, especially if those commands involve hurting or attacking other people. If a schizophrenic communicates that he has been ordered or commanded to commit an act of violence, action must be taken immediately to stop him from carrying out the violent act. For instance, some schizophrenics have claimed in the past that they were commanded to kill, and the consequences of not obeying the command were so terrible that they had to do it. For instance, a schizophrenic could say, "I was asked to kill my children; otherwise they would be destroyed by aliens that are invading the earth." The schizophrenic may see the vivid picture of these scary aliens (visual hallucination). She may really believe that she is doing her children

a favor by killing them before the alien gets to them. The most common types of hallucinations are auditory (hearing) and visual (sight or seeing) hallucinations.

A person with schizophrenia may also have *social and occupational dysfunction*. This is primarily the inability to function very well socially and occupationally. The victims of this illness may not be able to go to work. If they work, they may have difficulty organizing their work and their lives. Basic activities of daily living like showering or brushing their teeth may become very difficult tasks. They may also have very poor interpersonal skills. They may not be able to make eye contact, or initiate a conversation. They may find it very difficult to warm up to people or make friends. They may also be very isolated. People who are uninformed about the nature of their illness may just see them as weird, cold, or eccentric.

*Speech disturbance* is very common with some schizophrenics. They can be very incoherent with their speech. They may not be able to carry on a simple conversation that makes sense. Sometimes, they may sound like they are speaking under their breath with little or no speech production. This brief and uncommunicative speech is called *poverty of speech*. Their speech could be very rapid and difficult to understand at times; this is called *pressured speech*. They sometimes make up new words that may have no meaning to the person listening to them. This is called *neologism*. They may also repeat or echo what others are saying; and this is called *echolalia*. They may also mix up phrases or jumble words together in a meaningless or illogical manner. The listener may not be able to comprehend what they are trying to communicate; for instance saying, "cow, orange, fireworks, cars, children, telephone…" This is referred to as *word salad*. A schizophrenic may sound like somebody with a private language, and this language is only understood by the person speaking it.

Schizophrenics can be relatively withdrawn from others, and have a typical look about them. They may have a *flat affect* (an expressionless look), and look like they are wearing a mask all the time. They may look like they are incapable of experiencing any emotions and sometimes look helpless. They may also look like they have absolutely no joy in their lives. They may respond inappropriately in an emotionally charged situation. For instance, they may laugh at the news of the death of a loved one or a close relative like a sibling or a parent.

Bizarre behavior and repetitive behavior are very common with schizophrenics. They may pace up and down the hallway for hours. They may also assume a robot-like or *catatonic state* for hours. The catatonic state is not very common; it is rarely seen.

*Winds Against The Mind*

Schizophrenics may be fixated on something or on a person. They may stalk a particular person, believing that they have a special relationship with that person. A schizophrenic may believe that he is married to a queen or a famous person, and he may stalk that person, and not be able to understand or comprehend in his delusional state why the person is not intimate or close to him. Schizophrenics may be very concrete in their delusional thinking. For instance, a schizophrenic could say, "Buy me a fire extinguisher to put next to me when I sleep at night, and if I die before the morning and go to hell, I can extinguish the fire in hell with the fire extinguisher."

Schizophrenics may turn to drugs and alcohol to self-medicate. Using these illicit substances may produce a state of elation, or a high, that temporarily overrides or clouds their awareness. Lack of awareness may make them forget their problems temporarily. They will not have to deal with the symptoms of their illness in that period of time that they are under the influence of the illicit substance.

Some of the early signs of schizophrenia in adolescents may include not wanting to get up in the morning (especially to go to school), sudden drop in grades, lack of motivation to succeed, loss of interest in life, and loss of interest in other people. They may also have some irrational beliefs and magical thinking. For instance, they may truly believe that they have extraordinary abilities, and they can save the world. They may also believe that they can make things happen just by thinking about them. A good example would be the delusional belief that they can find themselves in space just by thinking about doing so. Parents or guardians who notice any or all of these signs, or any other unusual signs, in their children for a period of time should get help for them. The onset of this illness is usually in the late teens or early twenties. It may strike in high school or during the college years when most children are away from home for the first time. Although the late teen years through the early twenties are a common time frame for this illness to strike, it must be pointed out that schizophrenia can strike at any age.

This devastating illness affects people in many societies. There are no parts of the world where there are no schizophrenics. The cause of schizophrenia is still very poorly understood. Many reasons have been given over the years for the cause of this terrible mental illness. One of the mostly widely publicized biological causes of schizophrenia is the malfunction of certain neurotransmitters in the brain. Neurotransmitters are chemicals in the brain that occur naturally. They help to conduct messages between brain cells, called neurons. When these chemicals occur in the right proportion, a person functions normally. In a schizophrenic, the

192

chemicals that are manufactured may be disproportionate, not in a normal balance. Certain chemicals may be overproduced, while others are in short supply. The brain cell that carries the chemical, which is called a neuron, can also malfunction, and other biological factors may also be involved.

From the current scientific knowledge, a person who is pre-coded to develop schizophrenia will develop it, no matter what. There is no preventive care known yet for schizophrenia. Heredity plays a significant factor in this illness. People with schizophrenia usually have family members with the history of this illness. Also in twin studies, identical twins are both more likely to develop schizophrenia than fraternal twins. Identical twins are supposed to be a mirror image of each other with the same genetic code, as opposed to fraternal twins who may not even look alike, and they are not expected to have exactly the same genetic code. In other words, genetic factor is much stronger with identical twins in developing schizophrenia than in fraternal twins.

The diagnosis of schizophrenia should be made strictly by a licensed clinician. The clinician must have sufficient medical knowledge, training, and certification in the area of psychiatry, psychology, medicine, or nursing. Such a clinician could also be any other properly trained and licensed clinician, who is qualified to make such diagnosis in that community. There is no definitive laboratory test available to diagnose schizophrenia. The diagnosis is primarily made based on the person's history, and the observations of the clinician who is making the diagnosis.

As sad as it sounds, living with schizophrenia is not a hopeless situation. Many productive and highly educated people living with this illness are making positive contributions to society. Also, many medications can be prescribed to correct the chemical imbalance in the brain. Different medications work for different people. The exact medication that would help a particular person will be determined by the symptoms the person is experiencing at the time of diagnosis, in addition to a comprehensive history from the client and the people around the client. Medication management may also require trial and error in order to find the perfect one that works well for each individual. It is recommended that only licensed clinicians prescribe any medication for the treatment of this illness. Self-medication could be very dangerous and destructive.

In addition to medication management, individual therapy is also recommended in the treatment of schizophrenia. Those who are battling this illness can learn different positive coping skills, and different ways to manage their illness during individual therapy. For instance, they could learn how to ignore the voices (auditory hallucination), and to ignore the unreal things they see (visual hallucination), and to be able to say to the voices or what they see, "I know that you are not real, and I will not respond to you."

Group therapy is also beneficial. It might be in the form of a support group for people living with schizophrenia in that community. Victims of schizophrenia are able to learn what other schizophrenics are going through, and how they are coping daily with this illness. Living with schizophrenia is like a full-time job for some of the victims of this illness. They are constantly struggling to sort out what is real from what is not real for most of the day. Support groups encourage openness, identification with others, and a sense of relief for the individual victims that they are not alone. These groups provide an emotionally safe environment where no one will be judged by anyone else. Usually group members can give mutual respect, understanding, and acceptance to each other.

Functional and social skill groups may also help with rehabilitation. Skills such as maintaining basic hygiene, interacting with others, and carrying on social conversations without disrespecting or interrupting others are all taught at such groups. Job training groups are also helpful to prepare schizophrenics for the job market. Being able to work and earn an income, no matter how small, could help the victims feel good about themselves, give a sense of purpose, and help to elevate their self-esteem.

Family support groups are targeted primarily for family members of schizophrenics. Family support groups are usually beneficial, especially for the family members of a person newly diagnosed with the illness. Most people know little about schizophrenia until it touches them personally. Learning how other families are dealing with schizophrenia can help them cope and accept the illness. Schizophrenia is physically, emotionally, and financially draining on the family.

It is important that the victims of this illness stay in treatment with the help of their clinician, and use their medications regularly as prescribed. All of the treatment approaches may be used in combination with one another to produce the best result. The most dangerous thing to do is not to get help. People with schizophrenia and everybody around them will benefit from the stability of the sufferer if this illness is properly managed and kept under control.

Finally, like many mental illnesses, schizophrenia is
victims of this illness tend to hide the illness from the
of being ostracized or abandoned by others. They may
escape further and further into their delusional or unre
a mental illness that is unfair to the people afflicted witl
with a normal functioning brain and have great drear
children. Schizophrenia is like a thief that sometimes ..  ..  ...
hopes, and aspirations of the parents or the family members of the victims.

It enslaves the victim's mind. Schizophrenics feel trapped, and some silently cry
for help. Unfortunately, this illness can completely take over the mind of its
victims, and leave them totally ignorant of their actions. If help is not quickly
sought in the delusional state, schizophrenics may respond to the altered sense of
reality by carrying out a horrifying act of violence against others. Later, they may
feel very ashamed of their inappropriate actions after the active phase of their
illness, and apologize. After they become stable and are in touch with reality, they
may wish they could change what they have done. Unfortunately, it is always too
late. It may also be difficult for family members and society at large to forgive
acts of violence by schizophrenics. Nobody wants to be a victim of an undeserving
or unjustified act of violence from other people, no matter how sick the other
person is. Some schizophrenics may direct the violence toward self and sometimes
commit suicide. Some get totally frustrated and exhausted from living with this
very sad illness, and the voices may sometimes ask them to commit suicide. It can
be hard to predict a pattern in their behavior, so people who live with or care for
schizophrenics must be vigilant. The degree of the illness and the level of
functioning vary with each individual. Some individuals have mild to moderate
symptoms, while others have severe symptoms.

Schizophrenia is misunderstood, and a lot of people are afraid of schizophrenics.
Unfortunately, it is not the fault of the schizophrenics that they have this illness,
but at the same time, the rest of the society also has a legitimate right to be
concerned about their own safety. The best approach is for society to make a
conscious effort to understand this illness. Many schizophrenics are not scary; they
can hold down a job and live a close to normal life. With increased knowledge and
understanding, people can aggressively work on getting help for schizophrenics
before they commit an extreme act of violence toward others or themselves.

## PART VII

# COMMON PROBLEMS RELATED TO EATING: EATING DISORDERS

## Anorexia Nervosa:
# AMY'S STORY

Igrew up wanting to be perfect, and I was very compulsive about everything. I was a straight-A student in school and always tried to please my teachers. I tried very hard not to be on anybody's bad side—I tried to please my parents, my friends, and everybody around me. I had a strong need for perfection and a very strong need to be in control of every situation in my life. There was one situation that I desperately wanted to control but could not control; it was the amount of time I spent with my parents. My parents' work required them to travel frequently because they were in the entertainment business. They left me at home with a nanny most of the time. I had a very wonderful, kind nanny, but still, she was not my parent. I missed my parents a lot when they were gone. I would get very anxious and sad whenever I would see them packing for the next trip. Even as a child, I tried to hide my feelings, and I kept my anger and sadness inside. I cried myself to sleep many nights, wishing my mom could read me a bedtime story. I would visualize that my parents were next to me at bedtime and it would help me go to sleep.

At the end of school days, other children got picked up from school by their parents. They would run to the car and hug their mom or dad, but I got picked up by my nanny. I always wished my parents would pick me up, too, and I could run and hug them, just like the other children. My parents would come back from their trips with lots of gifts for me, but it did not make up for their being gone. Whenever they came back, they spent the little time in between their next trip catching up on their social life in the community. They organized a lot of parties and went to a lot of parties as well. My parents were not alcoholics, but occasionally when they both drank a little too much, they got into verbal arguments. My mom especially could not handle alcohol; I remember she always acted funny with very little alcohol. I would say my mom would drink mainly to fit in with her social circle. I hated it when my parents argued. You could tell that they loved each other very much, but the occasional arguments upset me. When I was younger, I would go to my room and cry, but when I grew a little older, I would try to play a peacemaker between my parents. I was very resentful of their arguments. I would say to myself, "First they were gone and now they came back home only to argue instead of spending time with me." I harbored an inner resentment toward my parents, but I never showed it to them. I suppressed all my emotions instead.

I was involved in different sports—soccer, basketball, and volleyball. I also took piano lessons, ballet, and gymnastics. My obsession with being perfect nearly was getting out of control; I just did not know how to forgive myself if I were not perfect. I would get really upset if I made any mistakes during practice, and continuously berated myself over my errors. When I reached early puberty and began developing as a young woman, I hated myself. I believed that I could no longer be good at anything if I put on more weight and had all these changes in my body. I was extremely worried about weight gain and initially devised a way to control my weight by skipping one meal a day. I talked about food a lot, but not because I wanted to eat it. As I grew older, my fear of gaining weight became worse and worse. Whenever I looked into the mirror, I saw a very fat person. Being able to control my weight gave me a sense of control over my life. It was as if something were planted in my brain that constantly told me that I was fat. Later I started skipping two meals a day and gradually turned to using diet pills.

I slowly stopped socializing with the outside world. In the past I would go out with friends. We would go shopping at the mall or go to the movies as a group. When I went out with my friends, they would always want to get popcorn, candy and snacks or "grab a bite to eat afterwards". At first, I usually said that I was not hungry and my friends did not mind. The skinnier I got, the more they started to ask questions or make comments. They would say things like "you never eat anything." Or "why aren't you eating again Amy?" Their comments bothered me and hurt my feelings. I decided that if I did not go out with my friends, then I would not have to worry about my friends bothering me concerning food. I did not want to go on dates either. I wanted to have a boyfriend like any other girl, but I did not want to deal with being taken to a restaurant or any type of activity where I would have to see food.

Within a few months everybody noticed the drastic changes in my weight, and I could sense that people were talking about me, but it could not stop me from not eating. My schoolmates and friends would constantly comment on how skinny I was. I got so angry that I stopped talking to almost everyone at school. I felt like if they wanted to talk about me all the time then I did not need them. My teachers were worried and asked to see my parents. I very defensively told my teachers that my parents were not available, but they could see my nanny if they wanted. My nanny was equally worried about me, but she could not tell me what to do. I was too adamant and stubborn to take any instructions from her. She would try to force me to eat, and I would explode into anger. The mere thought or sight of food created a lot of stress and fear in me, and got my heart racing. I spent an unreasonable amount of time in the exercise room working out. We had a very well equipped exercise room in the basement of the house. I would keep exercising until I felt so dizzy that I would pass out. I was obsessed with weighing myself and always felt a big sense of relief whenever the scale showed I was losing weight. I walked around feeling lifeless most of the time, but I could not be bothered. My menstrual cycle became irregular, but I was not worried about it because I was not sexually active. In fact, I was very happy. I would prefer my menstrual cycle to go away because I never accepted it, psychologically or mentally. I always wished I did not have any monthly periods.

My parents came back from one of their very prolonged trips and noticed how wasted I looked. I lost so much weight that I looked like a skeleton and my hair was thin and falling out. They were totally shocked. My parents confronted me about my weight, and I was very defensive. My mom was especially devastated. She cried bitterly, repeatedly saying that she did not know where she went wrong. She even started throwing things around her room out of frustration. My parents had mistakenly thought that by providing me with a lot of material comfort, I would be okay. They completely forgot about emotional comfort.

My mom would put me in front of the mirror with her and would ask me if I saw what she saw. In my mind I thought we must have been looking at two different people because I only saw myself as a fat person. I was very convinced that nothing was wrong with me. People stared at me everywhere I went. I hated the staring but I could not stop starving myself. Eventually, my parents were able to convince me to go to the doctor's office with them, and I reluctantly agreed to go. The doctor diagnosed me with anorexia nervosa, a type of eating disorder, and I was checked into a treatment center.

Treatment for me initially was a torture. I considered running away from the treatment center many times. In my mind, I was convinced that I was fat, and I could not understand why everybody was trying to make me gain weight. I could not see what they saw, and my mind could not register what everybody was saying to me. In other words, I just did not get it.

My treatment lasted for three long months, and I was lucky my parents could afford to pay for it. It was a long road to recovery, and I was relieved to go home. I have had two minor relapses since my first hospitalization, but nothing like the initial episode that resulted in my first hospitalization. I must confess that I still have a chronic fear of food and a fear of gaining weight, and I continuously struggle with my fears. I am using the coping skills that I learned at the treatment program to change the way I think and see myself. I was also diagnosed with underlying depression, so I was in treatment for both depression and an eating disorder. I was placed on some medications for the treatment of the depression as well.

I am so glad to say that I am making progress. I am eating healthy without starving myself. I am also interacting again with the outside world. I have lost some friends because they did not understand my illness, but the friends that I have kept have been very helpful. My relationship with my parents has also improved. I followed up with therapy at an outpatient treatment program. The inpatient and outpatient treatment, and several family sessions we had with my parents brought out a lot of hurt and pain that I kept inside of me growing up. The emotional neglect by my parents obviously affected me more than I thought. This was partly responsible for my struggle with anorexia nervosa. I could not control my parents' trips, but I could control my weight. The sad thing about this illness is, you do not feel cured of the illness, but you can always control it. You feel like your brain is tricking you whenever you look into the mirror. Your brain continuously tells you that you are fat because you only see a fat person in the mirror, even when you are lifeless and almost disappearing. The goal is to control the illness by not giving in to the deceitful thoughts, and not believing what you see in the mirror. I have to struggle constantly with reprogramming my thinking, and this is emotionally draining. I do not feel sorry for myself or walk around with self-pity, but I am still baffled about how I ended up this way. I try to focus my energy on recovery and thankful for every day that I am here. I always tell myself it could be worse, and I realize everybody has issues that they struggle with, which may not necessarily be anorexia nervosa. If your story sounds like mine, please get help. Do not allow anorexia nervosa to cut your life short. There is help out there; it is never too late to get help.

# Quotes of Encouragement...

As the wind blows harder and Amy's story sounds familiar to you, remember the following:

*"Don't forget until it is too late that the business of life is not business, but living."*

~ *B.C. Forbes*

Anorexia nervosa can kill; the disease will deceive you and push you to your grave; your brain will trick you and convince you that you are fat until you waste away. Life is a precious gift that must be protected by a strong desire to live; fight for your life before it is too late. Death is irreversible. *(LB)*

*"Talk back to your internal critic. Train yourself to recognize and write down critical thoughts as they go through your mind. Learn why these thoughts are untrue and practice talking and writing back to them."*

~ *Robert J. McKain*

The manifestation of anorexia nervosa is primarily your thoughts that translate into the way you see yourself. Look for the inner strength to recognize these deceitful and destructive thoughts; confront them and recognize these thoughts as lies. Be mindful that they can only destroy you, and talk back to the thoughts through the same mind that produced them. Tell the man in the mirror that he is not real. *(LB)*

*"Remember you will not always win; some days the most resourceful individual will taste defeat. But there is in this case always tomorrow— after you have done your best to achieve success today."*

~ *Maxwell Maltz*

Anorexia nervosa can be a continuous struggle for the victim, so be grateful for daily victory over the disease. Take one day at a time; the secret to living is not to give up. Life is worth fighting for. Don't allow your struggles or your failures to speak to you, because you fail only when you stop trying. *(LB)*

*Winds Against The Mind*

## Bulimia Nervosa:
# MARGARET'S STORY

I had two sisters who could eat anything they wanted and not gain a pound, but everything I ate just seemed to stay on me. I had always been a little chubby compared to my sisters. I believed that I was being punished when we were growing up for not being as slim as they were. Mom would allow my sisters three scoops of ice cream, and allow me to have only one. It was definitely an unpleasant experience for a child, and I resented it. There were always a lot of "fat" jokes around my house. To my surprise, Grandma and other family members seemed to talk a lot about weight, too. Most people in my nuclear and extended family were very insensitive to the overweight women in the family. Being skinny was apparently more valued than any personal success or achievement.

We usually had Thanksgiving at our grandparents' house every year; everybody seemed to watch the plate of every overweight member of the family when the food was being served. If anybody who was considered overweight took large servings, there would be a lot of giggling, eye-rolling, and rude comments being made immediately in the room. Stories of academic success, professional success, and other great achievements were played down, but stories of successful weight loss were celebrated at the dinner table.

I felt as if I were being raised in an environment where being overweight was considered a disease. I was not considered as pretty as my sisters because I was not as slim as they were. My mother hurt me the most when she would brag about my sisters' looks when we were little girls, without any consideration of the fact that I was standing right next to her. I even heard her talking to a friend one day on the phone about how I was not as pretty as my sisters because I did not take after her looks. She joked that I looked too much like my father. I was so upset, that I wanted to walk up to her and ask her why she married my dad when she did not want her child to look like him. Instead, I walked to my room and cried my eyes out. My grandma was not much help either; obviously she liked my sisters more than me and treated them much better because they fit the image of the beautiful grandchildren she wanted.

I decided to channel my energy to other things, and I succeeded at it. I worked very hard in school and kept my grades up, and I was involved in Girl Scouts, the school band, softball, and basketball. The school that I attended did not make it easier on me because coming behind my older sisters was like torture. Students and teachers would tell me all the time how pretty my sisters were with absolutely no compliments to me. The most annoying part was that they expected me to be happy about these comments. I had no resentment toward my sisters, but I was jealous of them because of the insensitive attitude of everybody around me about my looks. No one commended me for being a good student, although my sisters were not. They were not failing students—just mediocre or average. Nobody complimented me for being good in the school band or on the basketball team. In fact, some students made fun of me, saying that I looked like a boy. It was common for me to hear on a regular basis that I was not as pretty as my sisters. When one of my older sisters graduated from high school, she was overwhelmingly voted the homecoming queen, primarily because of her looks. My mom bragged so much about it that I was annoyed. The older I grew, the more painful it was to listen to all of the rude comments about my weight and about how pretty my sisters looked.

By the time I knew what was going on, I was already using food to cope. I initially told myself that I might as well be fat and happy, but my mom tried to control everything I ate around her. Whenever she noticed any little increase in my weight, she would get on my case and develop a lot of anxiety. Almost immediately, she would start counting my calories and cutting down on my calorie intake and my food. I got overwhelmingly positive comments from my mom for any slightest weight loss. I finally figured out that there must be another way around this calorie counting, so I started binging and purging. By the end of middle school, I would put my finger deep into my throat in order to induce vomiting after a big meal. I was very pleased with myself that I found a way to keep my weight down without controlling what I ate. When I started binging and purging, I stopped gaining weight. I felt very much in control that I could eat large portions of whatever I wanted (binging) and make the food come out by vomiting it (purging). I would hide food in different places in my room, such as inside my closet, drawers, under my bed and inside my pillow. I would also hide food in my locker at school. I felt a sense of relief every time I vomited my food after eating. As I kept the weight down, people were suddenly more complementary about my looks. I started to get more attention from the boys and other girls would tell me how pretty I looked. In fact I remember a time when my parents had one of our family friends over for dinner. She said "Wow Margaret! You are not that chubby little girl you used to be, you are starting to look more and more like your sisters everyday."

Gradually, I went from just inducing vomiting to adding over-the-counter medications to purge. I felt more and more in control. One day after I had eaten tons of junk food, I went into the hallway bathroom in our house to throw it all up. As I was barfing, my sister knocked on the door to see if I was alright. I told her I was okay, that I probably ate something bad that had upset my stomach, and made me throw up. She believed me, but from that moment on, I started to get worried about others finding out what I was doing. I decided that I would no longer throw up in the hallway bathroom anymore. Since I did not have a private bathroom in my room, I devised other ways to hide my purging. I would throw up in containers and plastic bags when nobody was around and dispose of it without anybody knowing or suspecting. With time, I started feeling sad and guilty, and the abuse was showing on my body. Unfortunately, I could not make myself stop. I would wake up with swollen eyes, and I was late to school, basketball practice, and band rehearsal. I was falling asleep in the classroom and felt very tired most of the time. I realized that my behavior was destructive, especially because my teeth were getting decayed and discolored. I realized later that it was from the continuous contact with my stomach acid due to induced vomiting. It would cross my mind to stop this behavior, but I was in total denial. I told myself that as long as I was in control, everything was okay. My mom suspected that something was going on, but she was in total denial as well. She was more interested in my keeping my weight down. She would rather close her eyes to anything else that might be happening, as long as I was not overweight. I was always feeling dizzy; I would pass out and quickly regain consciousness. Somehow nobody saw me when I would have the fainting episodes; I always regained consciousness very quickly, and I was so relieved that I had not been caught.

One fateful evening, we had a big basketball game against one of our rival teams and a big party at my high school. There was a lot of food everywhere — pizza, hot dogs, hamburgers, popcorn, and drinks. I was very excited, and I was having the time of my life with all of the festivity. I went into one of my binging frenzies, eating everything I could lay my hands on. Suddenly, I was in a panic, and I got worried about all the food I had been eating. I went to the bathroom to induce vomiting and came back out to join the rest of my friends. I was chatting as usual and socializing, and that was the last I remembered. I suddenly collapsed. My friends called 911, the emergency number, and an ambulance rushed me to the hospital. I woke up and found myself on the hospital bed with my parents and my sisters at my bedside. I was asking everybody what happened to me and how I ended up in the hospital. "You collapsed at the basketball game," they said, "and you were rushed to the hospital." I felt a sense of shame and a sense of relief at the same time. I felt ashamed because all of the people I was hiding the illness from were now aware. On the other hand, knowing that I could not hide the illness anymore gave me a sense of relief, because I had tried to stop in the past but I could not stop on my own. The doctor later explained to me that I passed out because I had what was called fluid and electrolyte imbalance from the continuous self-induced vomiting.

I voluntarily told my parents how I had been hiding food in my room and taking medications to induce vomiting. My mom was not totally unaware of what was going on with me, but she did not know that I would go to such a great extent to keep my weight under control. She had an emotional conversation with me after my recovery; she said to me that she actually thought she was being a good mom by making me aware of the need to keep my weight down. She apologized for everything she did to worsen my eating problem and explained that she did not intend to hurt my feelings. She truly thought she was helping me. After the conversation, I realized that everything my mom did was done out of ignorance. She also mentioned that she dealt with the same issue growing up with my grandmother, and she remembered how she was hurt by it. Sadly she forgot all too soon and could not believe she did the same thing to her own child. My mom was very sorry about all the pressure she had put on me to lose weight.

The good news is, I am in recovery and I am grateful for a second chance to live. I have not had any relapses since my last hospitalization. Part of my recovery process was to go to therapy on my own and also with my family at times. For the first time, my parents realized how dysfunctional our family was, especially about weight issues. My mom also realized for the first time that she did not have the perfect family she thought she had. I was very glad that my sisters were involved in the therapy as well. I was worried about them because they relied too much on their looks, and had already integrated this principle of 'what is beautiful is thin' as their idea of beauty. I have learned to eat healthy food, to love myself for who I am, and to focus on my strengths instead of my weaknesses. I constantly say to myself that everybody cannot be a beauty queen. The tone has changed in my house since my diagnosis with bulimia, and my extended family, especially my grandma, now watches their comments and their attitudes about weight and food. My illness and my struggles were blessings in disguise. There are no more jokes about weight or fat, and everybody is more sensitive, more caring, and more supportive of one another. I now have a wonderful boyfriend who is caring and supportive. Sometimes, I still struggle with the thought of wanting to binge and purge, but I have learned to control it and stay focused. I also try to avoid eating by myself. Eating with others always puts me in check. Binging and purging was something I did mostly in secrecy. If your story sounds like mine, do not wait until you end up in the hospital. Please get help before it is too late.

# Quotes of Encouragement...

As the wind blows harder, and Margaret's story sounds familiar to you, remember the following:

*"The choice is yours. You hold the tiller. You can steer the course you choose in the direction of where you want to be — today, tomorrow, or in a distant time to come."*

*~ W. Clement Stone*

You have to confront this mental illness called bulimia and seek immediate help. You cannot afford to procrastinate, because it could be too late for you. When you assault your body with eating and purging, you can throw your body into chemical and electrolyte imbalance and even die. The choice is yours; there is no doubt that it is a mental struggle, but don't be a helpless victim. *(LB)*

*"No one on earth can hurt you, unless you accept the hurt in your own mind."*

*~ Vernon Howard*

Many people have fallen victim to eating disorders like bulimia because of unkind words and actions of others, especially from those who are supposed to protect them. Don't allow the wounds to stay with you forever or to shape the course of your life or destiny. Don't accept an everlasting hurt and pain and don't give anybody permission or power to scar you for life. *(LB)*

*"To begin to think with purpose is to enter the ranks of those strong ones who only recognize failure as one of the pathways to attainment."*

*~ James Allen*

You may find yourself relapsing in your battle with bulimia, but don't ever give up. It is okay to fall, but it is not okay to stay fallen. Stay strong and keep trying until you get it right; you fail only when you quit trying. *(LB)*

## Binge Eating Disorder:

# JOSEPHINE'S STORY

B y the time I was seven, my family had already moved at least seven times. My parents were never married. I have two brothers, and we were all born out of wedlock. When I was around three years old, my dad just left, and we never heard from him again. My mom had drug and alcohol problems. I remember coming home from school in first grade and finding my mom sleeping completely naked on the living room floor. She was too drunk and too high on drugs to even cover up. She smelled so badly it made me sick in my stomach. I went to the bedroom to get a blanket to cover her up, and I was very sad. My mom could not care less about us; she entrusted us to the care of any stranger who would watch us for her, or she would just take off and go for days leaving us to care for ourselves.

As a child, on many occasions I watched the apartment managers order our belongings to be thrown out on the street because of back payment in rent. One of my most vivid, bitter memories was coming back from school one day in kindergarten and finding all of our belongings on the street. My two most precious belongings at that time were my dolls. One was porcelain; the other was plastic. My porcelain doll was broken and completely shattered; the plastic doll was all damaged and muddy. Unfortunately, it rained that day. I cried very bitterly because my dolls were my best friends. I played with my dolls and talked to them a lot, although they could not talk back to me. I used to sleep next to my dolls at bedtime because they gave me a sense of security and companionship. I cried very bitterly for my dolls for days, because the loss of my dolls to me was like losing two precious lives. My mother salvaged what she could from the rest of our belongings, and we moved to the homeless shelter. We later moved from a shelter to a rented trailer home.

Food was not always readily available to us, and when it was available, it was not healthy but inexpensive junk food. Mom was physically and verbally abusive, especially when she was drunk and high on drugs. I was full of imagination as a child, and my imagination used to give me a sense of hope for the future. I always imagined a Cinderella story that somebody like the fairy godmother would show up one day to rescue my brothers and me. Also, I was sexually abused by the different boyfriends that my mom brought home. I was scared to tell her about these episodes because she would not believe me. She always got enmeshed in unhealthy relationships with her boyfriends. There were always a lot of drugs, a lot of alcohol, and a lot of physical and emotional abuse in the house. My brothers and I were too scared of her to say anything about her relationships with her boyfriends.

When we looked sad, Mom was quick to tell us that she had some physical needs as well, and we were not the only reason for her existence. She would threaten to put us in the custody of the Department of Human Services and send us to foster care if we made her angry. She told us a lot of horrible stories about foster care. We were so scared to go to another place worse than the hell we were already living in that we kept quiet and just did whatever she wanted.

By the time I was a teenager, I was already sleeping with my mom's boyfriends. Whenever Mom was gone and I was alone with her boyfriends, they exploited me for sex. Her boyfriends gave me money and bought little things for me after they had sex with me. The money and the gifts were big treats for me at that time, and I was very happy to have them. My mother brought different boyfriends home to come and live in the trailer with us. The average length of stay for most of them was about one to six months, and then they left. The relationships were always very toxic with lots of fights. The landlord who rented the trailer to us even took sexual favors from my mom in exchange for rent. The trailer was the first stable, long-term accommodation we ever had because it was paid for by sex instead of cash.

I ended up running away from home by age fifteen. By the time I ran away from home, I had already had three crude abortions, and one of them almost cost me my life. I lived with different men, prostituted myself, and went into similar dysfunctional relationships just as my mom did. I hated myself, and I saw a very ugly person every time I looked at myself in the mirror. I ate all the time and I did not know why I could not stop eating. I gradually started gaining a lot of weight, but I could not even be bothered about the weight. I was able to get men who liked overweight women, so the weight did not matter to me as long as I could still get a man.

# Winds Against The Mind

I worked different odd jobs, but my favorite job was to work at a restaurant as a waitress, because the tips really added up to a substantial amount for me. After I gained too much weight, nobody would hire me anymore as a waitress in the restaurant. I was very upset because the only job I could get in the restaurant was in the kitchen, and I did not like it. I was complaining to a friend and a co-worker one day about how I missed the tips from being a waitress and how I could not pay my bills. She talked to me about losing weight, and I bluntly told her that I could not do anything about my weight. Eating made me feel better, and I was not ready to give food up. She then suggested that I could enroll in a school program that she was enrolled in. The program helped high school drop-outs to prepare to pass the GED ( General Education Development, an equivalent of a high school diploma) examination and get a high school diploma. Then the program helps its graduates enroll in a nursing assistant program. The program takes six months, and graduating students may be licensed as nurse assistants. My friend and I used to work together in the kitchen, and after getting this training, she made at least twice the amount of money she was making as a cook. I was so excited about the program. I was able to pass my GED and get my high school diploma. I also enrolled in the nursing assistant program and passed.

I started working immediately after the program. I was working two jobs and making a lot more money than I had ever made, except when I was prostituting myself. At that point, I thought my life was finally turning around, but the unfortunate part of my story was that most of the money I was making was going toward food. By the time I knew it, I had ballooned up, and I was so fat that it became a problem to carry myself. Despite the fact that I was drowning under my own weight, I still could not make myself stop eating. I developed a lot of health complications that were associated with being overweight, and by the time I knew what was going on, I was already on disability. I knew that I was gradually killing myself with food, and I would probably eat myself to death, but I still could not stop eating. I became a couch potato, eating more and more, and feeling good with every bite of food I put in my mouth. People would stare at me and make fun of me everywhere I went. It hurt my feelings, but not enough to stop me from eating. One day, I was watching the television and accidentally switched to this program where the hosts were talking about people who cannot stop eating. I felt insulted and wanted to change the channel, but something inside me would not let me. I sat there to watch the program, and it was as if they knew my story and my struggles. I sat there and cried for hours, realizing for the first time that I was using food to heal a deeper emotional pain. I called the help line that was flashed on the screen immediately, and this simple step was the beginning of my healing process.

My life has taken a different turn, I have lost more than one hundred and twenty pounds, and I am still losing more weight daily. I have a goal of a weight I will be comfortable with, and I do not intend to stop until I achieve that weight. I eat healthy food, exercise, and practice a healthy lifestyle now. I feel much better about myself. My energy level has increased, and I am not on a lot of medications anymore. I can now go to the store and buy clothes like every other person out there. I can run my own errands and buy my own groceries. The best part of the story is I have a well-paying job. I am also in therapy, and I am able to identify what my real problems are. I am also working through my problems learning to leave the past that I cannot change alone. Instead, I am focusing on the future that I can change. I am active in a support group; it is good to be in a position to help and encourage others and also to learn from other people as well. I can now walk down the street without being stared at by everybody. I am dating, going out with my friends, and really enjoying my new life. I wonder how many people are out there with a story similar to mine, trying to use food as a medication to heal. Please do not sit there and eat yourself to death. There is help out there, so do something about it before it is too late.

# Quotes of Encouragement...

As the wind blows harder and Josephine's story sounds familiar to you, remember the following:

*"Every experience in life, everything with which we have come in contact in life, is a chisel which has been cutting away at our life statue, molding, modifying, shaping it. We are part of all we have met. Everything we have seen, heard, felt, or thought has had its hand in molding us, shaping us."*

*~ Orison Sweet Marden*

Never judge people by their weight; don't call them weak, or look down on them because they are overweight. You only see the fruit, but don't know the seed. You have never walked in their shoes or carried their cross; if you cannot take away their pain, don't add to it. *(LB)*

*"Progress, however of the best kind, is comparatively slow. Great results cannot be achieved at once, and we must be satisfied to advance in life as we walk step by step."*

*~ Samuel Smiles*

There is no shortcut or crash program that can keep your weight off permanently. You did not gain the weight overnight, so don't aspire to lose it overnight. Walk through your program step by step; frustration sets in easily with an "on and off" battle with weight, but slow and steady always wins the race. *(LB)*

*"We cannot tell what may happen to us in the strange medley of life. But we can decide what happens in us — how we take it, what we do with it — and that is what really counts in the end. How to take the raw stuff of life and make it a thing of worth and beauty — that is the test of living."*

*~ Joseph Fort Newton*

To improve your physical or external well-being, first improve your internal or psychological well-being; see every hardship as an opportunity to grow. Don't entertain discouragement and guilt. Be the architect of your own success and turn the raw deal of life into gold. Be an over-comer; then you can enjoy both physical and mental well-being. *(LB)*

# General Understanding About Eating Disorders

A my, Margaret, and Josephine all suffered from eating disorders. Living with *anorexia nervosa*, *bulimia nervosa*, and *binge eating disorder*, are classic examples of the daily struggles and continuous battles that some people experience when it comes to food consumption. The majority of the people in most societies are able to eat normally, consume appropriate calories, and maintain appropriate body weight without any struggle or even thinking about it. Unfortunately, it does not come so easily for people with eating disorders.

An eating disorder is a serious problem with long-term psychological and medical consequences. People with eating disorders usually have other diagnosable medical conditions or mental issues affecting their responses to food. Most common are depression and anxiety. A history of sexual, physical, psychological, or mental abuse is frequently reported with eating disorders. A history of emotional neglect is also very common. People with eating disorders are usually prone to anger. They may have poor impulse control. Some are usually emotionally labile, (shifting quickly from being angry to being pleasant).

Eating disorders are a problem in most societies, but they are more prevalent and better diagnosed in the western world. They are also believed to be more common among females than males. The concept of "thin is beautiful" is edified in the western culture. It is seen in the modeling industry, television, magazines, schools, workplaces, and every section of society. This attitude may have contributed to the higher incidents of anorexia nervosa and bulimia nervosa in the Western world. Binge eating disorder is very similar to bulimia nervosa because people with both

217

disorders are compulsive overeaters. The major difference between binge eating disorder and bulimia nervosa is that binge eaters will not do anything to get rid of excessive nutritional consumption that exceeds their body requirements. On the other hand, bulimics continue to binge until they develop severe abdominal pain, and vomiting usually follows to relieve the abdominal pain.

Eating disorders are also common in the athletic world, especially if the particular sport places a lot of emphasis on thinness. Common sports and recreational activities that place a lot of emphasis on being thin include figure skating, gymnastics, track and field, soccer, and ballet.

There has been a lot of public discussion about the addictive properties of eating disorders. Some eating disorders have or share common features with addictive behavior, because the victims use food in a compulsive way for a mental or psychological advantage to treat psychological and emotional pain. Each of the three examples of eating disorders discussed has its unique symptoms, and the treatment of each is different from the other in some aspects. The symptoms at the time of diagnosis and the history of the clients are seriously taken into consideration in the treatment and management approach. Basic facts and understanding of the three types of eating disorders discussed will be explained independently.

## Anorexia Nervosa:

# BASIC FACTS & UNDERSTANDING

A*norexia nervosa* is not an appetite problem. Those who suffer from this eating disorder willfully restrict food intake and sometimes over-exercise compulsively. They may also engage in other drastic measures such as using diet pills in their efforts to lose weight. All these measures to lose weight are the result of a distortion in self-perception, with severe inner fear of becoming overweight. Self-starvation is a classic symptom of anorexia nervosa. There is a psychological or mental numbness to body sensations and feelings of hunger in order to control weight. The victims feel fat with a normal body weight, and still continue to feel fat when they are disappearing or emaciated. An individual with anorexia nervosa always see a fat person whenever she looks in the mirror. She is adamant and unwavering in her desire to lose weight. It must be noted that the word 'anorexia' simply means lack of or loss of normal appetite, but *anorexia nervosa* is an eating disorder. People with anorexia nervosa are commonly referred to as anorexics.

Many anorexics say that they are very compliant, and as children, they usually went out of their way to cooperate with others. They are usually very passive growing up, and always willing to please others. They tend to lean towards perfectionism. If something is not perfect in their judgment, it is not good enough. They usually harbor internal anger and resentment toward their families. These feelings are suppressed, and anorexics use food in establishing authority and defining themselves. Unfortunately, this is a negative way of asserting oneself.

There is the belief that the families of some anorexics are usually too controlling and too enmeshed with no boundaries. As a result, the anorexic child may not be allowed to grow and develop a sense of self, because of the constant struggle to please the family and significant others. Consequently she uses food for control to establish and assert self. The family setting may be dysfunctional, with lots of strife and a possible threat of separation of the parents. An anorexic child may use an eating disorder or self starvation as an illness to glue or keep the family together artificially since everybody must rally around the sick child.

Apart from family dynamics, the biological causes of anorexia nervosa are attributed to the malfunction or dysregulation of certain neurotransmitters in the brain. Neurotransmitters dysfunction is very prominent in many mental illnesses. Neurotransmitters are naturally occurring chemicals in the brain that help to transmit messages between the brain cells called neurons. Some of these neurotransmitters are responsible for appetite control. Other biological factors may also be involved. Anorexia nervosa is also believed to run in families, and as a result, genetic or hereditary factors are strongly indicated.

Anorexia nervosa is common among both youth and adults. Some people live with this problem all of their adult lives and into their older years. It is very easy to miss the diagnosis of anorexia nervosa in the older population. Society may easily assume that an older person or a senior citizen should not struggle with food or his or her weight. Unfortunately, if the distorted perception of self and the struggle with food has been a lifelong problem, old age may not necessarily make it go away. Some people may have one episode of anorexia nervosa with no recurrence, but this is atypical or uncommon. A clear majority of anorexics battle with a lifelong struggle from this disorder.

Some of the possible signs and symptoms to look for include a strict and rigorous exercise regimen, preoccupation or obsession with thoughts of food, pushing pieces of food around the plate at mealtime and not eating the food, talking a lot about food, and cutting food into tiny pieces at mealtime. Other symptoms include feeling terrified of gaining weight, attaching one's sense of self-worth and self-esteem to weight, avoiding eating with people, claiming to be fasting most of the time, using diet pills, and claiming to be fat while wasting away. The immediate family members or close associates are usually the first to notice these signs and symptoms.

Many medical complications resulting from anorexia nervosa may include the following: severe weight loss or emaciation (wasting away), bradycardia (decreased breathing or heart rate), hypotension (low blood pressure), cold extremities (cold feet and hands), lanugo hair (fine soft hair usually found in newborn babies) on the body, muscle weakness, amenorrhea (seizure of menstrual cycle), constipation (inability to have regular bowel movement), peripheral edema (swollen feet), kidney problems, and liver problem (fatty liver degeneration). When blood is drawn for laboratory values or test, it usually shows abnormal values, especially in potassium and calcium levels. This, in turn, could cause fluid and electrolyte imbalance (imbalance in the fluid and essential elements needed for the body to function), causing the body to eventually malfunction. For an individual to stay healthy, all the essential elements needed by the body to function properly must exist in normal or appropriate proportions, in addition to adequate body fluid. This is usually not the case with anorexics.

Anorexia nervosa is very difficult to treat because of the victims' distorted perceptions of their appearance and their weight. They cannot see or conceptualize that there is a problem. There is a common saying that a 'disease known is half cured,' but most anorexics do not know that they have a disease, much less that they need to seek a cure. A few anorexics that may even have some insights into their problems are very stubborn, adamant, and indifferent. They are not willing to make any changes at all. Common studies such as an EKG (electrocardiogram), is usually required. An EKG is used to measure the electrical activities of the heart and could reveal an irregular heart rhythm or irregular heart beat. This could be an indication that the heart is not functioning properly. An irregular heart rhythm could be very deadly if it is not taken seriously. If the anorexic continues to refuse treatment, or the people around her do not seek treatment for her immediately, she could develop serious cardiac problems. She could eventually die from heart failure.

Hospitalization may be required initially in the treatment for stabilization. Anorexics may require initial forced feeding to keep them from dying from starvation. They may not necessarily agree to eat or cooperate with any attempt to make them gain weight. The goal of the people around them and the people involved in their treatment is to help restore their body to normal functioning at all costs and replenish abnormal electrolytes and other elements. This may have to be achieved against the will of the anorexic at that point in time. After the initial medical stabilization, anorexics are assessed for under-lying psychological problems such as depression, unresolved anger, and anxiety. A combination of medical and psychological intervention has produced a much better outcome in the management of this disorder. In the United States of America, continuous changes in the insurance policies and reimbursement of care are making long-term treatment unaffordable for middle-income and low-income earners. Anorexia nervosa can be very expensive to treat. The treatment approved by most insurance companies is mostly outpatient care. Long-term hospitalization treatment is mostly available to those who can afford to pay for it; otherwise, the out-of-pocket costs could be very draining financially for the family.

Part of the goal of the treatment is to help the victims change the way they think, especially how they view themselves and the world around them. Being able to deal with the inner confusion and misconceptions is a great step toward recovery. Clinicians work with victims to help them realize the seriousness of their illness. Underlying anxiety associated with the intense fear of gaining weight is also addressed. Medication management is also an important part of the treatment. Although there are no specific medications to treat anorexia nervosa, however depression and anxiety are very common with anorexia nervosa, and both could be managed with medication and therapy. The medication to be prescribed must be determined by a licensed clinician, based on the client's medical history and comprehensive assessment.

Family members are usually involved in the treatment of the anorexic. The goal is to identify the family's contributory factors to the illness if there are any, especially problems with over-involvement and enmeshment (no boundaries) with the anorexic. Support groups are also available for the victim of this illness and their family. A good support group will promote positive growth for the anorexic. She can learn functional ways of living with the illness and also realize that she is not alone in her struggle with anorexia nervosa. Family members can also learn positive coping skills by joining a good family support group. They can learn how to live successfully with the anorexic and help her to manage the illness as much as possible without being enmeshed (having no boundaries). Unfortunately, anorexia nervosa may not always be curable, but the victims can learn to manage and control the illness and be able to live a normal life. Anorexia nervosa must be aggressively treated and not taken lightly. It is a killer and the victim can die from starvation if proper care is not taken.

Bulimia Nervosa:
# BASIC FACTS & UNDERSTANDING

Unlike people with anorexia nervosa who are totally clueless most of the time about how dysfunctional their eating behavior is, bulimics have a clear insight into their eating problems. A bulimic consumes an unreasonably large amount of food, usually larger than what most people will eat during a similar period and under similar circumstances. Basically, the behavior is characterized by recurrent episodes of binge eating, usually done within a discrete or certain period of time (for example, binging continuously within a two-hour period), followed by self-induced vomiting, fasting, excessive exercise, compulsive dieting, enema, misuse of diuretics or laxatives, or any other medication that could control weight. Bulimics hide their binge eating because they are ashamed of it. The binging is mostly done in secrecy, unless they are accidentally discovered. They may also hide food in the unusual places such as under their bed and among their clothes in the closet. The binging continues until they develop severe abdominal pain, and the binging is usually followed by self induced vomiting to relieve the abdominal pain. They could follow the self-induced vomiting with other dysfunctional measures such as dieting and fasting. The goal of the bulimic is to prevent at all cost the weight gain that could occur from their binge eating. While this behavior occurs more commonly in secrecy, sadly there are groups of high school and college students who will engage in "scarf and barf" parties, where excessive eating occurs and is followed by induced vomiting in a group setting.

Bulimics believe that they cannot voluntarily stop eating or control how much food they eat. They usually feel depressed after binge eating. They have the tendency to criticize themselves after engaging in the behavior. They feel powerless, worthless, and hopeless, lacking a sense of control over their eating behavior. Unfortunately, the feelings of helplessness propel the bulimic to go back to binge eating over and over again. The cycle of binging and getting rid of the food at all costs then continues with one episode after the other. Some bulimics may binge for days and subsequently engage in compensatory measures for days after the binging.

Bulimics usually attach their self-worth and self-evaluation to their looks, their body shape, and weight. As a result, they develop poor self-esteem because they are usually not happy with what they see in the mirror. Bulimics may also have problems with occupational, social, and interpersonal relationships.

Unlike anorexics, bulimics are not wasted and emaciated. Bulimics typically keep a normal body weight. At the worst, their weight may fluctuate because of the up and down episodes of the fasting and the binging. This illness is very time-consuming. It interferes substantially with the bulimic's life. Like other eating disorders, bulimia nervosa is more common among females than males. It is also very common among youth and young adults. It is a problem in many societies, but the incidence is more common and better diagnosed in the Western world.

The biological explanation for bulimia nervosa, among other factors, blames the illness on the dysregulation or abnormal regulation of certain neurotransmitters. Neurotransmitters are certain naturally occurring chemicals in the brain that affects our day-to-day functioning. If there is a problem with the normal level or regulation of the neurotransmitters that controls the appetite, a person can develop bulimia nervosa. Bulimia usually develops in early adulthood. Bulimia may not be curable, but it can be managed effectively with appropriate medication and therapy.

It is unfortunate that bulimia may not be diagnosed for a long period of time because the overt (visible) signs and symptoms of the illness may not be noticed for a while. This is primarily because bulimics, unlike anorexics, usually maintain normal body weight, and when the body weight fluctuates, it could be taken for normal day-to-day dieting. The ability to hide the food and the behavior also makes it very difficult for the significant others to pick up on the early signs of the illness. Sometimes, bulimics are discovered after collapsing in a public or a private place. This could happen due to fluid and electrolyte imbalance in the body from the self-induced vomiting. Bulimics also make up stories to cover up their behavior. They play down the early signs and symptoms of the illness as flu or stomach cramps. Bulimics, like other eating disorder sufferers, always have some underlying psychological or mental issues that must be addressed in therapy. Most common problems are depression, anger, anxiety, labile mood (mood swings), substance abuse problems, poor impulse control, self esteem issues, compulsivity, and stealing.

The diagnosis of bulimia nervosa must be made by a licensed clinician. The clinician is usually trained in the area of psychiatry, psychology, medicine, or nursing. The clinician could also be qualified and certified in that particular community to treat eating disorders. This behavior must have been going on for a period of time. This determination is made based on the client's history and the professional knowledge of the clinician making the diagnosis. The clinical presentation at the doctor's office or the emergency room usually alerts the clinician to the illness. Sometimes, a visit to the dentist may expose the bulimic. Bulimics develop dental caries and erosion from the acid reflux that is always in constant contact with the teeth enamel from self-induced vomiting. A dentist may be the first to alert the parent of an adolescent that his or her child is suffering from bulimia.

Some of the other symptoms bulimics present include gastric dilation or rupture (stomach rupture), peripheral edema (rebound fluid accumulating in their feet especially if they are using diuretics), muscle weakness, scars and calluses on hands (from sticking their finger inside their throat to induce vomiting), and abnormal laboratory values causing fluid and electrolyte imbalance (for example, low levels of potassium and sodium in the body). An EKG (electrocardiogram) is also performed on the client to study the electrical activities of the heart. EKG could show abnormal activities of the heart, and this abnomality could be life threatening if it is not taken seriously.

Treatment must be aggressive after the diagnosis of bulimia is made to prevent sudden death or brain damage. The goal of the therapy is to combine psycho-therapy with medication intervention. Bulimics need a lot of education about modifying and changing their behavior. The self-esteem issues must be addressed in therapy as well. Working through the self-esteem issues will help to improve their interpersonal and social relationships with others, and will also improve self acceptance. Part of the therapeutic goal should be to help bulimics change the way they think so that they could see their world in a positive way. Changing their thought processes and having a better self-understanding in addition to medication intervention should produce positive results. Medication intervention should be determined by a licensed clinician only, after an extensive and comprehensive history from the client. There are no specific medications to cure bulimia, but other psychological problems associated with bulimia such as anxiety and depression can be treated with medication. Bulimics should not attempt to self-medicate because they have the tendency to become addicted to medications.

Some bulimics have a family history of neglect, lack of nurturing, sexual abuse, physical abuse, and chaotic family relationships. All of the situational and psychological or mental stressors in the life of a bulimic must be addressed as part of the healing process in therapy. Some therapeutic sessions should also include family sessions with the bulimic and the members of her family. The goal is to encourage the client and her family to address any negative family dynamics or issues. It is also an avenue to educate the family on how to live with and provide functional support for the bulimic. While being supportive, family members learn to still maintain boundaries and not enable the behavior of the bulimic.

Family members can also join independent support groups for families of bulimics. They can learn how other families are coping with the illness and manage to stay together effectively as a family. Bulimics can also join a good support group for bulimics only. They can share their stories freely with other members of the group. They also learn from the experiences of others. A group like this provides a safe environment in which to learn positive ways to cope with bulimia. It provides the atmosphere for bulimics to learn that they are not alone in their daily struggles.

# Binge Eating Disorder:
# BASIC FACTS & UNDERSTANDING

B inge eating disorder is very similar to bulimia nervosa, because people with binge eating disorder and bulimia nervosa are both compulsive overeaters. The major difference between the disorders is that binge eaters do not purge after over-eating. They become excessively obese and worry less than bulimics about getting rid of the weight, even if they hate the way they look.

It must be mentioned that not everybody who is obese is necessarily a binge eater. Some people have other underlying medical conditions or hereditary factors that may be responsible for their weight. The focus of this discussion is primarily about people who are obese because of compulsive overeating.

Like bulimia nervosa, binge eating disorder is characterized by recurrent episodes of binge eating and the consumption of an amount of food that is greater than most people would eat in a similar period of time or circumstance. Binge eating is usually accompanied by a sense of powerlessness and lack of control. Binge eaters believe that they cannot voluntarily stop eating or control how much they eat. They feel hopeless and helpless. They usually eat more rapidly than normal people do. They continue to eat even when they feel uncomfortable and full, primarily ignoring the fact that they are not physically hungry. They usually feel guilty, depressed, and disgusted with their behavior after overeating. They usually do not use any inappropriate compensatory behavior such as purging, fasting, exercise, or compulsive dieting to lose weight. The behavior is distressful for them, usually creating a lot of anxiety.

Depression is very common among binge eaters. Food is comforting, and is used to soothe an underlying emotional pain or distress. There is an unconscious psychological or mental belief among binge eaters that "if I eat, the pain will go away." Unfortunately, the food will not take the pain away. The pain will still be there after the large food consumption. The prognosis or hope for cure for binge eaters is much better than that of anorexia nervosa or bulimia nervosa. Usually, when the underlying triggers are identified and dealt with, binge eating becomes much easier to manage for the victims.

The greatest concern about binge eating is the possible health complications that could arise from obesity. Binge eaters usually have a sedentary lifestyle because of their weight, and a sedentary lifestyle is very unhealthy for anybody, especially binge eaters. Some health concerns that may arise could include breathing problems from the excessive body weight on the heart and problems with other internal organs like the liver and the kidneys because the organs are being overworked. As a result, they may develop shortness of breath or difficulty with breathing, apnea (sudden stop in breathing), and eventually, heart failure. Their kidneys could also fail, resulting in a diagnosis of renal failure. Binge eaters may also have diabetes, hypertension, high blood cholesterol, skin diseases, and body odor resulting from skin overlap. They could also have incontinence of urine and feces (inability to control urine and bowel movements), and general aches and pains. The medical problems resulting from excessive weight gain alone call for quick professional intervention, and this is why obesity cannot be ignored. The laboratory values usually show abnormal results when checked reflecting those abnormalities described above. Some of their laboratory values may be life threatening and dangerous if nothing is done to control the weight.

Many binge eaters always have a long history of major depression, a history of neglect, physical and sexual abuse, and psychological and emotional abuse. There is usually a history of improper bonding or complete lack of nurturing from the parent or the parental figure. Many binge eaters have reported eating more food when they feel down in the dumps or when they experience a negative mood.

If there is no underlying medical condition responsible for a person's weight gain, the diagnosis of binge eating disorder is easy to make because it speaks for itself. Looking at binge eaters, one easily notices that something is wrong because of the excessive weight that they are carrying. A bulimic, on the other hand, could have a normal weight.

A multidisciplinary approach is necessary for a successful treatment of binge eating disorder. This would require treating the medical as well as the psychological or mental problems. Depending on the extent of the obesity, changing or modifying the behavior through therapy and putting the client on a balanced diet with sensible calorie intake could work magic. If the obesity is life threatening, diet pills and surgical interventions such as stomach resection or lap band may be necessary to control the weight. The decision to perform the surgical procedure and the choice of which approach to use must be made by a qualified physician or clinician, based on the history of the client.

In addition to the dietary modification, the underlying psychological problems like depression and anxiety are treated with medications and therapy. The medications to be prescribed must be determined by a licensed clinician only, based on the comprehensive history and health assessment of the client. Part of the treatment goal for a binge eater is to allow the client to set a target weight and have an input on how to achieve the targeted weight. Exercise should also be a part of the treatment regimen. The weight loss should be a process. The rapid weight loss approach usually results in failure. Empowering the client and giving him or her positive reinforcement for the progress that is made is very important.

Support groups, such as Overeaters Anonymous, are also helpful. By joining the support group, binge eaters can gain inner strength to deal with their problems just from realizing that they are not alone. Meeting other people who have struggled with and won the battle against overeating and weight could be encouraging. A good support group would always provide the right atmosphere for sharing, learning and growing.

Finally, family therapy and family support groups may also be necessary to help the victims in recovery. This is especially important when childhood neglect, lack of nurturing, and emotional, physical, and sexual abuse are involved. Being able to work through the bottled-up anger and negative feelings through therapy would be crucial to a healthy recovery.

Binge eating is a problem in most societies, but it is more prevalent in some societies than others. It could be worse where food is cheap and readily available. It is unfortunate that binge eaters are under a lot of pressure in the western world where they are heavily stigmatized or seen as weak for being obese. It may not be seen as too much of a problem in a culture where obesity is not viewed as a disease. It is important that the rest of society who are not obese should try to be compassionate, and be mindful of the fact that an obese person is most likely feeling miserable already. It is not fair to make these people more miserable if we cannot help them feel better. Human kindness and compassion can make a difference in the lives of those who are a little different from the majority of the society. This is a lesson that should be taught across the board to all ages. With a little kindness and encouragement, binge eaters can gradually work on losing weight effectively and keeping it off.

## PART VIII

# COMMON PROBLEMS RELATED TO ANXIETY: ANXIETY DISORDERS

## Post-Traumatic Stress Disorder (PTSD):
# MRS. FORTUNE'S STORY

I am a sales representative, and my job required frequent trips out of town. My wife and I have been married for ten years with three wonderful boys. After ten years of marriage, she started behaving strangely in bed, and I could not be intimate with her anymore. She started complaining of having flashbacks of childhood memories of sexual molestation by her grandfather. Initially, I tried to be understanding, but after a while, I got very frustrated with her. I was extremely angry with her because my emotional needs were not being met in my bedroom. I started asking myself several questions. "What sort of sexual abuse issues is she allowing to affect a marriage of ten years? Why did the memory not bother her this much before we got married? And what about those years when we had our three children?"

I was just not going to buy whatever she was telling me. I was resentful of her actions and could not understand why she would not get over whatever happened to her in her childhood. I was raised in a very old-fashioned home, and sex was not something we talked about publicly. I found it very difficult to talk to anybody about what was going on with my wife. I got to a deadend with my emotional frustration and sexual deprivation so I decided to have extramarital affairs on my trips out of town. I rationalized that it was okay for me to have extramarital affairs. After all, it was not my fault. I concluded that my wife was crazy, and she had totally lost her mind. As long as my emotional needs were being met outside of my house on my trips, we could still remain married and raise the three boys in a stable home with both parents, and look like the ideal family for the public. I was too angry to have any guilt about my actions; I decided that it was going to be her problem only and not mine. I made sure I had some fun and satisfied my sexual desires on my trips. I didn't suspect that she was having an affair from the way she was behaving. I was convinced that no other man would want to come near a grown woman who was behaving so strangely, crying in the bedroom when a man came close to her.

I went on a business trip one day and as usual met a woman at the meeting who interested me. We connected from day one and carried on conversations as if we had known each other for years. Thinking she might be someone with whom I could have an affair, I began to flirt with her. The lady told me she was in psychiatry; I then cracked a joke to her that if she treated mental problems, maybe I needed to take her home with me to fix my wife because my wife was crazy. I told her that my wife really needed a 'shrink' because she was losing her mind. She cracked a joke back at me that maybe she could help fix my wife, so that my wife would not be so crazy. I told her no, that my wife's problem was too complex, and my wife was out of touch with reality.

The lady continued to ask questions, and we kept the conversation going. She kept making me more and more comfortable with the dialogue; she encouraged me to volunteer more information, and she gave me some real-life examples of different issues that people deal with in marriages. She finally said, "One of the most difficult issues is sex. Is that the problem or part of the problem?" she asked. I felt very uncomfortable and kept quiet for a second. I found myself suddenly relaxing and justifying that it would be safe to confide in her. After all, I may never see her again after the conference is over. I decided that maybe I could trust her and tell her about my wife because she was very knowledgeable about marital problems. She might have a suggestion for me on how to solve this problem that was indirectly destroying my marriage. I went ahead and told her that my wife complained about some flashbacks from some sexual abuse as a child, and I was initially supportive, but I did not understand why she could not get over it and move on with her life. I told her that I did not allow it to bother me anymore because what she was talking about did not make any sense to me. "Why now? How long do I have to put up with it?" I asked. I then confessed to the woman that I had been having extramarital affairs, and I was actually trying to get together with her for a possible affair. I confessed to her that I had an ulterior motive in trying to be friendly with her, but that the conversation had taken another turn.

She analyzed the psychological implications of what my wife was going through and how terrible such an experience could be for anybody mentally. She convinced me that it was more serious than I had thought and that what my wife was experiencing sounded like an untreated post-traumatic stress disorder. The conversation with her was an eye opener, and she suggested that I seek professional help for my wife immediately when I returned home.

I felt very sorry for my wife after listening to this woman, and felt very bad about the way I had handled the situation so far. My wife and I sought professional help as soon as I returned home from that trip. My wife broke down, crying at the therapy session as she told her story. My wife's father divorced her mother when she was three; the only father she grew up knowing was her stepfather, who happened to be a very wonderful man. Her mother had three more children with her stepfather. Her grandparents on her mother's side lived very close to them, and her grandparents were her babysitters. The closeness to the grandparents was intended to be a babysitting blessing, but it turned out to be a curse. She remembered the abuse vividly from age four.

She narrated her stories as follows, "Grandpa started the abuse initially by touching me inappropriately on my private part and also encouraged me to touch him inappropriately on his private part. I was innocent and thought Grandpa could do no wrong so I did whatever Grandpa said. It later advanced to other inappropriate sexual acts. Grandpa loved to go to the basement to do woodwork and repair things around the house. He would ask me to come along to the basement with him, and that was where most of the abuse took place. Grandma was always upstairs, either knitting or cooking. Grandma would run some short errands at times or go to meetings and leave me with Grandpa. Having just the two of us in the house was like a treat for Grandpa. He seized the opportunity to carry out all of his exploitative sexual acts with me. After every indecent act, Grandpa would give me treats and money. I had a piggy bank in the basement, and I saved the money in the piggybank. Grandpa told me not to tell anybody; he brainwashed me that what he was doing with me was something special between the two of us, and nobody must know. He also told me that Grandma would be very jealous if we told her and she might die, that I must not tell Grandma if I did not want her to die. I was too scared to lose my Grandma, so I never told her.

"As I grew older, I realized that my sexual relationship with my grandpa was wrong, but I did not know how to stop it. I was afraid to tell my grandma because she loved Grandpa and trusted him so much and finding out would have truly killed her, or so I thought. I was also too afraid to tell my parents because Grandpa came across as the most wonderful person in the world, and it would be hard for anybody to believe such a story about him. He put forward a very fake front that would make you think that he could not hurt a fly. I concluded in my mind that nobody would believe me, especially my mother, so I decided to keep the secret to myself. The abuse went on until I was about nine years old, and I looked for all the strength in me to tell Grandpa one day that I did not want to be special to him like that anymore. The abuse stopped. As I grew older, I felt a lot of shame and guilt about the abuse. I felt like it was my fault and I must have caused it. I also blamed myself for receiving the treats and the money from him. I felt guilty that I betrayed Grandma. How could I have done this to her? She was the best grandmother in the world. I felt like the most horrible human being that ever walked the face of this Earth.

"Three years after the abuse stopped, my stepfather's company gave him a promotion offer to head one of their new offices in another state, so we moved. I was extremely relieved that I would not have to see Grandpa so frequently anymore because I had grown to hate him, but I could not show it. I had to suppress the pain and the anger. I saw Grandpa only during the holidays. Still, coming home on holidays always made me want to throw up, so I was looking forward to becoming a young adult when I would not have to go with my parents anymore. When I was fifteen, Grandpa suddenly died of a heart attack. I was relieved that I would not have to see him again. I remember standing next to his dead body during visitation at his funeral and whispering to it that I hoped he would burn in hell. I was sick at my stomach when different people came forward to talk about how wonderful he was. I was relieved that he died, and he would never be able to hurt another child again. I said to myself that I would bury the memories with him, and move on with my life, but I was wrong.

"The memories kept coming back, and I kept fighting them and suppressing them. Something snapped after ten years of marriage, and I lost the battle to fight and suppress the memories. The flashbacks got worse and the video of all the sexual abuse with Grandpa kept replaying itself in my mind. My whole life was affected; I was feeling depressed, anxious, and was waking up with dreams of being raped. Whenever my husband tried to be intimate with me, I felt like I was going to be raped again and I could not attempt or enjoy intimacy with my husband anymore."

That was my wife's story. She was immediately diagnosed with PTSD (post-traumatic stress disorder) by the therapist. After knowing the truth of what happened to my wife, I felt very selfish and inconsiderate for cheating on her. I had no idea how much she went through with her horrible grandfather. It was so unfortunate that the person who was supposed to protect her was the perpetrator.

The therapist insisted that we had to tell my wife's parents as part of the healing process for my wife. My wife was reluctant, but I insisted that we had to let her parents know. To my surprise, my mother-in-law jumped up and 'hit the roof.' She got extremely angry and accused my wife of losing her mind. My mother-in-law told my wife that she would do anything to protect her father's name from being tarnished by her. My wife was devastated about her mother's reaction.

My mother-in-law called her sisters and angrily told them what her daughter had said about their dad. She was shocked when one of her older sisters confirmed that she had been sexually molested for years by their father, my wife's grandfather, the same man who had molested my wife for years. My wife's aunt said she had not told anybody. My wife's aunt told her sister, my mother-in-law, that she had kept her distance from their parents in a very diplomatic way and made sure that her children were never left with her dad, knowing what she had gone through with him as a child. My wife's aunt said she never took chances with her children around her dad at any time when he was alive, and she never talked about it because she could not afford to hurt her mom. My wife's aunt believed that her mother would have died from the information if she had found out about the abuse. Every victim tried to protect this wonderful mother and grandmother who had unknowingly married a child molester.

Apparently, my wife's grandpa picked his victim; he picked one particular child in the family at a time and carried out the abuse with only that child. His strategy was probably to create doubt if the victimized child ever talked about it. He figured it out that since he was not doing it to all of the other children, it would be easy to deny it and get away with it. Obviously, his evil scheme must have worked for him because only one of his daughters was abused, and my wife was the only grandchild with the same experience.

Another distant relative who had stayed with my wife's grandparents as a child also came forward with the same accusations after hearing about my wife's story. My mother-in-law was very sorry, and she worked very hard to make it up to my wife. My wife's grandmother was advanced in years, and my wife's family had a meeting after all the truth came out and arrived at the conclusion that Grandma would not be able to take the news. There was a consensus that the news should be kept away from her. It was decided that if Grandma found out the truth when she got to heaven, then she could deal with it then and there.

The healing process continued for my wife and me with therapy. Things are gradually returning to normal in our bedroom. We learned a great lesson from my wife's story, and we are very protective of our children. We always think an abuser or a child molester is a stranger out there, but the molesters or perpetrators are usually the people we trust; they are the people in our close circle, the people who are supposed to protect us.

PTSD is real; it is not imagined. We can all adversely re-live bad life experiences and be imprisoned by our minds. Please be receptive to get help if you need it. It can be very difficult to suppress the bad experiences and make them go away; it may be impossible for you to stop the storage in your brain from playing back the video of your life trauma. You may have to get professional help to have your life back. Do something about PTSD — it is never too late.

# Quotes of Encouragement...

As the wind blows harder and Mrs. Fortune's story sounds familiar to you, remember the following:

*"Never forget that life can only be nobly inspired and rightly lived if you take it bravely and gallantly, as a splendid adventure in which you are setting out into an unknown country, to face many a danger, to meet many a joy, to find many a comrade, to win and lose many a battle."*

*~ Anne Besant*

A classic danger in life is the sexual exploitation of an innocent child. If this happened to you, know that it is not your fault. You were a powerless victim; rise above the self-blame and guilt, get help, and don't be trapped for life. Fight the trauma with determination to live a peaceful and fulfilling life, and all the positive forces of the universe will come to your aid to help you win your battle. *(LB)*

*"Return to the root and you will find the meaning."*

*~ Sengstan*

Don't dismiss it or play it down if somebody you know is experiencing PTSD; don't be judgmental because you are not walking in their shoes. Be a helper and not a critic. Help them to get to the root of the problem, and you will find the meaning. Get them psychological help and work with them so that they can be free from living in fear. *(LB)*

*"Our trials, our sorrows and our griefs develop us."*

*~ Orison Sweet Marden*

The truth is; our trials, griefs, and sorrows, develop us only if we allow them to develop us, they could equally destroy us if we allow it; Don't allow unfortunate life experiences to destroy you, especially if you are a victim. Be good to yourself, it is not your fault, you have not caused the unfortunate experience, neither could you have prevented it. *(LB)*

*Winds Against The Mind*

## Post-Traumatic Stress Disorder (PTSD):
# MR. HUNTER'S STORY

Jimmy and I grew up in the same neighborhood, rode the school bus together to school, and played on the same baseball team. We lived in a small community. Our parents became very close friends because Jimmy and I were like brothers. We took turns spending the night at each other's houses. We got into trouble together and got spanked together. We shared many great moments and memories. I remember one day at age seven, I was riding my bike down a steep hill like a typical seven year old. I lost control and was thrown off the bike. I hit my head on the concrete and became unconscious. Thanks to Jimmy, who ran to get help, I survived, but I might have died if help was not sought immediately. I was rushed to the hospital, and it took me a while to recover. I could tell so many stories of good and bad times with Jimmy.

After high school, we both decided to enroll in the army. Jimmy came from a family of servicemen; his father, both grandfathers, and uncles were all in the military. We had both wanted to serve our country since we were little. Our decision to serve was not a surprise to both of our families. Another added advantage was that the military had a lot of great benefits and also helped with the tuition payments for higher education. Both of our parents would not have been able to send us to college unless we took a loan.

A year after our enrollment in the military, we found ourselves on the way to the battlefield. Jimmy and I narrowly escaped many close encounters with death, until this fateful day. The enemies opened fire on us, and Jimmy was killed, a short distance from me. When the sound of the gunshots stopped, I moved next to Jimmy and shook him. He was covered with blood, and I looked at my hands—they were covered with Jimmy's blood. I kept shaking him, but he was dead. I had seen many dead bodies on the battlefront, but it never crossed my mind that I would be kneeling down next to Jimmy's dead body one day. I wished I could have saved him the way he had saved my life when I had a wreck on the bike at age seven. I wished I had the magic to wake him up, but he was gone forever. I walked around lifeless like a zombie for days after Jimmy's death; there was no time to mourn any loss because we saw dead bodies everywhere, and you could not be sure if you would be the next. I was shot in the thigh shortly after Jimmy's death and sustained a very bad injury. I wished I could die too, just like Jimmy, but it was not my time to go.

I was sent back home to the military hospital. I had multiple surgeries and went through rehabilitation before I could walk again. I had an honorable discharge after my injury.

I went through a process of mourning over Jimmy's death after I left the military. For the first time I did not know what to do by myself or for myself without Jimmy. I realized then how lonely I was without my best friend. Everything in our little town reminded me of him; we had gone everywhere together. I started having nightmares about the war with people getting killed and dead bodies everywhere. I would wake up in the middle of the night in panic and sweat. I would dream and see Jimmy in the dream, crying for help, but I could not help him. I would see myself trying to touch Jimmy's hand and to pull him to safety, but I was never able to touch his hands in the dream. He always drifted away. I woke up many nights hyperventilating, struggling to breathe, scared, and in a panicked state. I spoke to my parents about my experiences, and my father advised me to try to settle down and have a family. My father thought if I had other things to occupy my mind, I would be able to get over my nightmares. I took my father's advice and married the girl I was dating at that time. I wished Jimmy were my best man or at least one of my groomsmen at the wedding. We observed a moment of silence in honor of Jimmy at my wedding.

My wife and I decided to start a family shortly after the wedding, and our first child was a boy. I was ecstatic at the birth of my son, and I named him Jimmy, in honor of my best friend. Despite my new life, new wife, and new baby, my nightmares still would not go away. My wife would still wake me up in the middle of the night on several occasions because I continued to scream and fight in my sleep as if I were still on the battlefield. She would say to me many times "Honey, you are at home, not on the battle field." The situation was getting worse, and I was almost getting scared of going to sleep at night.

By the time I knew what was going on with me, I had turned heavily to alcohol to cope. Initially, I drank in moderation, usually with friends, and nothing out of control. As time went on, I found myself drinking heavily, especially at night with the hope that I would be able to sleep better. I started going to bars and found myself picking fights at the bar when I was drunk. I was gradually losing control of my life, and becoming more and more irresponsible.

Two years after our first child, we had another son, and I was too drunk to witness his birth. My wife said she called me on the phone to come to the hospital when she was in labor, and I told her I was on my way. I have no recollection of my conversation with my wife. I must have been too drunk and probably blacked out when she talked to me. I became physically and verbally abusive to my wife, and I could not be a father to my children anymore. I was getting multiple tickets for driving under the influence of alcohol, and I was getting locked up in jail on and off. I was getting into public fights more and more and had several bruises from the fights. Despite my heavy drinking, the nightmares and the flashbacks would still not go away.

I looked at myself in the mirror one day after I was released from jail on a driving under the influence of alcohol arrest (DUI), and I was disappointed at the person I saw in the mirror. I did not even know this person anymore. I asked myself 'What happened to me? How did I come this far from a responsible person to an alcoholic?' I took a minute and reflected on my life: I was raised in a strict, religious family by two wonderful and responsible parents. We were not wealthy, but we did not lack anything that was needed for us to have a decent life. My siblings and I had clean clothes and food on the table, and we were able to participate in recreational activities. My parents were always there for us. We did not have any excess money to throw around, but we did not lack. We were a regular, happy, middle-class family. Here I was in front of the mirror, looking pitiful, a completely irresponsible alcoholic who could not take care of himself, not to mention his family. I decided at that point that enough was enough. I had been a disgrace to my parents, and nothing but a pain for my wife and my children. I decided to put an end to it all and end my life.

I went and got my gun, loaded it up and decided to kill myself. As I was about to pull the trigger, I decided to put the gun down to write a note of apology to my wife and my children and explain to them why I had to do this. I hoped that my children would be able to forgive me when they grew older and read the note. I was not expecting anybody at home at that time of the day. My wife's routine was to pick the children from the daycare after work and come home; it was unusual for her to be home at that time of the day. I had planned it in such a way that I would be dead for at least three hours before my wife could come home and find me.

Somehow, God was determined to save my life and to give me a second chance. I heard the door open as I was writing the note, and I stopped writing the note immediately. I wanted to pull the trigger before my wife could come inside the house; I did not want anything to stop me from killing myself. I suddenly heard the innocent voice of my older son calling 'Daddy, Daddy, where are you?' My hands went numb. I could not go through with the decision to pull the trigger, and I could not make myself do something so terrible around my family. I sat on the bed with the gun in my hand. My wife came to the room and found me with a loaded gun and an uncompleted note written to her and the children. She was terrified, and she carefully took the gun from me and called for help. My wife had come home at that time of the day because our younger son had a fever, and the daycare had called her to come take him home. She had left work, picked up both of our children because they were in the same day care, and gone to the pediatrician's office. She came home early because the daycare would not take a sick child back. Their trip home was what saved my life.

I was taken to a local hospital, and later ended up in a mental hospital. Finally, I was diagnosed with post-traumatic stress disorder as a result of my experience during the war, and especially from watching my best friend get killed close to me. I was also dealing with major depression. All along, I was using alcohol to treat my pain and the stress of re-living the war experience continuously in my dream. I was released from the hospital with a better understanding of what my problem was, and I started an intense psychotherapy and medication therapy in the hospital. I was discharged to an outpatient treatment program, and also attended a support group with other war veterans who had similar experiences. I was also placed on some medication for the treatment of my underlying depression and anxiety problems.

Whenever I think back on the pain I caused my family, I always feel like beating myself up. However, I try to look at the positive side. At least I am still here to make a change. I do not drink anymore, I have a decent job, and I am a better father and a loving husband. I always reflect on how long it took me to get help; if only I had known then what I know now. I know there are many people out in the world dealing with similar issues but not getting to the root of their problems. If your story or the story of someone you know sounds like mine, do not try to fix it on your own. Please get help. Post-traumatic stress syndrome is real; it is not all in your mind or is your imagination going crazy. You have been psychologically and mentally traumatized, and what you are experiencing is a result of the trauma. There is help out there. Sometimes, help will not come to you until you go to get the help.

# Quotes of Encouragement...

As the wind blows harder and Mr. Hunter's story sounds familiar to you, remember the following:

*"There are many truths, of which the full meaning cannot be realized until personal experience has brought it home."*

~ *John Stuart Mill*

We sometimes find it difficult to understand why some people go through trauma and are unable to move on with their lives; when we have a similar experience, our perspectives quickly change, and we have a new appreciation for what the other person is going through; we owe it to each other to be considerate and sensitive when people around us have been traumatized. PTSD is a horrible experience, and we don't have to wait to know the personal hell the victim is living in before we help and extend kindness. *(LB)*

*"When something (an affliction) happens to you, you either let it defeat you or you defeat it..."*

~ *Rosalind Russell*

Trauma and hardship are all part of the challenges of living; sometimes they sneak in on us, and sometimes we see them coming. Working through these experiences is part of our credits toward graduation from the school of life, and what we make out of these experiences will determine if we sink or rise, drop out from this unique school of life or graduate. We need to have a mindset to work through the storm and to come out a winner, so that one day we can encourage others with our past experiences. *(LB)*

*"I have known it for a long time but I have only just experienced it. Now I know it not only with my intellect, but with my eyes, with my heart, with my stomach."*

~ *Hermann Hesse*

No amount of explanation, textbook information, or education can make us understand a situation more than the person who experienced it. Living with PTSD takes over your entire being; the goal is to rise up to this elephant called fear and to be ready to defeat it. The battleground is in your mind, and the war must be won in your mind as well. *(LB)*

## Post-Traumatic Stress Disorder (PTSD):
# MRS. LAUREL'S STORY

School was just out for the summer, and I was kind of glad that I would be able to sleep a little longer since I did not have to get the children ready for school very early in the morning. Around six o'clock in the morning, I heard the fire alarm come on and make a very loud noise. In the past, our children would wake up early on a weekend or during the holidays and put food in the oven for breakfast and go back to watch the TV or play video games. Like typical children, they usually forgot that they put food in the oven and the food would burn and the smoke would trigger the fire alarm to come on. When I heard the fire alarm, I said to myself, 'Here we go again, the children must have left food in the oven as usual.' I had stayed up very late the previous night trying to get some work done, and I was annoyed with my children because the alarm came on.

The house was a three level house—the middle floor, the upper level, and a basement. I ran downstairs, first to the kitchen to check the oven, and there was nothing in the oven. I went to the family room where my children usually spend a lot of time watching the TV, and to my surprise, they were not there. I went to the basement, checked the garage, went back, and checked the entire middle floor of the house, but there was no evidence of fire and the fire alarm did not go off. I went back to the third floor, which was the bedroom area, checking each room one by one. At this point I was getting very scared and nervous because of the strong smell of smoke in the house. My problem was my narrow thinking: I thought if there were going to be a fire in the house, it would probably be in the kitchen. I never thought in my wildest dreams that I could be dealing with a fire accident in the bedroom area of the house, so the last area I checked was the bedroom area. The very last room I opened was my ten-year-old son's room, and half of the room was in flames with my son sleeping on his bed. I dragged him out of the room, alerted other family members in the house that my son's room was in flames, grabbed my nine-month-old baby from his crib and ran out of the house.

We called 911, the fire and emergency service, and they arrived on time to put the fire out. Our neighbors rallied round us and they were very supportive. The smoke damage was extensive; plus the water damage from putting out the fire added more damage to the house. It was all like a bad dream. Suddenly we had no clothes to wear and a lot of our valuables were all burnt or smoke damaged. We had to stay in a hotel temporarily, and we later moved to an apartment. It was a big life adjustment because we had been used to the comfort of having a lot of room and space.

After we settled down in the apartment, we went through a period of sadness. We decided to do the inventory of our damaged property ourselves to see what we could salvage, and it was even more traumatic. A lot of the family pictures were lost, especially the children's pictures when they were younger, vacation pictures, birthday parties, and school activities. I found myself mourning all the precious memories and valuables that I could never get back. It was very painful and heartbreaking. You hear about fires all the time. You see them on the news, but somehow you always think it will never happen to you. At the back of your mind, you unconsciously believe that it only happens to other people, forgetting that you are one of the other people, and it can happen to you as well.

The renovation was estimated to take three to six months, but it ended up taking nine months because of contractor problems. When the renovation was completed, the house was nicely done, and it was uplifting. We were all excited to move back to the house. My problem started as soon as we moved back; the memory of the fire kept re-playing in my mind. I was waking up in the middle of the night with dreams that the house was on fire again and I would smell strong, thick smoke despite the fact that there was no smoke. In a panic state, covered in sweat I would run through all three floors of the house searching for the source of the fire. Initially, my husband thought it was something temporary and it would go away, but instead it got worse by the day. I was having more and more sleepless nights and was feeling so tired. It became very difficult to get up in the morning and function. I left a standing rule in the house that everybody must leave their doors wide open at night. I was obsessively checking all the bedrooms after each nightmare episode. My children complained that they got scared many nights when they sensed any movement in their rooms, only to turn around to see that it was their mom. They complained of having their sleep interrupted because of my continuous room checks, and the sleep interruption made them feel tired in the morning too.

My problem did not stop with the nightmares. The sound of a fire truck or an ambulance threw me into a panic state and triggered my memories of the fire. I would pull to the side of the road on the highway and sit in the car for more than half an hour before I could join the highway traffic again. Just because I heard the sound of an ambulance or a fire truck, my brain would re-play the memory of the multiple fire trucks that parked in the front of my house on the day of the fire. I would instantly re-live the traumatic memory of the fire.

Life became very stressful for me because I could not make the nightmares and the ambulance and fire truck triggers go away. I came to appreciate the pain of others who had faced more severe situations. After all, we all escaped and nobody died or sustained a permanent injury in my family, but I was still this traumatized. Having this experience made me even more empathetic. It also helped me to reflect on the stories of others who faced greater trauma or sudden destruction.

I remember a friend telling me the story of a woman she took care of in the mental hospital, who had a nervous breakdown because she lost one of her two sons in a fire. She was able to save one of her sons, and when she went back inside to save the second son, the fire was too strong. Her son was screaming, "Mommy, Mommy, Mommy, help me!" but she could not save him, and the boy died in the fire. The woman suffered from a severe post-traumatic stress disorder, and she would wake up from her sleep repeatedly in the middle of the night, with nightmares of the fire and her son shouting for help, but she could not save him. She was constantly hearing her son's voice re-playing back in her mind and shouting for help day and night. She had a mental breakdown and required hospitalization.

My friend told me that some of this woman's family members were critical of her when they visited her at the hospital. They usually brought her son who had survived the fire to visit his mother. They would get very agitated and angry with her, saying she needed to get herself together, get out of the hospital, and take care of her son who was alive. They constantly nagged her that she should be happy that one of her sons made it, and she was irresponsible to have a nervous breakdown from the episode. Her family members were very impatient with her and got her very upset whenever they visited. They just could not understand why it took her such a long time to be able to function again.

Judging others is a sin we are all guilty of, and it is easy for all of us to judge other people when we are not walking in their shoes. The woman finally pulled herself together, but it took her a very long time to work through her loss and trauma. It was difficult for the people around her to understand that she was not ungrateful for the son that lived. She just suffered severe post-traumatic stress syndrome from the event that took the life of her other son. My friend who shared the lady's story with me had also had a traumatic experience as well that involved the loss of a child.

Having had a similar experience herself, she tried to explain to the woman's family members that not everybody who experiences trauma could get up the next day, erase the experiences from their mind, and continue to have a normal life. The healing process is different for different people. They needed to give the woman time to work through her trauma instead of making her feel worse and guilty for not appreciating the fact that she has one son alive. With professional help, the woman eventually moved on with her life and functioned normally again. She was able to take care of her son who made it out alive. She would call the hospital occasionally to thank the staff and let them know she was doing well.

To go back to my story, my nightmare experiences and fears of fire trucks and ambulances continued for several months. On top of that, nobody was getting enough sleep in my house at night because I continued to wake up frequently, screaming out in my dreams. Finally, we decided to have a family meeting, and the family came to the conclusion that we should put the house up for sale and buy another house. The family thought that if we moved to another house, the nightmares would go away. It was at this point that I decided to seek professional help. I loved my house and the neighborhood, and there was no guarantee that the problem would go away even if we moved to another house. The thought of leaving our house was very distressing for my children because they had their little clique of friends in the neighborhood.

I asked my family for six months to get myself together, and I promised that if there was no improvement after six months of seeking help, we would consider moving to another house. I used a multidisciplinary approach for help. I turned to my faith as a Christian and looked for strength in the Scriptures to help me. I also went for professional counseling. Eventually, I got over my fears.

We have been back in the house for more than eight years now, and my life is completely restored to normal. Looking back and reflecting on my experiences, I am very grateful that there is help for post-traumatic stress disorder, and it is possible to have a normal life again. There is no list of specific traumatic situations that would trigger post-traumatic stress disorder. Victims of earthquakes, floods, accidents, tornadoes, war, physical abuse, parental neglect, and any other event that could traumatize the mind may suffer from post-traumatic stress disorder. Do not think it is your fault, or view what you are experiencing as a sign of weakness if you have suffered or are suffering from post-traumatic stress disorder. If this story sounds familiar to what you are experiencing, please get help. It is never too late to get help.

# Quotes of Encouragement...

As the wind blows harder and Mrs. Laurel's story sounds familiar to you, remember the following:

*"If you wish to know the road up the mountain, ask the man who goes back and forth on it."*

*~ Zenrin*

Getting together with other people who experienced or are experiencing PTSD is a great step toward recovery; this could be best achieved by joining a support group, sharing notes, and expressing feelings without being judged. Learn positive ways to cope and know that you are not alone; these are a few of the benefits of joining a support group. *(LB)*

*"A very crucial experience can be regarded as a setback — or the start of a new kind of development."*

*~ Mary Roberts Rinehart*

Identify PTSD for what it is, seek professional help, and activate your inner strength. Strive to turn the traumatic experience into an opportunity to grow rather than regress. Remember that you have not asked for this trauma or caused it to happen, and be determined not to allow the trauma to deprive you of the joy of living. It is not easy but it is possible to grow from a traumatic experience with strong determination. Don't forget that you are still here—you have outlived the trauma, so activate your willpower to out-live the negative memories as well. *(LB)*

*"A clear understanding of negative emotions dismisses them."*
*~ VERNON HOWARD*

Part of the steps towards healing is to understand PTSD as a negative emotion produced from a negative experience. A clear understanding of the emotions will obviously help to understand how to manage these emotions. A healthy approach is to learn to dismiss the negative emotions. Say to your fears loudly that "I am safe now, and I am not going to be afraid anymore." *(LB)*

# MRS. SHEPHERD'S STORY

The first time it happened to me, I thought I was going to die. I was unable to breathe, and I was gasping for air. It was a very scary feeling. I asked my husband to call the ambulance. I was convinced that I was having a heart attack. The ambulance arrived, and I was rushed to the hospital. Every possible test was conducted on me, and I was kept on a twenty-four hour overnight stay for observation at the hospital. Every test came back negative, and the conclusion was that since nothing was medically wrong with me, I was probably experiencing a panic attack.

I was very angry and upset with the hospital staff. I was convinced that they did not know what they were doing. I was so sure in my mind that something serious must be wrong with me. The physician who attended to me at the hospital instructed me to follow up at my primary care doctor's office, which I did. I went to my doctor's office with so much anger and frustration, telling him that I had a heart attack, and the people in the hospital were incompetent. They could not detect it or come up with the right diagnosis. I threatened to sue the hospital staff for a misdiagnosis if I eventually found out that I had had a heart attack. My primary care doctor also ran a series of tests and sent me to a heart specialist. At the end, he concluded that nothing was wrong with me, and he would have to agree with the hospital's findings. He said we would wait for a while and see if it was a one-time incident or if the symptom would repeat itself. About a week after I got a clean bill of health from my primary care doctor, I experienced the same symptoms. It was a choking feeling, with chest pain and stomach pain. I was covered in sweat, and I asked my husband to take me to a different hospital. Again, after every test was conducted, they could not find anything wrong with me. At this point, I began to feel a sense of embarrassment, and I did not want to go back to the same hospital or my doctor's office anymore, but I was still convinced in my mind that I was going to die and nobody would be able to determine the cause of my death.

I devised another plan and started visiting different doctor's offices, making sure I covered my tracks. I did not volunteer my previous history or diagnosis. I was shopping for a doctor that would be able to diagnose this illness that I believed was going to kill me and was being played down as a panic attack. I was convinced that my problem was a life-threatening situation, and nobody was picking up on the right diagnosis. All of the different physicians that I visited concluded that I might be experiencing panic attacks without comparing notes, but the panic attack explanation sounded too simple for what I thought I was going through. To me it felt like closeness to death every time it happened. The attacks became more and more frequent, and I was worried about when the next one was going to come. I would feel dizzy and lose consciousness at times when I had the attacks. I became terrified and got scared of the possibility of having the attack in a public place.

Gradually, I stayed more and more at home out of fear, and eventually quit my job and refused to leave the house. I gave my reasons for quitting my job as health-related. I lived in a big city and had to take a subway (underground train) to work. I asked myself this question, 'What if I accidentally fell over into the train track after an attack and got run over by the train?' The other option was to drive to work, and that was not even an option for me. I was worried that if I had an attack and lost control of the car while driving, I would endanger my life and the lives of others. I concluded that I made the right decision to quit my job. I refused to go to the grocery store and the mall to shop. I could not believe that I would ever give up going to the mall because it was my favorite thing to do in life, especially since our children were grown and gone.

Before I knew what was going on, a year had passed by since I put myself under a self-sentenced house arrest. My husband was extremely frustrated with me; he did not know what to do but he gave me unconditional support. I kept my problems a secret from my children and my family. I announced to everybody that I decided to take an early retirement, and everybody was happy for me. The problem gradually got worse, and my husband was so worried that I would not leave the house under any condition. He encouraged me to do something about the situation. I told him that my plan was to seek professional help from doctors in another state with the hope that they would be able to come up with a better diagnosis. My husband insisted that I had to follow up on my plan if I strongly believed that it would solve my problems, but I was not going to listen to him. As long as I was inside my house I was okay and felt safe.

After almost two years of my self-imposed house arrest, we had our first grandbaby. Our daughter was counting on me to help her with the baby after the delivery since I was retired. My fears got worse when she was closer to delivery, and I had more frequent attacks. The fact that I would have to leave the house to go and help with the baby was killing me. The children noticed that I was not leaving the house, but they rationalized that I was probably enjoying my retirement to the fullest. I had worked very hard all my life, and they thought I deserved all the enjoyment I could get.

My daughter and my son-in-law were so excited to call my husband and me to announce the arrival of their new baby girl and our first grandchild. "We named her after you, Mom," my daughter said with excitement. I was so happy, and I cried for joy. I was saying to myself that I was so lucky this deadly disease that nobody could diagnose did not kill me before the birth of my first grandchild. I sent balloons, flowers, and a gift basket, then came the time for me to go and see the baby in the hospital. My anxiety spiked up, and I had bouts and bouts of panic attacks. The chest pain felt so horrible. I told my husband that I simply could not go with him. I frantically told him that it was impossible for me to leave the house, unless he wanted me to die.

My husband went to the hospital alone to see the baby. He was very angry with me that I would not even visit my first grandchild. He ran completely out of patience with me, and he could not be himself and watch me live the rest of my life in a cage. He even threatened to file for a divorce or move out of the house unless I agreed to get help. He made the threat out of desperation to make me seek help; in his mind divorce was not an option for him.

After a few weeks of arguments, I decided to compromise and get help. My husband set an appointment with our family doctor and literarily dragged me to the appointment, despite a lot of resistance from me. Our family doctor was the very first doctor that initially suspected that I might be having panic attacks. I was angry with him the first time I went, and I had not been back to his office for almost two years. He thought that everything was okay with me and that was why he did not hear from me again. He had no idea that I had put myself under house arrest. What made the situation difficult for me to accept was that the panic attack explanation sounded too simple. What I thought I was experiencing felt close to death. I was convinced that whatever was going on with me must be very deadly. The doctor emphasized again that the symptoms of panic attacks often present in such a way to get the victims thinking that they are dying of a heart attack or facing a life-threatening illness. He explained that millions of people suffer from panic attacks every day, and the illness could be successfully managed with medicine and therapy. I was started on medications, and the doctor warned me that some of them could be addictive, and I would have to be weaned off the medications gradually as soon as the symptoms subsided. I was also referred to a specialist for intense therapy.

Finally after a few months, I had my life back. My husband had to break the news of what had been going on for more than two years to our children, and they were shocked. I was hiding the problem from the children all along because I strongly believed that I did not have a correct diagnosis. I was waiting until I got the correct diagnosis before breaking the news to my family. My daughter and my son-in-law who had a new baby were very unhappy with me until they found out the truth about my struggles with panic attacks. I had promised to help them out with the new baby, and they were counting on my help. Unfortunately, I did not see the baby for the first six weeks of her life because of my irrational fears. I was able to visit my granddaughter after I started treatment.

Years have gone by since my last panic attack. I am now a free person. I have five beautiful grandchildren, and I am able to enjoy all of the seasons of the year with my family without locking myself up in the house. My husband is also retired, and we are enjoying our retirement to the fullest. We are taking vacations and are fulfilling all the dreams we had for our retirement. I have learned to appreciate life even more, and I try to make up for all the years and months I lost to this illness. The truth about a panic attack is this: it is real. If it is not treated, it could totally paralyze a person's life. The symptoms truly felt like deadly symptoms, and it was difficult for me to believe that there was nothing terminal going on with my body, such as a real heart attack. The good news is there is treatment for panic disorder; nobody should be living with it and not get treated. If my story sounds familiar to you, do not ignore the symptoms, get help.

# Quotes of Encouragement...

As the wind blows harder and Mrs. Shepherd's story sounds familiar to you, remember the following:

*"You gain strength, courage, and confidence by every experience in which you really stop to look fear in the face... The danger lies in refusing to face the fear, in not daring to come to grips with it... You must make yourself succeed every time. You must do the things you think you cannot do."*

~ *Eleanor Roosevelt*

Panic attacks will keep you in a cage like a bird; you have to confront these irrational fears every time they present themselves. For you to succeed and to overcome dreadful bouts of panic attacks, you must do the exact things that you dread repeatedly until you are no longer afraid of them. Confront your fears, and they will leave you alone. *(LB)*

*"What is needed rather than running away or controlling or suppressing or any other resistance is understanding fear; that means, watch it, learn about it, come directly in contact with it. We are to learn about fear, not to escape from it."*

~ *J. Krishnamurti*

Your freedom lies in understanding why you are having these irrational fears and what is bringing on the fears. Once you get to the root of the tricks your mind is playing on you, you can work toward getting professional help. You don't have to escape from your fears; reverse the role and make your fears escape from you. Don't be trapped — life is short. *(LB)*

*"Your brain shall be your servant instead of your master. You will rule it instead of allowing it to rule you."*

~ *Charles E. Popplestone*

The fear that is producing continuous panic attacks originates from your mind. Your mind and your brain are one and the same—look for the inner strength to take control of your mind. You cannot be a slave to your own mind; get help and free your mind; you have only one life to live. *(LB)*

# Phobia:
# LUCY'S STORY

Since I was a child, I never liked closed spaces. I remember how reluctant I was to go to the basement of my house as a child because it was too closed in and very claustrophobic for me. I remember feeling dizzy, as if the walls and the ceilings of the basement were going to close in on me, and I got so scared anytime my parents sent me on an errand to do something in the basement. I would play outside and see a flying plane, and I would run inside the house at the sight and the noise of the plane. I always felt that the plane might drop from the sky. The thought of flying in a plane would not even be a consideration for me, I told myself over and over as a child. I had no doubt in my mind that there was no way I would be flying that high in the sky. Luckily for me, I did not have to worry about flying while I was growing up. My parents were the second generation of their family in America. We did not have many extended family members; the few family members we had lived nearby. Finances were also a big factor; my parents did not take us on any family vacations because we could not afford it. They were busy working hard, trying to make ends meet and sending us to school, with the hope to live the American dream fully one day. I must also add that we did not miss taking vacations at all because there was a lot to do for fun in the big city where we lived.

By the time I graduated from college, I realized that I had never been on a plane. Finally, a situation came when I had to go on a family reunion trip. A group vacation package was put together by a travel agent, and everybody in the family was scheduled to fly on the same plane for this family vacation. I was so scared, I had to take medication to calm me down and help me to go to sleep on the plane. This was the only condition that would make me even get on the plane. Unfortunately, things did not work out as I expected; the flight turned out to be a very rough flight, and this just made a bad situation worse. The sleeping pill did not help at all. I was wide awake throughout the flight, and I was so terrified that I decided to come back from that trip on the bus instead of flying back with the rest of my family. I was just so glad to get off the plane, and I promised myself never to get on another plane again. It took me a whole day to come back on the bus, but I didn't care. I was just not going to get on a plane ever.

I also had phobia about going on an elevator. My phobia about an elevator was multiple. First, I was afraid of the height if I had to ride in an elevator in a tall building, and second, I had a fear of being in a closed space when inside an elevator. Throughout my college years, I avoided going on elevators. Some of my classes were in tall buildings, but fortunately they were not more than three or four floors above the ground level. I always made sure I left my dormitory early enough to allow myself to climb the stairs instead of riding on the elevators. On days when I was late to class, I would choose to go on the stairways and enter the classroom late rather than ride the elevator and be in class on time. Whenever my friends and classmates tried to convince me to go on the elevator with them, I gave the excuse that going up and down the stairway was my way of getting my exercise for the day. I never liked any building that was more than two floors, but I could still cope with a few floors off the ground if I could climb the stairs instead of riding an elevator.

Finding a job was not a problem for me after graduating from college because my field of study was very lucrative. The biggest problem for me was going after the best job opportunities; I restricted myself because of my phobia. Any interview or job opportunity that would require flying or working in a tall or high-rise building was taken off my list immediately. I passed up great job opportunities, but I was still able to get a good job that would not require flying or riding an elevator. I went on to get a master's degree in my field, and unbelievable job opportunities with great benefit packages opened up for me in other parts of the country. I turned down the offers because I was very close to my family. Accepting a job that would take me far away from my family would require flying back and forth to come home, and that would be too difficult with my phobia, I rationalized. Hopefully something that would be worth my moving would open up within a driving distance. I finally settled down to a wonderful job in the same city with my parents and my extended family.

Life was great for years because I was able to work my life around my phobias. Finally I met a wonderful young man and we got along very well from day one. A few weeks into our relationship, I reluctantly discussed my phobias with him, worried that they might turn him off. To my surprise, it was not a big problem for him and I was so relieved. He proposed to me within six months of our relationship, and within one year we were married. We went to a beautiful resort within driving distance for our honeymoon because I refused to fly. On our way back, we stopped at an amusement park, and my husband went on wild rides at the park. I was so terrified and sick at my stomach to watch him on the rides that I would close my eyes and open my eyes only when he got off the ride and tapped me on the shoulder. When we bought a house, I made sure we did not buy one with a basement because of my fear of closed spaces.

Life was great after marriage. We were two professionals, each of us on six-figure salaries. My husband and I had only one restriction on our lives, and that was to work around my phobias. Every time my husband suggested that I get help, my anxiety level would go up, and I would get very angry with him. I used a guilt trick on him; I would say to him that "you were aware of my phobias before you married me." I was so afraid to get help since, getting help would require me to fly or go on elevators eventually. I concluded in my mind that this would definitely kill me. I decided that I was going to navigate my life without going on elevators or the planes. My husband would crack jokes that more people get killed in cars than on planes, and I would tune him out or ignore his jokes.

After three years of marriage, we decided to start a family. We had saved a lot of money in three years and had paid down a lot of our debts and college loans. My husband also got a new and better paying job. My husband's new job was on the fourteenth floor of a tall building, and I refused to visit his new office. We both decided that I should stay at home, and I should consider going back to work when our children are of school age. We had three children close together, and I was extremely busy. I still continued to live life around my phobias.

By the time our oldest child was five years old, he was already talking about going to Disney World and going to Nickelodeon Studios. He would come home and talk about all the beautiful places his friends were visiting, and he asked us over and over again when we would go. My anxiety would go up every time he talked about visiting places that required long trips, especially a trip to Disney World. It would take three days on the road with three little children to drive to Disney World from where we lived. I knew my husband would definitely not agree to such a long driving trip. He would tell our son that our trips depended solely on when Mommy was ready to go, and that would only be when Mommy was ready to go on the plane. The children would ask if we could drive, and my husband would explain to them that the distance was too far to drive. I used to get very upset with my husband. I felt that he was not very understanding and supportive enough of my fears. I was also upset that he would joke about my phobias around our children.

## Winds Against The Mind

My oldest son would ask me why I did not want to go on a plane. It became an embarrassment, and I denied my problems to my son simply because he could not understand what phobia was at that age. I realized that I had to come up with something to tell him because he kept asking to go to Disney World. Finally, I had to tell him that we had to wait until his youngest sister turned four, so that she could enjoy the trip as well. Our youngest child was only one at that time. My son trusted me and looked forward to when his baby sister would turn four. Every year when his sister got a year older, he would get very excited because that meant one year closer to go to Disney World. When my youngest daughter turned three, it dawned on me that I had to get help rather than putting the entire family in bondage because of my phobias. I was so afraid of letting my son down when his sister turned four after waiting for three years to go to Disney World. I was worried that he might grow up and not be able to trust me. I came to the conclusion that it would be really selfish on my part to deprive my children of having great childhood memories of fun trips and family vacations because of my irrational fears. I finally sought help, and my husband was relieved.

After several months in therapy plus medication management to control my anxiety, my life was changed. I could fly in planes and ride on elevators. I could go to my husband's fourteenth floor office to take him out for lunch, and I could go on rides with my husband and my children at the amusement parks. Finally, we took a family vacation to Disney World, and it was one of the best trips of our lives. Life is more fulfilling without phobias, and I feel refreshed that I can do a lot more with my family without restrictions or catering to my fears. The thought of being able to take any job that I want whenever I am ready to go back to the work force is also exciting. For the first time, I do not have to worry about what part of the country the job is in, whether it is in a high-rise building or on what floor the office is going to be. I have decided not to look back on what I have missed; instead I look forward to the life ahead of me. The greatest relief is my family is not in bondage to my phobias anymore. Nobody should have to live with phobias for the rest of his or her life, because there is help for phobia. If your story sounds like mine, please do not live in bondage. Do something about it—get help.

## <u>Quotes of Encouragement...</u>

As the wind blows harder, and Lucy's story sounds familiar to you, remember the following:

*"To fight fear, act. To increase fear—wait, put off, or postpone."*
                                        *~ David Joseph Schwartz*

The biggest mistake is to postpone the need to confront your phobia. The best wisdom is to act immediately and not allow phobia to control your life; phobia is an irrational fear, and avoiding the object you fear can be time-consuming. By the time you know it, you find yourself planning your entire life around escaping your feared object; you don't have to live with phobia—get help and get yourself out of bondage, and give yourself a chance to live a free and happy life. *(LB)*

*"It is an old psychological axiom that constant exposure to the object of fear immunizes against the fear."*
                                        *~ MAXWELL MALTZ*

One of the interventions to beating phobia is by constant exposure to the object feared. With constant exposure the brain re-programs itself to see no need to be fearful of the feared object. *(LB)*

*"Do what you fear and fear disappears."*
                                        *~ David Joseph Schwartz*

There is no shortcut to dealing with phobia; do what you fear, and the more you do it, the less anxious you become; in the long run, the fear will finally disappear or at least become manageable. *(LB)*

## Obsessive Compulsive Disorder (OCD):

# SHARON'S STORY

I believe I had the obsessive compulsive personality traits growing up. As I grew older, I probably developed obsessive compulsive disorder. I was a straight-A student throughout my educational career. Any grade that was not an A was not good enough for me. I remember I had a school project to build a castle in fourth grade; I worked on it for three days non-stop with my mom's help. The castle looked beautiful and when it was almost completed, my mom even took a picture of it. I looked at the castle one morning and thought it was slanting, so I decided to tear it down immediately. My mother was very upset with me because she had spent a lot of time helping me with the project. As little as I was, I tried to explain to her that a castle cannot have a defect because the king and queen live in it. I told my mom that a slanting castle was considered a big defect, and we did not want the king and queen to die, so we had to fix it. My mom did not accept my argument because she thought the castle was very beautiful for a fourth grade project. I had to build another castle all over again without her help.

I also remember working on a group project in high school with some classmates. I spent hours on the project and kept other students working for hours until everybody got burned out and frustrated with me. I was also very meticulous about my room at home; everything was properly arranged. You would even wonder if anybody lived in my room. I also dusted and cleaned my room all the time, and I felt much safer in my room than in any other part of the house. I was lucky to have a private bathroom attached to my bedroom. I kept my bathroom spotless all of the time because I was afraid of germs. My parents did not notice that something was wrong with my behavior in my teenage years; they were just very grateful that I was not a messy teenager like their friends' children.

# Winds Against The Mind

One day I watched a program on TV about dust mites in pillows. It was explained during the program that dust mites were tiny invisible creatures living in the pillows, and they could produce allergies. I washed my bedcovers, comforters, and pillows so much that my parents had to buy new bedding sets for me very frequently. When I was in college, I would write and rewrite essays over and over again, believing that they were not good enough each time. I barely had four hours of sleep at night because of my obsession with perfect work and perfect grades. I realized that a lot of people were not willing to partner with me in group projects. I did not think anything was wrong with me until I asked my best friend if she would like to be my partner on one project, and she bluntly refused. She made a comment that college could seem overwhelming when doing a project with someone like me because I was too obsessive compulsive and too much of a perfectionist for her liking. She said the project would never be finished. I felt very offended but quickly dismissed her comment and justified it in my mind that she was a lazy student anyway, and she was not making as good grades as I was.

I graduated from college at the top of my class and was able to secure a good job. After college, I married a man who was totally clueless about my obsessions. He just thought I was a neat freak, and it was okay with him if I was obsessed with neatness. My problem got worse by the day, and I realized that it was more than a personality trait. It was obviously obsessive compulsive disorder.

I had all these rituals on my head that I had to follow rigidly on a daily basis. My rituals were very time consuming, and I realized they were not sensible for me to do. Unfortunately, I could not make myself stop doing them. With one foot in front of the other, I had to count a certain number of steps before going out of the door. If I did not count the steps, I would become anxious. I repeated the same steps over and over again to make sure they were perfect. I had to wake up very early in the morning, at least three hours before work, to have enough time to perform certain rituals to keep me germ-free. Keeping up with my rituals was easy to cope with when I was single because I was on my own, but it became very complex and annoying to my husband when I got married. My husband did not understand why I needed so much time in the bathroom every morning before work. It was a struggle for him to get me out of the bathroom in the morning so that he could at least have a chance to use the bathroom and get ready for his own job.

I would wash every item I used or touched over and over again, and I would also wash my hands insanely. There were times that I would finish a bar of soap to shower in one day; I was trying to make sure I had no germs or bacteria left on my body. I went through the rituals of disinfecting the bathroom every night in preparation for a shower in the morning. I strictly did not touch any doorknob without a handkerchief or a paper towel. I heard it somewhere along the line on the television that the easiest way to get germs is by touching a doorknob. I carried packets of facial tissues with me at all times to open the door knobs. I also had some rituals at home such as obsessing with stoves and the security alarm system. I would come back to the house over and over again to check the stove and the security alarm whenever I had to go out. My brain would be telling me that the house might catch fire because I did not turn off the stove, and a thief might come in and raid the house because I did not set the security alarm. I got worse by the day and picked new obsessions each day.

I woke up one morning and could not keep any food down. The first thought that came to my mind was food poisoning, and I went to the doctor's office. The doctor decided to do a pregnancy examination on me, and I laughed hysterically because I had been told that I could not have a baby because of some problems with my womb. To my surprise I was pregnant, and my husband and I were so excited. My husband was especially relieved; he thought if I had a baby to occupy my mind, I would be able to get rid of my "strange habits," as he called them. My husband referred to my obsessions as strange habits, because he could not really understand the reasons behind such behavior. Instead of the expected improvement that my husband was looking forward to, I added the obsession of trying to follow a perfect diet during pregnancy. I tried to rationalize in my mind that if I did not follow a perfect diet, something might go wrong with the pregnancy, and the baby would die. I was so rigid about the time of the day I ate. I had to have certain types of food and certain quantities of food at specific times of the day. I also had a rigid schedule for drinking milk because the doctor recommended that I drink a lot of milk. I ignored my hunger pangs during pregnancy to keep to my rigid schedule.

My husband was very worried about my rigidity, but fortunately for us, our son survived. After he was born, I picked up another obsession, which was to keep him within my eyesight always and to watch him all the time. I would rationalize in my mind that if I did not keep him within a safe distance, something could happen if I was away and he could die. Before I knew what was going on, I had planned out an entire lifetime for our son in my head. I planned to keep him at home until he could go to school. I planned to volunteer in his school and also be a room mother, so that I could make sure he was within a reasonable distance to me. I planned to go on every field trip, and he would not be spending the night with his friends because something might go wrong.

S    As the list of my obsessions grew, it was becoming more and more difficult to cope with the compulsion and the rituals needed to feed the obsession. I was keeping myself awake almost around the clock to watch our son. Occasionally, I would nod off from exhaustion, and I would wake up with a lot of anxiety, scared that he might be dead. I realized that I was not rational, but I could not make myself stop. I wore myself out completely from trying to watch the baby day and night. Life became unbearable, and finally I had a nervous breakdown. I was admitted to a psychiatric (mental) hospital. I begged to keep my son with me at the hospital, but the hospital staff refused to allow me. They constantly reassured me that he was okay with my husband. My anxiety level grew out of control, and I was so worried that my son might die. I was given some medications at the hospital that knocked me out and put me to sleep for long hours. That was probably the first time I had gotten a decent sleep in years. After about three days of doing nothing but sleeping, I started an intensive treatment program.

The doctor identified my problem as obsessive compulsive disorder. He also identified that I had anxiety problems and depression that were undiagnosed. I was started on some medications and behavior modification to help to deal with my obsessions and compulsions. The staff helped me to work on changing the way I think and the way I see and interpret my world. I was discouraged from dwelling on my obsessions and also trying to feed into the compulsions.

By the time I left the hospital, I was a better person. I followed up with my outpatient treatment program, and life is much better now without obsessions and compulsions. I can function normally at home for the first time, and I went back to work. My child is in a daycare, and my husband has his wife back. I am just glad to be able to enjoy life again as a normal human being. Obsessive compulsive disorder is very draining and time consuming. It drains you completely of your energy until you have none left in you. Something in your brain tells you to do something and if you do not do it, you become afraid something terrible will happen. You know in your mind that your thoughts are not rational, but the compulsion is so overpowering, you cannot make yourself not respond to the obsessive command and thoughts. You find yourself repeating a process endlessly over and over again. I believe nobody should live with this disorder; it is a total handicap. The good news about obsessive compulsive disorder is that it can be managed and controlled with treatment, and you do not always have to give in to the compulsions. If my story sounds familiar to you, get help and stop compromising your life.

# Quotes of Encouragement...

As the wind blows harder and Sharon's story sounds familiar to you, remember the following:

*"Are we controlled by our thoughts, or are we controlling our thoughts?"*
*~ Raymond Holliwell*

Your battle with OCD is simply a battle with your thoughts, and you are losing the battle. You have allowed your thoughts to control you. You have to fight the irrational fears and do the exact opposite of what your thoughts tell you not to do. Become rebellious; don't wash your hands when your thoughts scare you about germs, and don't check your stove when your thoughts scare you about a fire. The only way to win the battle with OCD is to rebel against the thoughts that create these fears in your mind. Sooner or later you will discover that the thoughts are empty threats, all lies, and tricks of the mind. There is no imminent danger to you; to win the battle you have to control your mind. *(LB)*

*"The man who acquires the ability to take full possession of his own mind may take full possession of anything else to which he is justly entitled."*
*~ Andrew Cárnegie*

You are not free until your mind is free. With OCD, your physical being is in jail because your psychological being is in jail; your physical being cannot be free from jail until your psychological or mental being is released from prison. The mind and the body work together, and one is not free of the other. For you to be in full control of other areas of your life, you must first be in full control of your mind. Get rid of the irrational fears, and don't allow OCD to limit your life. *(LB)*

*"One of the great discoveries a man makes, one of his great surprises, is to find he can do what he was afraid he couldn't do."*
*~ Henry Ford*

Be aware that OCD is an irrational fear that must be ignored, and once you refuse to entertain the fears, you will discover a new world of no restrictions, a free world, a world that is not so dangerous, and a world where you can do all the things that your mind scares you not to do. *(LB)*

*Winds Against The Mind*

## Generalized Anxiety Disorder:

# PAULA'S STORY

I did not understand why I worried all the time; all I knew was I was constantly worrying about something, and I could not make myself stop. When I was a child, my father's job required for him to travel a lot. My worries started then. I remember staying up most of the night quite often just because I was worrying about my father's safety. All sorts of thoughts would fly through my mind, "Supposing he gets into a wreck and dies? What is the family going to do, and how are we going to survive?' I was always relieved to see him come back home safely, and felt very sad when he had to leave again. Missing him made me sad, but what bothered me the most was the fear of something happening to him.

One day, I overheard my parents talking about the possibility of my daddy losing his job. I was so scared and so worried because Daddy was the major bread winner and mom was a stay-at-home mom. As usual, I was worried about what we were going to do if he lost his job and how we were going to pay the bills and buy food. I figured it out in my mind that we might have to move in with Grandma and Grandpa, which I was not excited about because they have a very small house. These were some of the questions and debates that went through my mind continuously.

Eventually, everything was restored to normal at his work, and he never lost his job. I also worried about my mom and the possibility that she could die, although she had no physical illness or any life-threatening condition. I would be so terrified from my worries, thinking that if she should die, the family would fall apart. I worried about my siblings, my friends, and even my teachers at school. My worry list was virtually endless. It was always tough for my mom to get me up in the morning to go to school because I would have spent most of the night looking at the ceiling in my bedroom and worrying about different things. I was always very tired from not sleeping well at night. Unfortunately, nobody realized what a personal hell I lived through as a child.

Despite my worries, I was able to keep my grades up in school. I survived young adulthood and made a transition into an adult chronic worrier. I went to nursing school and became a registered nurse and got married. My first marriage ended up in a divorce partly because of my excessive worrying. I practically drove my first husband crazy, although the marriage was plagued by other problems. I remember having enormous quarrels with my first husband whenever he came home late, despite the fact that his lateness was justified and job related. I worried that something terrible probably happened to him at work or on the way home, and I would become agitated by the time he showed up. The marriage finally ended up in a divorce. My first husband was glad to get out of the marriage and was even more relieved that we had no children together.

I got married a second time and started a family immediately; we had two children. I desperately wanted to have children with my first marriage, but it did not happen. Even with two children and a very busy life, I still could not stop worrying. I would worry about my husband, my siblings, my parents, my job, and everything I could possibly think of. After leaving work, I would get home and worry about my patients. I would call the hospital, asking the nurses who worked the shift after me about the patients. It was so bad that whenever I made a call to my work, nobody wanted to answer my call, and everybody avoided me. Other staff would crack jokes to me to go home and spend my time away from work with my family and to stop calling. If I got to work the next day and some of my patients were already discharged, I would spend an enormous amount of time worrying about how they were doing at home. Worrying became my second nature, and I did not get enough sleep at night. I spent most of my day drinking coffee and getting very easily irritated with everybody.

I worried about my children constantly. Whenever they were in school, I would worry about something happening to them. I would worry that they might choke on their lunch, or they might get injured during physical education, or they might be abducted on a field trip. All these thoughts would usually fly through my mind, and I would call the school and find a flimsy excuse to talk to their teachers just to be reassured that my children were fine. Sometimes I sensed the frustration in their teachers' voices. I was probably the only mother who called so frequently.

Maybe it was a psychological issue for me; I did not know. I tried to understand why both my first husband and my second husband had jobs that required traveling just like my father. My first husband was an area manager of big departmental store chain, and his job required covering several stores in a one-hundred mile radius. My current husband is a pilot. I wondered if I was unconsciously trying to duplicate my father by marrying men with traveling jobs, so that I could shift my worries from my father to my husband.

I continued the same pattern of worrying with my second husband, but he dealt with it very well by just ignoring me. If he came back late from a trip because his flight was delayed, I would quarrel with him as if it was his fault that his flight was delayed. If he went on a trip and did not call me as soon as he arrived at his destination, I would go berserk with my worries, leave several messages on his phone, and page him several times.

My parents were in their late seventies, and they lived alone. I would worry about a thousand things that could go wrong with them, especially because my mom had diabetes. I would worry about the possibility that my parents could fall, that my mom's blood sugar could be out of control or that my dad might develop a stroke because he had high blood pressure. I called and checked on my parents frequently, and they enjoyed it. My parents were just grateful that they had such a caring child, but they would have probably felt sorry for me if they had known that I spent most of my time worrying about them.

After a while, my co-workers became inpatient with me and reported to my boss that I called the hospital too much after my shift, asking about the patients, and it was very distracting for them. My boss had a discussion with me about the situation, and I told her that I had been a chronic worrier all my life, and I worried about anything and everything around me. I explained to her that I did not know why I worried so much for no obvious reason. My boss suggested that I should seek professional help. She was able to identify with me, because she dealt with a similar issue in the past. She clearly stated that we come across to others as very caring people at first, but with time everybody gets fed up with us.

I consulted a therapist and I was diagnosed with generalized anxiety disorder. I was put on anti-anxiety medications and also attended therapy sessions. I practiced relaxation techniques and tried to replace my irrational worries with rational and calm thoughts. I have to remind myself that despite all my worries over the years, none of the things that I worried about has happened. My parents are still alive, well advanced in years and still going strong, and my husband is doing well as a pilot, and his plane has not crashed, and my children have grown to be very healthy teenagers. Obviously my worries were pointless. They were unnecessary mental exercises. I joined a support group and found out that there are many people out there like me who spend their time worrying all round the clock unnecessarily.

Life is much better with professional help—I sleep better, I feel better, and I am not driving everybody around me crazy. It is unfortunate that a lot of us with anxiety disorder do not get help; we accept the illness as normal, thinking we are supposed to feel the way we are feeling. If your story sounds like mine, get help and stop worrying. There is a lot more to live for than spending a lifetime worrying.

# <u>Quotes of Encouragement...</u>

As the wind blows harder and Paula's story sounds familiar to you, remember the following:

*"This is where you will win the battle—in the playhouse of your mind."*
~ *Maxwell Maltz*

When you subject yourself continuously to unnecessary worries, you have allowed your mind to become a battlefield, and the ammunition and weapons helping to carry on the battle are your irrational fears, manifest in your constant worries. You have the choice about whether to make your life a permanent battlefield full of restlessness and agitation, or to seek the alternative. Identify this unnecessary war that you are fighting within yourself, and make peace with yourself by throwing your worries out of the window. *(LB)*

*"Courage is resistance to fear, mastery of fear—not absence of fear."*
~ *Mark Twain*

We all experience some level of anxiety in our day-to-day lives; mild anxiety may be helpful for us to be able to achieve our goals and to complete our tasks; anxiety becomes a problem when it takes over our lives. Our goal should be to master our fears by having a good understanding of what triggers our anxiety. We should be able to rationalize that excessive worries and anxiety are counterproductive. When fear and anxiety get out of proportion, we must have the courage to resist them and not be controlled by them. *(LB)*

*"Confront your fears, list them, get to know them, and only then will you be able to put them aside and move ahead."*
~ *Jerry Gillies*

Excessive worrying is an irrational fear; take an inventory of your fears, reflect on them, and realize that none of your fears came true. Acknowledge that your fears are irrational; they are a wasteful mental exercise and are an unnecessary self-torture. Set them aside and move on to a healthier life that is free of worries. *(LB)*

*Winds Against The Mind*

# General Understanding About Anxiety Disorders

A nxiety disorder is one of the most common and one of the least diagnosed mental illnesses. It is also one of the most under-treated mental disorders, because many people with anxiety disorder do not seek professional help. They believe they are supposed to feel the way they feel, and they are supposed to live with the way they feel. Everybody must have experienced anxiety somewhere down the road in life, and whenever we perceive a threat, we may become anxious. For instance, a college student may be anxious about a test because of the perceived threat or fear of making a bad grade and failing the class. For us to have a better understanding of anxiety disorder, we must be able to make a distinction between fear, normal day-to-day anxiety, and an actual anxiety disorder.

*Anxiety disorder* may be classified as irrational fear with no basis for the fear, whereas a rational fear has a source of threat to the person. People experience fear when there is a recognizable external source of danger to the person. For instance, when someone goes camping and suddenly faces a lion—such an experience would definitely provoke a lot of fear. The intensity and the duration of a person's fear may be proportionate to the source of the danger. For instance, seeing a snake three yards away may invoke a different reaction from seeing a lion three yards away. Fear produces changes such as rapid respiration (rapid breathing) and rapid heartbeat. Fear triggers a redistribution of blood from the other parts of the body to the muscles to prepare the body for what is called a "fight" or "flight" response to the threat. "Fight" or "flight" response is the body's ability to confront or fight the fear immediately, or to immediately run away from it.

We experience normal day-to-day anxiety to serve as a push or motivator for us to accomplish some of our goals. We may get anxious if we are stuck in the traffic and are running one hour late to work because of the fear of losing our job and losing an hour's worth of pay. Normal day-to-day minor anxiety that we experience could enhance our productivity.

Anxiety disorder may not necessarily involve an obvious threat to the person experiencing the anxiety. For instance, a person who has phobia of snakes and passes out from seeing a snake on the television is obviously experiencing an intense emotional reaction to a situation that does not produce immediate threat. This is a classic example of *phobia*, a type of anxiety disorder. This reaction could be considered irrational.

Another classic example of irrational fear is experienced by people suffering from *obsessive compulsive disorder*. They have an intrusive thought which interferes with their ability to concentrate, and they feel compelled to fix the situation by performing a compulsion or ritual to relieve the anxiety. For example, a woman who is on her way to work may repeatedly return to the house to check the stove because of the fear of setting the house on fire. She knows fully well that the likelihood that the stove might be on is zero, yet she still goes back to check the stove at least ten times before finally going to work. Her brain has convinced her to check the stove continuously, despite the fact that the stove is off. This reaction is obviously irrational, but she still feels compelled to do it.

Some people may also experience a *panic attack*, which is an overwhelming feeling of doom and anxiety of such a great proportion that it mimics a heart attack. Usually there is no underlying trigger or provocation for this feeling or this attack. When it becomes overwhelming and frequent to the point of debilitation that the person experiencing the panic attack cannot carry on normal day-to-day functioning, it becomes a *panic disorder*.

People who have experienced a traumatic event may re-experience the trauma or the experience through irrational fears from intrusive recollection of the experience, daydreams, and nightmares. This is called *post-traumatic stress disorder*. People who have been in terrible wars or a severe accident may experience post-traumatic stress disorder. A young man who was saved from a severe car wreck may have continuing dreams that he was in a car wreck, waking up in sweat and totally terrified by the dream.

Generalized anxiety is not regarded or perceived as a problem because we all need a little bit of anxiety in our day-to-day functioning. It becomes a problem when it interferes with our ability to function socially, occupationally, and emotionally. It is then classified as *generalized anxiety disorder.*

Post-traumatic stress disorder, panic disorder, phobia, obsessive compulsive disorder, and generalized anxiety disorder will all be discussed separately because each disorder has its unique symptoms. The treatment of each disorder is different, based on the symptoms and the history of the client.

## Post-Traumatic Stress Disorder:
# BASIC FACTS & UNDERSTANDING

*Post-traumatic stress disorder,* commonly referred to as *PTSD,* is usually experienced by people who have experienced, witnessed, or survived a traumatic event that is outside of the range of the common day-to-day experience. This event would involve an actual threat of death or serious injury to the person traumatized or to others. The experienced event provoked a response of intense fear, helplessness, or horror, and this experience is persistently replayed in the mind of the victim. The re-experiencing of this event can be in the form of painful dreams, images, nightmares, flashbacks, thoughts, perceptions, feelings, illusions (for example seeing a toy gun as a machine gun), and hallucinations (false sensory perception in the absence of an external stimuli). Hallucinations can be in different forms; for example, it could be visual, auditory, or olfactory; for example, a military veteran who returned from a deadly combat may be seeing dead soldiers (visual), smelling bodies of dead soldiers (olfactory), or hearing the voices of dead soldiers (auditory).

Examples of common unfortunate life experiences that could cause PTSD include sexual abuse, rape, torture (for example, prisoners of war), severe assault, bombings (such as Oklahoma bombing), victims of September eleventh twin tower attacks, fires, severe physical injuries, flooding, and hurricanes (such as hurricane Katrina and hurricane Rita), earthquakes in the bed of the ocean resulting in the loss of lives (such as the Tsunami), the death or deaths of people in military combat (such as the Vietnam and Persian Gulf wars), train or plane crashes, severe car accidents, shooting incidents, or mass murders (such as the tragic incident at Virginia Tech University).

PTSD victims usually experience physical and psychological symptoms such as sweating, palpitations (rapid heartbeat), confusion, a feeling of impending doom, fear of death, insomnia (inability to sleep), hyper-vigilance (excessive alertness), exaggerated startled response (such as jumping up at a slight touch), difficulty concentrating, and nightmares. They may experience what is called psychological numbing, in which they may become cold emotionally. They may be unable to show any affection toward other people or significant others. They may be unable to experience joy or pleasure, and may have diminished interest in day-to-day activities. PTSD has serious consequences on the family; it may cause divorce and abuse in families if no help is sought for or by the victim.

People suffering from PTSD may avoid people, places, or activities that remind them of the traumatic event. For instance, somebody who narrowly escaped death from a severe flood or hurricane accident may not want to go back to live in the same district or the same neighborhood. They may avoid conversations or talks about the trauma. People around them may describe them as strange because they feel detached from other people. They may have diminished interest in usual day-to-day activities. They may forget or be unable to recall part of the details of the traumatic event.

Another area of the life of PTSD victims that may be severely affected is their social interaction. They may have problems trusting others, and also have severe difficulty in getting along with others, especially at work. Interpersonal relationships are always seriously affected. The severe and uncomfortable anxiety they experience may push them to turn to substance abuse to self-medicate. It is an unconscious effort to numb the pain and to make the pain go away. Unfortunately, alcohol and drug abuse usually complicate the illness, leading sometimes to spousal and child abuse, and an inability to hold a job. If the traumatic experience is such that others died and the PTSD victim survived, he may feel very guilty about surviving and feel unworthy to live. Victims may be afraid to make commitment, invest in a family, or work on relationships. This is because they believe that it is a waste of their time, and something tragic may happen again. Depression is very common, and alcohol and drugs are commonly used by victims to treat the depression.

The situational cause of PTSD always speaks for itself, but there is always the big question as to why some people have PTSD after experiencing a traumatic event, and other people experience the same traumatic event but do not develop PTSD. Unfortunately, there is no one conclusive answer to this question. This is a question that is still generating a lot of clinical research. With what is known so far, many factors are believed to be responsible in determining who will and will not develop PTSD. These include a good support system and early intervention in confronting and getting help after a trauma. Other biological factors may also be involved.

Biologically, it is believed that the effects of the trauma or the stress affect the chemical balance or equilibrium of certain naturally occurring chemicals in the brain called neurotransmitters. The shift or the dysregulation of the neurotransmitters produces the physiological and the mental effect of re-experiencing or re-living the traumatic experience over and over again as if it has just happened at that particular time. Other biological factors may also contribute to these problems.

PTSD can affect anybody—man or woman, child or adult, young or old. PTSD is present in every culture because traumatic events happen in every culture. People in different cultures may react differently to traumatic experiences based on their cultural beliefs and cultural training. Some people experience PTSD shortly after the traumatic event, and some may not experience the PTSD for years. It is poorly understood as to why some people re-experience the trauma immediately and why some re-experience the trauma much later in life.

It is unfortunate that people who are experiencing PTSD may not be treated kindly by the rest of society. Others are easily turned off by their behavior and may consider them as irresponsible or dysfunctional people. It is also unfortunate that many people with PTSD do not get help because they cannot identify or understand what they are experiencing. People with poor social support and poor coping skills are not likely to do well in coping with PTSD as compared to people with good family, social, and community support. Some people may also turn to their religion to cope with the trauma. Some of the victims always feel that they can deal with the situation on their own. If there is no improvement over a period of time, professional help must be sought.

A conclusive diagnosis must be made by a certified clinician who is professionally qualified to make such a diagnosis in that community. These usually include a specialist in the area of psychiatry, psychology, nursing, and general medicine. Several factors are taken into consideration in making the diagnosis, especially a comprehensive history of the client. There are special clinics established by the government of the United States of America to treat veterans of war with PTSD. There are also qualified clinicians and treatment programs in different communities that could help the general public with the treatment of PTSD. The goal of the clinician is to help the victim of PTSD see the world differently and to understand that they could not have been able to do anything to prevent the event that produced the trauma from happening.

In addition to therapy, medication management is also helpful. There are many medications available to help the client cope with and minimize the symptoms of anxiety, depression, irritability, anger, intrusive recollections, and flashbacks. The type of medication to be prescribed is determined by the individual's history, and a comprehensive health assessment by the clinician. The symptoms the client is experiencing at the time of the assessment are also taken into consideration.

Support groups for victims of PTSD are also helpful. Victims share their experiences with others who have survived the same or similar trauma. Victims realize that they are not alone, and they are not abnormal—they are just traumatized. Victims also learn how others are coping with the illness. The importance of a good support group should not be underestimated because a support group is very instrumental to recovery from PTSD. The family members of the victim must also seek professional help, and attend a joint help session with the victim if possible. It is important to deal with possible issues of neglect, physical, and psychological abuse from the victim of PTSD toward his family.

## Panic Disorder:
# BASIC FACTS & UNDERSTANDING

A *panic attack* is a sudden overwhelming feeling of intense and disabling anxiety or fear and apprehension, resulting in physical and psychological symptoms in the victim. Some of the symptoms may include palpitations (rapid heartbeat), sweating, chest pain, dizziness, feeling choked, fear of dying, fainting, feelings of losing one's mind, numbness, shortness of breath, trembling, overwhelming feelings of doom, tension, and extreme irrational fear. An average person has experienced at least one episode of a panic attack somewhere along the line in his or her life. Such sporadic experiences of panic that we may have experienced or have happened to us every once in a while does not constitute a panic disorder. If panic attacks become recurrent to the point of incapacitation, and the victim is unable to carry on the normal day-to-day activities, the diagnosis of panic disorder is made. It is primarily characterized by a crescendo or bouts of fear and apprehension in the victim and the victim in turn manifests several physical and psychological or mental symptoms in response to the frequent panic attacks.

Some people are able to pinpoint or identify the time they had the very first panic attack; it could be at a time they were under a lot of stress. For instance, the stress of starting a new job can trigger an attack. This type of stress is called situational trigger. The majority of the people suffering from panic disorder cannot pinpoint a particular stressor or trigger, but they usually have a recollection of the very first time they experienced a panic attack. The first experience might have occurred while they were engaged in a daily routine activity like shopping, driving to work, or being at the movie theatre. The sensation comes all of a sudden, and they may feel as if they are about to die from a heart attack. If they have subsequent attacks or bouts of attacks after the first one, they may believe that they have a life-threatening illness and also fear for their safety pending the next attack. They might make life changes to be sure that they are in a safe environment when the next one strikes.

Victims of panic disorder may end up with self-imposed house arrest, believing that their house is the only safe haven or the only place where they are free from harm. They may initially go doctor shopping, which is visiting one doctor after the other in an effort to get a confirmation that they have a deadly illness. The significant others or family members may get frustrated and resentful of the victim because the disorder interferes with the equilibrium or the day-to-day functioning and maintenance of the family. For instance, the disorder can put tremendous stress on the significant other, such as the spouse, if the spouse suffering from panic disorder suddenly quits his or her job. This could, in turn, put undue financial pressure on the family. It may require one spouse working two jobs in order to support the family.

As usual with many mental illnesses, the biological causes are identified with an abnormal level or dysregulation of certain neurotransmitters in the human brain. Neurotransmitters are certain naturally occurring chemicals in the brain. The proportions or levels in which these chemicals occur in the brain affect our mental functioning. Too little or too much of some of these neurotransmitters can produce overt manifestation of certain commonly experienced mental problems. There are some other biological factors that could also be involved.

Panic disorder can strike at any age. Some people may experience it in the early adolescent years, some in the adult years, and some when they are much older or become senior citizens. It is important to seek professional help in order to make sure that the bout of panic attack is not caused by an underlying medical problem. For example, somebody with the history of heart attacks or heart problems may develop panic attacks from excessively worrying about death. In such a situation, both the medical and the psychiatric conditions must be addressed. A knowledgeable, licensed, and qualified clinician in the field of medicine or mental health should make the diagnosis.

Medication management and therapy are essential in the treatment of panic disorder. The choice of medication to be prescribed must be strictly determined by a licensed clinician based on the client's comprehensive history and health assessment. Unfortunately, some of the medications used in the treatment of panic disorder are addictive. This is one more reason why a client should be under the supervision of a licensed clinician when on medication. Some of these medications are carefully tapered off when the disorder is resolved. Medication treatment for panic disorder may require a combination of medications.

In addition to medication, individual therapy is also important in the treatment of panic attacks or disorder. Part of the goal of the therapy is to help improve the quality of life of the victim by helping the victim to think differently and to see the world differently. The world must not be seen as a dangerous place. A client must be encouraged to change his or her behavior and to give up their fears. The therapist may help the client realize that his fears are irrational, that he can gradually resume normal functioning and have a fruitful life. Deep breathing exercises may also help to relieve anxiety in a person suffering from panic attacks.

A support group is also very important. Clients learn from others in the group and share their experiences with one another since they are all experiencing similar symptoms. Being able to talk about their fears in a non-judgmental environment could be very therapeutic and healthy to the mind. They can discuss different ways to cope and learn new ways of not giving in to the fears. Support groups also provide a sense of relief to the victims of panic attacks when they realize that they are not the only one on the face of the planet struggling with this particular mental disorder. Family members of clients with panic disorder may also need family therapy sessions with the clients. It is also important for family members to join an independent family support group where they can learn how to live with their family member who is suffering from panic attacks. The family could also learn to help the victim make a healthy and successful transition to a normal and functioning life, without being enmeshed with the victim or encouraging dependency.

## Phobia:
# BASIC FACTS & UNDERSTANDING

A *phobia* is a persistent irrational fear of a specific object, activity, or situation that causes the person experiencing the phobia to have a compelling desire to avoid the feared object, the feared activity, or the feared situation at all costs. The person experiencing the phobia recognizes that the fear is excessive, irrational, and unrealistic; nevertheless, he cannot make himself stop from going to the greatest lengths to avoid the fear. When the compelling desire to avoid that which is feared interferes with a person's ability to function on a daily basis, the diagnosis of phobia is made.

People battling phobias can encounter *anticipatory anxiety*, which means already getting anxious just from the thought of encountering the object that they fear. For instance, somebody who is scared of snakes and is going on a field trip to a zoo may be experiencing dizziness just from the thought of visiting the zoo and the possibility of seeing a snake in the zoo. It must be noted that not every phobia requires treatment. If avoiding the feared object does not interfere with the person's quality of life significantly, the phobia can be ignored. For instance, somebody who is afraid of water may avoid swimming, going on a cruise, a lake, a bridge, or to the beach. If he is afraid of going on a bridge, he may choose to live and work in a community where he will not have to go on a bridge, or he may find alternative route to his destination that would not require him to go on a bridge. This may not severely interfere with that person's overall quality of life, although it is still perceived as an unhealthy limitation on the life of that person. On the other hand, when the object feared paralyzes a person with phobia and puts limitations on certain important areas of that person's life, the phobia must be addressed with treatment of some sort. A good example would be that of a person who works in the media and suddenly develops sociaphobia (fear of public places). He or she may find it very difficult to be in public places. Definitely such a phobia must be addressed because it interferes with that person's means of making a living. A television anchor going around to interview people would definitely not be able to make a living with extreme fear of going to public places.

There are numerous types of phobia, but some common examples are:

- Acrophobia or fear of heights
- Agoraphobia or fear of open space
- Claustrophobia or fear of closed space
- Glossophobia or fear of talking
- Hematophobia or fear of blood
- Hydrophobia or fear of water
- Monophobia or fear of being alone
- Mysophobia or fear of germs
- Sociophobia or fear of public place
- Xenophobia or fear of strangers
- Zoophobia or fear of animals

*Acrophobia* or fear of height may cause the victims to avoid living or working in a high-rise building. They may also have difficulty going on a plane or going on rides in amusement parks. *Agoraphobia* or fear of open space may cause the victims to avoid open spaces. For instance, they may not be able to go to a rally or an amusement park. They may not even want to get out of the house and may end up locking themselves up in the house for years if the illness is not treated. *Claustrophobia* or fear of closed space may make the victims avoid closed space, especially if there is a perception that there may be no escape if something should happen while in that environment. Such people may not want to go to the attic, closed basement, ride in an underground train, go in an elevator, or go into a tunnel. *Hematophobia* or fear of blood can make the victims pass out at the sight of blood. People who have a phobia for blood may avoid choosing a profession that would put them in constant contact with blood. For instance, a person who desires very much to be a nurse or a doctor may choose to be a teacher to avoid contact with blood.

*Hydrophobia* or fear of water can make a person avoid driving on a bridge, taking a vacation by the sea or a lake, going to a huge water park, or even going near a swimming pool. They may never dare to learn how to swim or to encourage people close to them like their spouse or children to learn how to swim. *Mysophobia* or fear of germs may cause the victims to be afraid of germs or dirt to the extent of going extra miles to keep their environment free of germs. They may continuously disinfect their environment and invest a lot of money in buying different cleaning products. They may also avoid places where they believe they could catch germs such as a hospital. They may never be able to use a public restroom or toilet. *Sociophobia* or fear of public place may cause its victim to avoid going to public places. They may be afraid of humiliation or embarrassment in a situation where they must interact with other people. They may develop severe anxiety in social setting and avoid public speaking or eating in a public place. They may chronically seek isolation to avoid social interaction. *Zoophobia* or people afraid of animals may not like the sight of any animal, including domestic pets. They may develop severe anxiety if a cat or a dog comes close to them. They may avoid situations that could put them in contact with animals, such as not visiting a friend or family who has a pet. Going to a zoo or taking their children to a zoo would definitely not be a consideration for them.

The cause of phobia is poorly understood. There are different ongoing studies in the scientific world about the cause of phobia. Biochemical theory points to an excessive production of certain neurotransmitters. As mentioned earlier in the discussion of other mental illnesses, neurotransmitters are some naturally occurring chemicals produced in the brain. Excessive or insufficient production of certain neurotransmitters could cause overt manifestation of mental illness. Other biological factors may also be involved.

Phobia affects men and women equally, and anybody in any age group can experience phobia. Phobia affects people in most societies. Individual reaction or the degree of anxiety experienced may be different from culture to culture, based on cultural training or cultural reaction to fear.

Professional help must be sought when phobia interferes with or imposes limitations on a person's life; otherwise, the phobia can be ignored and not aggressively treated. Treatment is recommended only in severe situations. A qualified clinician must be consulted for the treatment of phobia. Part of the treatment goal is to help the people experiencing phobia change the way they think about the object they fear, or change the way they see the object that produces the fear. As a result, they can react differently, get rid of their fear, and change their behavior in regard to the feared object.

A very widely used technique in the treatment of phobia is called *systemic desensitization*. A person experiencing phobia is presented to the stimulus or the object that is producing the fear gradually until that object no longer produces fear or anxiety in that person. For instance, a person who is afraid of snakes is first asked to visualize a snake, then look at the picture of a snake, then watch a snake on a television, then watch a live snake in a cage, and finally touched a non-poisonous snake in cage until the person is no longer afraid of snakes. Another technique that may be very stressful for the client is called *flooding*. With flooding, a person is repeatedly exposed to the feared object or stimulus until the anxiety response decreases; for example, making somebody who is afraid of the elevator go up and down in the elevator several times continuously until he is no more afraid of going on the elevator. Flooding may be very stressful for some people. It is better done in a controlled, supervised environment with a professional. Flooding may not be a good option for everybody battling with phobia because the stress reaction to the object feared may outweigh the benefit of treating the phobia.

People with phobias may also participate in group therapy or support groups. Group members could share their experiences of how they managed to live with and eventually conquered their fear. Learning from one another and providing support to one another is always beneficial to people struggling with phobia.

## Obsessive Compulsive Disorder:
# BASIC FACTS & UNDERSTANDING

In understanding *obsessive compulsive disorder* (OCD), the reader must understand what an obsession is and what a compulsion is. *Obsessions* are unwarranted persistent thoughts, impulses, and images that a person perceives in his or her mind to be senseless and intrusive, but the person is unable to make them go away or to ignore them. For instance, a person who believes that he is going to get germs from touching a knob would have an intrusive thought of getting germs pop into his mind every time he touches a door knob, and would become anxious and obsessed with the fear of getting germs. Obsessions produce severe anxiety in the person experiencing the obsession, and he performs a compulsion or a compulsive act immediately to relieve the anxiety.

*Compulsions* are basically ritualistic, repetitive behaviors that a person engages in to neutralize the anxiety provoked by an obsession. A person is constantly and uncontrollably driven to perform the compulsion in order to neutralize his irrational belief that something dreadful or catastrophic would happen to him if he does not perform the compulsive act. A person who has the obsessive thought that he would contract and be infected with germs by touching a doorknob performs the compulsive ritual by rushing to wash his hands every time he touches a door knob. He believes that if he does not wash his hands, he will die from an infection from germs he was in contact with from the doorknob. A person going through the rituals of obsession and compulsion is said to be suffering from obsessive compulsive disorder, commonly called OCD.

Giving in to the compulsion is primarily meant to bring a permanent relief of the tension and severe anxiety provoked by the obsession. Unfortunately, performing the compulsion only produces a temporary relief of the anxiety, and the obsessive thought immediately repeats itself. As a result, the compulsive act must be repeated over and over again, and the person goes around in circles. A lot of anxiety builds up whenever a person with OCD tries not to give in to the compulsion, and he or she will eventually give in. The behavior becomes an infinite task, very time consuming and incapacitating. A good example is that of a person running in and out of the house several times on his way to work, checking to see if the stove has been turned off. Despite the fact that he knows that the stove is off, the thought keeps popping into his head that the stove may still be on and he may burn the house down. He keeps responding to the thought by running back to the house to check the stove over and over again. He knows in his mind that his action is irrational, but he cannot stop it.

Everybody must have experienced an obsession or compulsion somewhere down the line in life; it becomes a disorder when it interferes with activities of daily living or ability to function. When people have to accommodate the obsession and the compulsion into their daily routine to the point that it slows down or completely shuts down other areas of their lives, they need to seek professional help. There are many certified clinicians who could help with the treatment of OCD.

OCD can affect everybody—man or woman, child or an adult, young or elderly, rich or poor. In most cases no precipitating factor could be found for the disorder. OCD can start gradually and progressively get worse. Again, the biochemical theory in the development of OCD has focused on the dysregulation or abnormal regulation of the neurotransmitters, which are naturally occurring chemicals in the human brain. Excessive production or insufficient production of some of these naturally occurring chemicals has been found to be responsible for many mental illnesses, including OCD. Some special types of x-rays of the brain also point to some abnormality in the frontal lobe (the frontal portion of the brain) of a person with OCD. Other biological factors may also be involved.

The diagnosis of OCD must be made by a certified, knowledgeable and licensed clinician in the medical or mental health related field who is qualified to make the diagnosis in that community. It must be noted that a person may have obsession with compulsion or a compulsion without an obsession. To meet the diagnosis of OCD, the obsession and the compulsion could exist together or it could be obsession or compulsion only. People with OCD sometimes suffer from some other mental illnesses such as depression. The daily struggle of dealing with a nerve-wracking and time-consuming disorder like OCD is enough to throw anybody into depression. OCD can cause so much distress to the point of interfering with occupational and social functioning. Some people with OCD are totally paralyzed by the disorder to the point of isolating self from the rest of the world, and they may eventually die from the disorder. For instance, a person who locks himself up in the room because of fear of being contaminated by germs may eventually die from starvation, social isolation, and lack of communication with the outside world.

There are many medications used in the treatment of OCD; the appropriate medication for an individual must be determined by a licensed clinician. The underlying depression that could accompany OCD can also be treated with medication. As mentioned earlier, it is not very likely for a person to be a happy OCD client. Therapy is also important in the treatment of OCD. Some clients do well on therapy alone, and some are able to cope and to stay in recovery by using a combination of medication and therapy. Part of the treatment goal in therapy is to help the client change the way he thinks and responds to the obsession and the compulsion. In addition to changing the way he thinks, he must also modify his behavior in response to the obsession and the compulsion.

One of the behavior modification intervention used in the treatment of OCD is called *flooding*. For instance, somebody who is afraid of touching doorknobs and washes his hands excessively after touching a doorknob may be kept in a treatment facility for three days with no option to leave. In that three-day period, he would be mandated to open doors and to touch doorknobs without being allowed to wash his hands. He would be under strict supervision until he becomes less anxious and less sensitive, and he is able to open the doors without washing his hands every single time he opens a door. Flooding is a continuous or massive exposure of the client to the anxiety-provoking situation or object of fear, until he becomes less sensitive to it. Flooding may produce excessive anxiety in some people; it must be used with caution under professional supervision. Another treatment approach is called *response prevention*. For example, somebody who is afraid of setting the house on fire and is constantly going back and front to the house to check if the stove is off would not be allowed to go back to the house to check the stove. This means he is not responding to the obsession until he is accustomed to ignoring the obsession. Any of the treatment approaches should be under the supervision of a certified clinician.

Relaxation exercise and techniques may also be beneficial for people with OCD. The goal is to take their minds off their obsessions and compulsions. For example, somebody who checks the stove obsessively could set his mind on going for a long leisurely walk, using it as a distraction and a form of relaxation. The long leisurely walk allows him to refuse to give in to the compulsion of checking the stove. Whenever he has the obsessive thought that the house will catch fire, he will ignore it and his focus would be the walk. Active or passive exercises, music, a warm bath, and meditation are all common examples of healthy ways to relax and to ignore the obsession. Depending on the individual, it may require an extended time of therapy before some people with OCD could learn to relax and to give up their obsession and compulsion.

Support groups may also be very helpful for people suffering form OCD. A good support group is like a family. The people in the group come to the realization that they are not alone in their struggles with OCD. Each member would have an opportunity to grow and to learn from one another as they all contribute to the group positively.

Another type of obsessive behavior called *obsessive compulsive personality disorder (OCPD)* is usually confused with obsessive compulsive disorder *(OCD)* that was earlier discussed. To help the reader understand these two disorders, let's look at the differences between the two. Obsessive compulsive disorder (OCD) is an anxiety-related problem, whereas obsessive compulsive personality disorder (OCPD) is a personality-related problem. Unlike people with OCD, people with OCPD do not have to deal with the continuous intrusive thoughts popping into their heads (obsession), and the compulsive ritual in response to the thought (compulsion) which is the hallmark or a constant struggle in the case of OCD.

On the other hand, OCPD people are preoccupied with perfectionism, orderliness, efficiency, mental, and interpersonal control at the expense of flexibility. They are their own taskmasters. They drive themselves crazy in an effort to create perfection in everything. They are preoccupied with details, rules, lists, orderliness, and organization or schedules to the extent that the major point of the activity is lost. The preoccupation of OCPD people with perfectionism interferes with their ability to complete tasks. For instance, if they have a project due, they may work on it so long that it would become almost impossible to get to the final product. They never believe that whatever effort they put into the project was good enough at any point in time. They are constantly busy trying to achieve perfection until they lose track of what they are supposed to do.

OCPD people usually turn others off because of their inflexibility and preoccupation with perfection. They may end up being alienated from others because nobody wants to work with them. They do not know how to relax or to enjoy freedom. They could be excessively devoted to their work to the exclusion of leisure. They do not take vacations or even take their weekends off. Every second is occupied in their world. They have no time for friends or socialization, despite the fact that there may be no economic justification for their excessive work. They are very rigid and are unable to deal with spontaneity. They are overly conscientious and scrupulous. They are very strict about matters of morality and religion. They can be very stubborn or seriously influenced by their inflexibility. They must have their way or no other way.

OCPD people may be insensitive to the feelings of others, and they may not be able to warm up or to express emotion to others. Since they cannot relax, they may end up living an emotionally barren life. They may not be able to discard worn-out or worthless objects; they are usually pack rats. They hold on to worthless objects even when there is no sentimental use or value attached to the objects. They do not believe that others can do things as well as they can do them. As a result, they cannot delegate responsibility. They are always overexerted from trying to do everything on their own. They may be miserly to others and themselves. They hoard everything, including money. They worry too much about future catastrophes and of destitution or possible lack in the future. This line of thinking is used to justify hoarding and miserliness.

People with OCPD can be very difficult to live with because life to them is strictly about lists and order. For instance, every can must be labeled in the cabinet and arranged in a certain way. Every towel must be folded and arranged in a certain way, the bed must be made in a certain way with no wrinkles every morning, the shoes must be arranged in a certain way, and the list goes on endlessly. They get very upset when things are changed in their environment. They see things only in one way, and they expect the rest of the world to compromise. Their inability to tolerate change could make life very stressful for them. For instance, if they have to go to another part of the world with a time difference of seven hours, they may be in serious distress when compelled to change their personal habits such as reading the newspaper, drinking coffee, and having a bowel movement at a certain programmed time of the morning.

OCPD people usually want to extend the day beyond twenty-four hours. They are always stressed out, and they never have enough time to finish anything. Since OCPD is a personality disorder, it is usually difficult to change. It takes a lifetime for a person to form or develop certain personality traits and to learn certain behaviors, and it may take a long time to unlearn and modify such behaviors. Professional help may be needed in the treatment of OCPD.

On the "healthy" end of OCPD is the *obsessive compulsive personality trait*. People with the traits have some similar characteristics of people with OCPD but they are not excessive. People with obsessive compulsive personality traits could be very successful because they are detail oriented and organized without taking everything to the extreme. They could be successful scientists, technicians, corporate executives, academicians, and straight-A students. They are usually an asset to any establishment because they have the zeal for excellence and distinction without driving other people insane.

OCPD has both genetic (hereditary factors) and environmental components to it. It is believed that if a child has controlling parents or controlling parental figures and the child was over-disciplined when growing up, the child could have OCPD as an adult. It is also believed that children whose parents have OCPD could have OCPD from learning this behavior from their parents or parental figures.

Diagnosis must be made by a licensed clinician who is knowledgeable in making such diagnosis. Medications have not been proven to be effective in the treatment of OCPD. The first line of treatment is not medication intervention. Gradual behavior modification may be helpful. The goal is to point out the maladaptive or dysfunctional behavior to the clients and to teach them an alternative or a more adaptive and less stressful way of achieving the same result. This is especially important in the areas of delegating responsibility. Another way to help people with OCPD is to help them see the world differently and think differently, without feeling as if they are losing control. It is important for them to learn interpersonal and social skills and realize that the world does not revolve around them or cater to their needs only.

Relaxation exercise and simple relaxation techniques may also be helpful for people with OCPD. Common examples are deep breathing techniques, listening to music, leisure walking, having a warm bath, and meditating. Group therapy can also be helpful, because a group setting may be a safe place for them to be confronted with their maladaptive behavior. They could also learn from others and share their experiences with others.

## Generalized Anxiety Disorder (GAD):
# BASIC FACTS & UNDERSTANDING

The major characteristic of *general anxiety disorder (GAD)* is excessive worrying and anxiety. People with general anxiety disorder (GAD) feel very helpless and unable to control their worries. They are usually tense and easily irritable. They may have difficulty concentrating or may easily go blank. There may be a legitimate reason for concern in the mind of the worrier, but the worrying is usually out of proportion to the reason for the concern. For instance, the wife of a pilot who worries every time her husband flies finds herself awake most of the night and is unable to function effectively or to concentrate during the day. Definitely, there is a legitimate reason for her to be afraid because people rarely survive a plane crash. However, the chance of a plane crashing is so remote compared to the number of car accidents on the ground. More people die everyday from car accidents compared to the possible death from a plane crash.

People with GAD may get on other people's nerves and may become very annoying with their out of proportion worries. Others may be very impatient with them and try to avoid them. They may be very difficult to work with because decision-making can be very difficult or almost impossible for them. They are usually restless and are keyed up most of the time. They are always on the edge, and always complain of feeling tired a lot. They may have difficulty falling asleep. They may wake up very frequently in the night and feel as if they did not get any sleep at all when they wake up in the morning. Their worry list is endless—they thrive on worrying, and they have to have something to worry about twenty-four hours a day. They could stress themselves out worrying about the weather, if it will be too cold or too hot, and worry about if it will rain and if the rain would be heavy or not.

They are afraid of making mistakes, and they anticipate future problems and worry about these anticipated problems. They may worry about picking the right clothes to wear to work in the morning, and worry all day long that their makeup might not have been applied properly. People with GAD are found in most societies. People could have the disorder at any age—as a child, as a young adult, as an adult, and in the older years of life.

Again, the biological cause of GAD is attributed to the dysregulation or abnormal regulation of certain naturally occurring chemicals in the brain called the neurotransmitters. Appropriate regulation of the neurotransmitters in the brain has a lot to do with our mental health and well-being. When there is an abnormality in the composition or level of certain neurotransmitters in the brain, there could be a visible manifestation of mental illness. Other biological factors may also be involved. There is a hereditary or genetic factor implicated in GAD. People with this disorder are likely to have a family history of relatives suffering from or who have suffered from this disorder.

It is very important to know that the diagnosis of GAD could be missed very easily, because people with this disorder usually function with it. The red flag is the level of anxiety of the victims, which usually affects their efficiency. Since GAD is poorly diagnosed, it is easy to overlook the signs and symptoms, play it down, or not to take it very seriously. Some people with GAD may have other psychological or mental problems that have not been diagnosed, such as depression. This could be detected during a comprehensive assessment with a clinician. Several reasons including childhood loss or separation issues are also attributed to the cause of GAD.

There is the tendency for people with GAD to self-medicate with alcohol and drugs. This is usually done in an effort to help them relax or calm down from their continuous worries. They may also be addicted to medications that would help them to relax and sleep. Usually, when GAD is treated, the drug abuse may cease. Every case of GAD may not necessarily need professional help. We all need a little bit of anxiety in our lives to be motivated, meet deadlines, get to work on time, pass our examinations, and carry out our daily activities. However, if anxiety compromises our efficiency, concentration, and sleep and makes us tired, keyed up, irritable and edgy, these may be more severe signs and symptoms of GAD. Professional help may be needed at that point. We must always remember that the intensity of the vegetative or the day-to-day symptoms of GAD are not always severe, and we must be very careful to not ignore them.

A certified, knowledgeable, and licensed clinician who could make such diagnosis in that community should be consulted. A very thorough assessment is usually done by the clinician, and the course of treatment would be determined based on the assessment of the clinician and the symptoms of the client.

Part of the treatment goal is to help change the way clients see the world around them, so their level of worrying is no longer out of proportion. If they realize that terrible things are not always happening to all the people they worried about over the years, and their anticipated disasters usually do not happen, they may be able to control their worries. Medication management is not the first option in the management of GAD. However, it may be necessary initially to control the anxiety, depending on the individual and the severity or the seriousness of the symptoms presented. Medication must be carefully introduced and carefully tapered off as soon as the symptoms improve. This is to prevent the clients from becoming addicted to the medications.

Relaxation exercises are also beneficial to people with GAD. Some commonly available relaxation exercises that can be practiced at home include meditating, reading, having a warm bath, watching a relaxing movie, and listening to soothing music. For example, listening to a music that depicts the sound of the ocean waves could allow the listener to mentally visualize sitting on a beach. This exercise could be very relaxing.

A support group may also be beneficial to the people with GAD. Their interaction with other members of the group can make them realize that they are not alone in their struggle with this disorder. Family therapy may also be beneficial for family members of someone suffering from GAD. It is always helpful when family members have a good understanding of what is going on with their loved one. It enables families to cope better. They can help to steer their loved one to the right path and call to his or her attention the excessive worries. Family members could also learn to ignore some of the worries and not feed into them. Recovery is always better and faster with good family support and family understanding of the illness.

# PART IX
# COMMON PROBLEMS RELATED TO CHILD AND ADOLESCENTS

## Conduct Disorder:
# JANINE'S STORY

J anine grew up as the sweetest little girl; she was adorable, and everybody loved her precious smile and warmth. She was the middle child, with an older brother and a younger brother. Janine never met a stranger; she was a sociable and outgoing child. When she was in middle school, around age twelve, we started to notice some changes in her, such as telling frequent lies. We got many notes from the teachers because she was getting into fights at school. Her grades were dropping, and she was not doing her homework or studying for her tests. She was also skipping classes to hang out with or to be around her friends.

Initially, we thought she was going through the typical preadolescent struggles, and she would get over it. We set firm limits with her and took away a lot of privileges. As parents, we did not think we had too much to worry about, because we believed we did the best we could by teaching our children good values and modeling good behavior to them. We spent constructive time with them; they were not neglected, and we were able to provide for all of their basic needs. We just automatically assumed that they should be fine and would grow up to be responsible adults.

As Janine grew older, the problems grew worse. She was obsessed with boys, and was preoccupied with being popular and being accepted in her school by her peers. She constantly talked on the phone to her friends far into the middle of the night. We tried to monitor her time on the phone as much as possible, but when we would go to bed, she would find her way back to the phone and would stay up half of the night talking. Our first shock came when she was fourteen; we got a call from a police officer from a mall telling us that she had been caught shoplifting. She was arrested for stealing, but was released to us later by the police officer. She had to go to juvenile court and had to do community service. The judge was lenient on her because she was a first-time offender; she had no previous history of stealing in the public. It was such an embarrassment for us as parents that our child was caught stealing. Other people who knew our family walked onto the scene when she was being questioned and arrested by the police because the mall was a public place, and the city where we lived was not a very big city.

The situation got worse from then on, despite our efforts to set firm limits with her. She became very rebellious and argumentative. She was not even willing to accept any personal responsibility for her behavior. She would make statements like "All teenagers shoplift; I was just the one who got caught this time, and it is not a big deal." What we identified as the biggest problem with Janine was her group of friends, and all of our efforts to separate her from her friends failed.

Janine went from making weak grades to failing outright in school. We started finding cigarettes and condoms in her school bag whenever we did a random search. Obviously she was sexually active, and she would not even entertain any discussion about her sexual activities with us. Whenever we brought it up, she would tell us that her sexual life was not any of our business. We sought professional help for her in an outpatient counseling setting, but there was no improvement in her behavior. Her psychiatrist recommended a short-term hospitalization for her, which she very much hated. She came back and acted remorseful for a few weeks, but went back to the same set of friends and started acting out again. We started finding bottles of alcohol in her room. She was coming home late and sneaking out of the house at night. My husband and I would be driving around the town at two o'clock in the morning, trying to find Janine. Eventually, she dropped out of high school. She started running the streets at nights, going to clubs and parties. She was arrested at one time in the company of her teenage friends as an accomplice to a crime for trying to rob a store. She had to spend some time in the juvenile lockup for it.

Janine's behavior was tearing the family apart. There was a lot of blaming and finger-pointing, despite the fact that we could not really pinpoint anything that we had done wrong raising her as parents. After all, her siblings who were raised in the same house were doing well; they had their own fair share of teenage troubles, but not anything out of control like Janine's. Our other two children were partially neglected because Janine became a drain on the family, but they handled it fairly well. Janine was in and out of the juvenile court system and had about five short-term inpatient admissions in a mental hospital. Janine exhausted all of the insurance coverage we had on her for hospitalization. At a point, everybody in the house was constantly quarreling with each other, without realizing that we were all reacting to the stress that Janine was putting on the family.

## Winds Against The Mind

As the pressure and the stress gradually got worse, Janine's younger brother started to show signs of depression. Janine's older brother dealt with the situation by staying busy and working very hard all the time. All of a sudden, our oldest son became the peacemaker in the house. He was always trying to appease everybody to make sure the family was not completely destroyed. I developed hypertension from worrying about Janine, and I was not sleeping well. I found myself complaining of pain all the time and no medication would make the pain go away. My pain was apparently emotional, not physical; all the pain was from my unsettled and troubled mind.

Janine became both a financial and emotional drain on the family. She was drinking, smoking, and using illicit drugs. She pawned a lot of my jewelry and valuables in the house to support her drug habits. She stole from us and her older brother. She even forged our signatures to collect money from our bank accounts. It was very difficult as parents to live with such terrible pain and disappointment and also try to carry out our regular routine of going to work and maintaining a family. You walk around all the time wondering what will happen next. Every time the phone rang, our hearts raced, wondering what the phone call was going to be. My husband and I gradually started slipping into depression because we did not know what to do next. Our oldest son came to us one day and said 'I have lost my sister, and I don't want to lose my parents.' At that point, we decided to seek professional help as a family.

In the course of the family session, the doctor recommended that we put Janine in a long-term hospitalization program. Her outpatient therapist had already suggested it, but when we looked into the cost, it was about fifty thousand dollars a year, and it was not covered by our health insurance policy. There was no way for us to come up with that amount of money; we already had huge debts from Janine's frequent hospitalization and insurance deductibles. Our family health insurance coverage was not one hundred percent reimbursement for services provided, and we had to work out monthly payment plans to pay the remaining part of the bill that was not covered by the insurance policy.

Finally out of desperation, my husband insisted that we had to give her a final and last chance at getting her life back on track. She had only a year until she turned eighteen, after which she might end up in an adult jail. We put all of our resources together; my husband took on a second job, and I took on a part-time weekend job. We even cashed out some of our retirement benefits and borrowed money on our house. Our oldest son even volunteered to help us out financially, but we refused to accept his financial help. He was literarily putting himself through college by working to pay his own tuition.

# Winds Against The Mind

Finally, we sent Janine away to a wilderness program. It was supposed to last for one to two years, depending on how much progress the child makes. The youth who participates in the program are usually evaluated after a year for their readiness to go home. Some get to leave, and some have to stay for two years, depending on how much progress they make. We prayed that one year would work for Janine because the thought of having to support her in the program for two years was not even conceivable for us as a family. It would almost be like putting us in financial bankruptcy. We knew we would do it if we had to, but it was not something to look forward to.

Janine was very angry about going to the wilderness program. It was a very structured program with full supervision. Among other things, the youth participants were taught how to cope with peer pressure, get their priorities right, treat themselves and others with dignity, and stay away from drugs and alcohol. Further, they developed a sense of values, became accountable for themselves and others, and developed positive self-esteem, as well as forging a goal and a vision in life for themselves. The program was intense, and we were impressed with its goals and outcomes. The goal was primarily to modify the behavior of the youth so that they could become responsible adults. Medication management was also included as part of the program if the youth needed to be on medication. We were only allowed one visit a month.

The first month when we visited Janine, she refused to talk to us because she was angry with us for putting her into the program. The therapist suggested that we stay away for one month, so we visited again the third month. We were so shocked at the new person who we saw on our next visit. Janine was making sense for the first time in a long time, telling us she had turned her life around, and she planned to be a better person. We took everything she said with a grain of salt, because we did not know if it was one of her usual tricks, or if it was real this time. At every visit, we had family sessions. In one of the sessions, Janine broke down and cried; she apologized for all the problems that she had created for us financially and emotionally. We were shocked to see a very remorseful Janine; it was like watching somebody else's child. She had never shown any remorse in a long time; she would blame everything on us and tell us it was all our faults. She had also frequently accused us of overreacting, saying that she was just like typical teenagers out there.

When it was getting closer for Janine to come home, we started having a lot of anxiety. We were not sure if the new person was going to be real or not. It was decided at the program that she was ready to go home after a year, so we brought her home to a warm reception. We gathered friends and family together to celebrate her coming home, and we had a toast to a wonderful life for Janine. It was very emotional for all of us, especially Janine. She broke down in tears and cried, promising to take a new turn for the better. She said she felt like the prodigal child, and she was grateful for the unconditional love shown to her. To our surprise, Janine changed her life around forever. She took a GED course (General Equivalent of Diploma) and passed her high school certification equivalent examination. She became more spiritual and became a youth leader in the community. Janine would tell her stories to different youth groups to encourage other youth to stay out of trouble. She enrolled in a community college and kept her grades up. She worked very hard and stayed completely out of trouble. She has become a source of inspiration for other teens in our community.

As a family, we went through a lot of hurt and pain, financial stress, and emotional loss. However, Janine's turnaround was the medication we needed to cure our hurt and pain. If your child is like our Janine, do not give up. There is a lot of help out there. It may take a couple of trials for your child to get it right, but the key is not to give up. Know that it is very convenient to give up, but you cannot give up. Remember you can make it if you keep on trying, but you must try, try and try, try and try. Stay with it until your child gets it right. Hopefully, it will not be too long.

# Quotes of Encouragement...

As the wind blows harder and Janine's story sounds familiar to you, remember the following:

*"The path is smooth that leadeth on to danger."*
                              *~ William Shakespeare*

Teenage truancy is always presented as fun; it is sometimes downplayed as what teenagers do. Fighting, stealing, drinking alcohol, using illicit drugs, and sexual promiscuity all feel and look like fun; unfortunately, these are pathways to destruction. Take an inventory and look at the possible consequences of your behavior: unwanted pregnancy, a child having a child, sexually transmitted diseases, addiction, jail, and the list goes on. Wake up from your deep sleep, because this is not fun, and it is a waste of your precious, youthful years. You are going to travel this road only once. It is impossible to gain back the lost years, take a moment to stop and think. *(LB)*

*"You are a product of your environment. So choose the environment that will best develop you toward your objective. Analyze your life in terms of its environment. Are the things around you helping you towards success—or are they holding you back?"*
                              *~ W. Clement Stone*

Choose your friends wisely, because the people you surround yourself with can make or break you. If you keep yourself in an environment of successful people, you are likely to succeed, but if you keep yourself in an environment of failures, you are likely to fail. What type of company are you keeping, and what type of friends are you surrounding yourself with? Don't forget that you are only young once, and everything has its season. Don't watch your life fly away in front of your eyes and let your season pass you by. *(LB)*

*"The little reed, bending to the forces of the wind, soon stood upright again when the storm had passed over."*
                              *~ Aesop*

If you have followed the wrong path and have made mistakes, be the come-back kid. It is never too late to turn your life around for the better. You cannot change the past, but you can change the present and the future. *(LB)*

<u>Autism:</u>

# DONNIE'S STORY

L ike many new parents, we were excited to have our son, Donnie. We felt prepared because we had waited for five years after marriage to have him. We were so happy about this baby that we drove everybody around us crazy! We read every book we could possibly read on babies, and we asked other parents as many questions as possible. When we found out that we were going to have a boy, our excitement doubled. It would not have made any difference to us if it was a boy or a girl, but we wanted a boy first if it was possible. We threw a small party to announce to our close friends and our family that we were going to have a boy. We planned to have two children hoping that one would be a boy and the other a girl. For us, this was fifty percent of our prayers answered. If the next baby turned out to be another boy, we would still love him very much anyway.

There was no dull moment in our lives for the nine months of the pregnancy. The joy was so great, and the delivery was a touching and memorable experience for us. Bringing Donnie to this world was a miracle for us. We took several pictures every week just to capture and to compare every developmental stage of Donnie. The pictures looked different every week as he grew older, which was very exciting. As he grew daily, we were hoping to see changes based on what we read in the books, but his growth process did not seem to match what we had read. The doctor and other parents assured us that not every child would follow textbook format for developmental growth, and there should not be any reason for us to be alarmed or concerned. Donnie was so adorable; we were too happy with him to have the time to focus on some of the early cues or signs of autism. The assurance from others that every child may not necessarily follow the textbook format of growth was good enough for us to not worry too much.

We started paying more attention as he grew older and he became more and more difficult to console when he cried. He also stiffened whenever we tried to hold him, and he did not like to be held. We noticed that he was not very affectionate or attached to us the way some other babies in his age group were attached to their parents. We loved to take his pictures at every opportunity we had, but we noticed that it really upset him every time we tried to take his picture. My husband played it off that he was trying to be a typical boy and be really tough. By the time he was two, it was obvious that his growth was not following typical developmental milestones. The doctor started preparing us for the possibility that he may be autistic, especially with a lack of speech at age two. We started getting a little scared, because we thought all along that whatever was going on with Donnie was temporary, and he would snap out of it.

As young new parents, we were not interested in learning about childhood developmental problems. It never crossed our mind for a second that something could be wrong with our child. As far as we were concerned, we thought the odds were in our favor as parents because we were young and healthy, and we continuously maintained a very healthy lifestyle. By the time Donnie was two and a half years, the pediatrician gave Donnie a conclusive diagnosis of autism. We knew very little about autism; we had the basic knowledge that it was a childhood developmental disorder and that was about all we knew. The doctor spent time with us, explaining the possible future challenges we would likely face in raising Donnie. We were so shocked and overwhelmed by the initial outpouring of information that was given to us. Since then, we have learned nearly everything one can learn about autism. Our knowledge grew very quickly because we live with somebody with autism, our own child.

Donnie would have the most terrible and violent temper tantrums with no trigger or basis for it; he would throw things around the house and bang his head on the floor. Donnie was a picky eater; he wanted to eat the same thing for breakfast, lunch, and dinner. Any little change in his environment would upset him. He liked oatmeal, and he could not understand why he was not allowed to eat oatmeal three times a day. We insisted and maintained most of the time that he should eat other food, but we would end every meal with oatmeal, or at least a little oatmeal with every meal to keep us from deviating from his routine. Oatmeal literally became a dessert for Donnie. Occasionally, we would not have any luck with making him eat anything other than oatmeal, and we would have to give in and let him eat oatmeal instead of letting him starve.

## Winds Against The Mind

We started noticing a lot of unusual behavior with him, such as rocking himself in a chair non-stop for hours. He preferred solitary play and did not want to be hugged or be around anybody. He would spin and rock back and front endlessly in a chair. He did not show any emotion; his affect (facial expression) was completely flat and expressionless. We took every early intervention advice to try to stimulate his interest, so when he showed a little interest in animal toys, we went and bought a puppy. He treated the puppy more like an object, and paid very little or no attention to it. We cuddled the puppy, and gave a lot of attention to the puppy in his presence to model affectionate behavior to him, hoping that it would get Donnie's attention and help with his socialization skills, but it was a failed effort. When the puppy grew older and started barking a lot, Donnie became very resentful of the puppy. He became very violent with the dog whenever the dog barked continuously. We later realized that the barking sound was affecting his nerves and his hearing, and we were forced to give the dog away.

We also discovered that Donnie found a way to take the telephone off the hook. Friends and families were always complaining that our telephone line was always busy. We did not realize that the ringing tone of the telephone was like a sharp knife cutting through Donnie's ear, which was why he found a way to take the phone off the hook. We had to shop for a telephone with very low and more soothing ringing tone. We constantly made adjustments around the house to make the world a less hurtful place for him. He hated the sound of the vacuum cleaner; we had to make sure we vacuumed the house only when he was not home. He enjoyed exerting his energy at the park whenever the park was not too busy and noisy. He loved the swing and the slides. He hated the sound of the washing machine and the dryer; the buzzing sound of the dryer when the clothes were dry made him very angry. The sound of the doorbell also got on his nerves, so we changed the doorbell to a more soothing, musical sound, and we continuously made every possible effort to accommodate him. Something as simple as the sound of the bathroom vent and the air conditioner irritated him.

He could not tolerate places with lots of noise, like an amusement park. It took some harsh experiences for us to figure out some of his dos and don'ts. We took him to see the fireworks on the Fourth of July one year; he hated it so much and reacted as if we were putting a knife through his throat. We had to take him back home as quickly as possible. He liked hiding in unusual places such as under the sofa, between the mattress and the box springs, and between the sliding closets doors that usually fold. We tried very hard to keep Donnie engaged, and made a conscious effort to interrupt him from escaping into his own private world. Living in his own world was exactly what he wanted to do all the time if we let him.

We realized that we had to prepare him for school and to encourage socialization as much as possible. We took him to speech therapy five days a week; we also went to social training and a behavior modification program. We gave him positive reinforcement whenever he responded to and got involved in his environment. One of the keys to our success with Donnie was that we took the warning from his therapist and his doctor very seriously that we must not allow him to be alone too frequently. The therapist emphasized that part of the symptoms of his illness was to shut the rest of the world out and to keep to himself in his own world. Keeping him engaged and involved was very draining on us, but we loved him so much that we would do anything as parents to help Donnie develop his socialization skills as much as possible. We kept Donne very busy and very structured until his bedtime.

Donnie's difficulty with communication made us result to trial and error most of the time in order for us to pinpoint his wants and needs, and it was especially difficult for us when he became aggressive. When he had some of the normal childhood illnesses like a headache, earache, or stomachache, he sometimes acted out because he could not communicate his problems to us. Donnie would walk around with a cut on his foot for days before we would finally notice the cut. We made sure we did a head-to-toe check on him daily. Donnie was fixated on the color green, and we tried as much as possible to buy mostly green clothes and green toys for him.

It was difficult to introduce any form of change to him, and making him accept that he could not wear the same clothes everyday was a big struggle. Donnie was very talented with drawing; he drew on everything in the house—walls, books, plastic bottles, clothes, and anything that he could possibly draw on. We spent a lot of time trying to work with him to draw mostly on a board and paper. Donnie's artistic talents really came out whenever he visited a place that interested him, or saw something that interested him. He would come home and reproduce what he saw in a beautiful art. He would see something on a billboard while we were driving and draw it exactly as it was on the billboard when we got home. We encouraged his artistic talents a lot. Donnie was also amazing with numbers.

With early intervention and unconditional love, Donnie did well, and he was able to mainstream into a regular school. We continued to keep him structured and involved with the rest of the world. We were very lucky with the wonderful teachers he had; they were always willing to work with him. He had some behavioral problems, especially with temper tantrums; we worked with him by setting firm limits and making sure there were no external triggers for his outburst. He got into a lot more trouble at lunch time in the school cafeteria, and we figured out that the noise in the cafeteria would trigger his outbursts. The teacher gave him an exception to get his food early from the cafeteria and to eat it at the back of the classroom. That took care of the cafeteria problem. He also got into trouble a lot at the gym whenever he experienced sensory overload; the noise in the gym irritated his nerves badly and made him act out. The gym teacher always picked up on the cue, and he would send him to the classroom where he quickly settled down.

We faced different challenges everyday with Donnie; one morning he went on a rampage of breaking things in the house because we ran out of oatmeal, and we could not give him oatmeal for breakfast. Donnie just could not deviate from his routine, and he would need a lot of preparation if there was going to be a change in his routine. We had to constantly prepare Donnie before school was out for the holidays and to reinforce it repeatedly to him that he would be on vacation soon, and he would not be going to school for some time. We also had to start preparing him long in advance to go on a family vacation.

Donnie has some limitations, but he has been able to live close to a normal life because of early intervention and extensive therapy. No matter how strong you are, you still wonder why this has happened to your son. It is a lot of financial and emotional stress. You give up so much in search of a close-to-normal life for your child. You also have to live with the rest of the world, because there are those who have no patience to understand your pain and your frustrations. We joined a support group and found out how lucky we are even with Donnie's limitations. There are a lot of other children with autism in the support group who are not responding very well to therapies and different interventions like Donnie. We found out that Donnie's autism is one of the milder ones. Donnie is responding well to medication and therapies.

To us, Donnie is our miracle, and we would not trade him for any other child in the world. We have learned a lot about life by being his parents. We love him unconditionally, and we are happy that Donnie is part of our lives. Despite the good and the bad times, we went on with our original plans to have another child. Our second miracle is a girl; we got exactly what we had hoped for. Our daughter's name is Charlene, and she is beautiful. We are grateful that she has no autism, and even if she did, we would not love her any less.

If you have an autistic child, do not give up or lose hope. Get help for your child. Behind the autism are wonderful beings and precious gifts from God. We hope and look forward to a day that there will be a cure for autism. We always allow Donnie to participate in research in search of a cure for autism. We hope that one day Donnie can look back and say, "I was one of the many autistic children who helped to find a cure for this illness."

# Quotes of Encouragement...

As the wind blows harder and Donnie's story sounds familiar to you, remember the following:

*"The hopeful man sees success where others see failure, sunshine where others see shadows and storm."*

*~ Orison Sweet Marden*

Raising an autistic child can be very challenging, but your mindset and your outlook about the situation will significantly influence your outcome; be hopeful and be determined to help your child to succeed and maximize his hidden potential in his own way. Don't give up, don't be discouraged, and remember that your child is special and special people need special attention. With perseverance, the sunshine will come after the shadows and storm, and when your child succeeds, you have succeeded as well. *(LB)*

*"One may walk over the highest mountain one step at a time."*

*~ John Wanamaker*

Raising an autistic child requires a lot of patience, so don't expect an overnight miracle—your miracle will come in stages. Be persistent; you may get frustrated, but don't stay frustrated. Remember it is not your child's fault; this is a journey you have to travel with your child one step at a time. The secret to helping your child unlock the puzzle lies in your dedication. Overdose on patience and perseverance. *(LB)*

*"Happiness does not come from doing easy work but from the afterglow of satisfaction that comes after the achievement of a difficult task that demanded our best."*

*~ Theodore I. Rubin*

Raising an autistic child demands the very best from both the parents and all the therapists involved with helping the child. It is definitely not an easy task; it requires a lot of time and energy to engage the child and to keep the child stimulated. Every little success the child makes is dependent upon the perseverance and the sacrifice of all involved. Reinforce and praise every little effort by the child, and the little step-by-step progress will bring you happiness and will make your effort and hard work worth it. *(LB)*

# Winds Against The Mind

## Attention Deficit Hyperactivity Disoder (ADHD):
# JUSTIN'S STORY

J ames and I were very young parents, and the best memory in our lives was the day Justin came into the world. We were very excited. We could not believe we had just had a child, it was a dream come true. We both screamed, "We did it!" All of the delivery room staff laughed hysterically at our announcement. Justin was handed over to us, and we cried for joy. Justin was a very happy baby; he came to the world with the expression on his face that he was happy to be here.

From the moment he could crawl, it became impossible to keep up with him. By the time Justin was ten months old, he was walking. He was such an active child, and it was almost like a full time job for us to keep up with his level of activity. I stayed at home with Justin until he was four, and it was the most difficult job I have ever had in my life. It was exciting and joyful to spend time with my son, but Justin was a handful. My husband came home every night to a very exhausted wife. It was impossible to make Justin take a nap or to slow him down. My husband would take over, and Justin would wear him out after a hard day's work. Justin would jump from one piece of furniture to another, and would constantly run from one end of the room to another. He was always in motion. He broke many things in the house such as cups, plates, decorations, and even the television at one time. We were very frustrated, and we talked to other parents about how active and restless Justin was. We did not know if Justin was supposed to behave the way he was behaving, or if our expectations were too high because we were new parents. Everybody played it down and told us that Justin's behavior was very typical of boys at his age. We were told that he would outgrow it.

I was very happy to send Justin to preschool when he turned four years old.

I went back to work, and my responsibility at my new job was much easier than keeping up with Justin. The preschool teachers started complaining that they could not get Justin to sit down and finish his coloring book, and they sent him home just about every single day with uncompleted work. Justin was also getting into frequent fights with other children because he could not wait for his turn at playtime. He was wetting the bed frequently at night, and was waking up very early in the morning. We could not understand why he seemed to require so little sleep. When Justin turned five, he went to pre-first grade. The problem got completely out of hand, and he was bringing home a bad note almost every day from the teacher. We were meeting with the teacher almost on a weekly basis. The teacher told us that Justin could not sit down to complete any task and he was easily distracted. He was very intrusive, and he would go from desk to desk, distracting other kids from doing their work. If Justin was reprimanded or corrected from doing something wrong, he would turn around almost immediately and would repeat the same behavior again.

From the time Justin was two years old, the only way we could take him out to a public place was to put him on a leash. We felt embarrassed about putting him on leash at age five, but we did not have a choice. On three occasions, Justin was almost run over by a car because he was not on a leash. It was as if it was impossible for Justin to walk; he was always running. Anytime we took Justin to a big department store, we would have the security guards looking for him within minutes of arriving in the store, except when he was on a leash. He would be running around restlessly and would quickly disappear from our sight. People gave us different advice on how to slow Justin down; some suggested that we cut down on his sugar intake, which we did. We saw a little improvement, but nothing significant.

When it was time for Justin to go to first grade, the pre-first teacher told us that he did not have enough maturity or social skills to proceed to first grade. My husband and I were so frustrated with Justin, we decided on the old-fashioned discipline, which was to spank him for every little offence or disobedience. We came to an unfortunate conclusion that our child was a "bad" kid. We took turns spanking him for every inappropriate behavior, but there was no progress or change with the spanking. Looking back now, I see now that our approach was purely child abuse. The spanking did not stop him from being restless; instead he became afraid of us and associated our presence with pain. Actually his behavior was worse with the corporal punishment or the spanking.

After repeating pre-first, Justin was promoted to the first grade. The first grade teacher just told us point blank that she could not handle Justin, and he was taking away constructive time from the other children in the classroom. We decided to try another school with a lower student/teacher ratio. We are grateful for the generosity of my in-laws, Justin's grandparents, who offered to pay for him to go to a private school with a smaller class size. Justin's problems continued, despite the lower ratio. The new teacher pointed out that we might need to get a professional help for him because he seemed to have all the classic symptoms of attention deficit hyperactivity disorder. She said Justin could not focus, sit still, or complete a task, despite the fact that he was getting more attention in a smaller classroom. Justin was also getting frustrated with our intervention of spanking him all the time. He was throwing more temper tantrums, and was feeling very sad and resentful of us. Obviously, Justin could not make any connection between the punishment and his behavior. He just thought we were very mean and wicked parents, and he became very resentful.

Other kids in the school did not like Justin either. Nobody wanted to play with him because he was very impulsive and impatient. His classmates reported him to the teachers frequently, so Justin felt rejected both at home and at school. He had a very poor self-esteem. He was also making bad grades because he could not settle down to complete his work, and the failure affected his self-esteem. He lacked total confidence in himself, and he started to actually believe that he was a bad and unintelligent kid.

We took Justin to see a psychiatrist at the suggestion of his new teacher and also out of our frustration as parents. The psychiatrist took an extensive history from us and gave Justin some age-appropriate tasks to do, but Justin could not complete any of the tasks. The doctor quickly diagnosed Justin with attention deficit hyperactivity disorder (ADHD). After the doctor explained the details of the diagnosis and the signs and symptoms to us, we thought he was showing us a documentary of Justin's life. My husband and I were very sad; we cried because we knew we had been cruel to this child simply because we did not know what was going on with him. We knew we were definitely guilty of child abuse; we were just lucky to get away with it. Justin was put on some medication, and he was also placed in a special program for behavior modification. We worked with the therapist to follow up at home on what was done during the therapy session. We reinforced Justin for positive behavior by giving him a treat or reward whenever he was able to complete a task or to follow directions. We set appropriate limits with him for disobedience or hyperactivity behavior instead of spanking him like we used to. Working with Justin is an ongoing intervention for us, and a lot of hard work; but we are grateful for the opportunity to help our child. Justin is doing very well; the process is slow, but we see some improvement every day. It is such a relief to see him get better.

My husband and I cannot help but wonder how many families out there are dealing with a child like our Justin and do not know what to do. ADHD is physically and emotionally draining for the child and the parents. The worst thing that could happen is not to know what to do about the disorder. If Justin reminds you of your child, get help for your child. When you help your child, you help yourself. Seeking help is a wise choice to make. Do not put your child through what Justin went through before getting the needed help. You can make life better for your child and yourself.

# Quotes of Encouragement...

As the wind blows harder and Justin's story sounds familiar to you, remember the following:

*"We increase whatever we praise. The whole creation responds to praise, and is glad."*

~ *Charles Fillmore*

Children with ADHD are often criticized very harshly and ostracized or alienated; unfortunately it kills their very fragile self-esteem and self-confidence. Gradually they start to believe and to see themselves as bad kids. Continuous criticism is counterproductive for these children; instead we should look for every opportunity to praise them for every little effort they make to cooperate with us and to respond positively to their environment. Positive reinforcement and continuous encouragement is one of the important keys to unlocking the best in the child with ADHD. *(LB)*

*"Two men look out through the same bars: one sees the mud and the other stars."*

~ *Frederick Langbridge*

You owe it to your child to ask yourself what you see when looking at your child with ADHD; is it the mud or the star? Your child becomes a star with your encouragement, and mud with your discouragement. Invest in your child to help bring out the very best in him. Your physical, emotional, and financial commitment will greatly influence the outcome for your child, and investing in your child is the best gift you can give to him. Your child is worth it. See your child as a star, not as mud, for if you don't believe in your child, who will? *(LB)*

*"Let me look upward into the branches of the flowering oak and know that it grew great and strong because it grew slowly and well."*

~ *Wilfred A. Peterson*

Patience and perseverance can work a miracle in bringing out the best in a child with ADHD. Don't focus on the challenges; instead focus on every little bit of progress, and watch your child grow from good to better and from better to best. With your dedication, the possibilities are unimaginable. *(LB)*

*Winds Against The Mind*

## Down Syndrome:
# SHIRLEY'S STORY

My husband and I tried to have children for more than ten years after we got married, but we could not. When I turned thirty-five, we decided to adopt. We adopted two children, a boy and a girl, and we were so happy. Our life was fulfilled, and the children brought so much joy to us. I never considered using birth control because I could never get pregnant. I did not see a need for it.

I was in my early forties when I got pregnant with Shirley. I did not even realize that I was pregnant. I did not know what it was like to be pregnant since I had never been pregnant in my life. I noticed that I was gaining weight and was feeling a little tired in the morning. I decided to go to my doctor for a physical examination to find out what was going on with me. She did a complete physical examination and told me she was going to do a pregnancy test. She said she suspected that I might be pregnant. I found it quite amusing, because as far as I was concerned, I was waiting for menopause. She took urine and blood samples from me and confirmed the pregnancy test as positive after doing a urine test in the office. She said the blood sample would be sent to the outside laboratory, and if it came back positive, then I was definitely pregnant. I did not say anything to my husband when I got home. I was convinced that the doctor was being ridiculous and did not know what she was doing. She called me the next day and confirmed that the blood pregnancy test was positive. I went the very next day to another doctor for a second opinion and had both urine and blood sample tests done, and the second doctor also confirmed that I was pregnant. I finally broke the news to my husband, and he was in total disbelief. I called my doctor and put my husband on the phone to talk to her. She confirmed the news and congratulated my husband. We were both hysterical and extremely happy because it had taken almost twenty

320

years before we got this miracle.

We told our older kids, who were seven and eight years old at that time, that they were going to have a baby brother or sister, and they were extremely happy. During the pregnancy, the doctor suggested that I take a test to make sure that there was no abnormality with the baby because of my age. When she explained that the procedure sometimes comes with a risk of losing the pregnancy, I refused the test. I was not going to take any chances after waiting for so long to get pregnant, and I was not about to lose the pregnancy. Shirley came to the world a week earlier than the estimated due date, and she was born with Down syndrome. Our love for Shirley was unconditional, but we experienced a sense of gain and a sense of loss at the same time. Why us? What did we do wrong? A lot of questions flew through our minds because we waited for so long for this baby. We had an idea what Down syndrome was; the doctor had mentioned the possibility to us before we had Shirley, but we never thought it could happen to us. We quickly got over our feelings, because we were more worried about Shirley; we did not know how good or bad Shirley's prognosis was. We were not sure of what the future held for her.

We went home and told our friends and family the news about Shirley. We also told our older kids that they were going to have a very special sister, who has Down syndrome. The children were just happy they were going to have a sister. Although we tried to describe Down syndrome to the children in age-appropriate terms, they did not quite understand what was going on with their sister. Shirley's diagnosis was very emotional for us, but we were still very happy with our miracle. We called friends and family to announce the arrival of Shirley, and the very first upsetting comment I got about Shirley was from one of my aunties who had always been very unkind with words; she said "Honey, that child will have to be institutionalized; there is no room for kids like her in our society." I cried very bitterly the day my aunty made that very cruel comment to me. I had just had this baby, and my body was going through a lot of changes. I would have thought that she would at least have had enough decency to keep quiet and refrain from commenting if she could not congratulate us or say something nice. I was even feeling guilty that it was my fault for bringing Shirley into this world, if she was going to have to face undeserved cruelty for being different.

The first health challenge we faced with Shirley was the diagnosis of a cardiac condition, and the doctor said she would have to have corrective surgery after she turned three months. It was so painful to watch her go through so much pain, but the surgery went well. She fully recovered from the surgery. Then we had to deal with bouts of respiratory infection, and we could hardly stay out of the pediatrician's office. Obviously because of the Down syndrome diagnosis, she was developmentally delayed. It took forever for her to crawl, and she did not walk until she was almost four years old. We did not treat Shirley differently from our other children. We took her to the park, the recreation center, and every other fun place where we took her older siblings. Unfortunately, society treated Shirley differently. Whenever she tried to play with other kids in public places, some parents would quickly pull their children away as if Shirley had an infection that was contagious. In fact, some people would look at her and look at us and shake their heads. Some people looked at us with an expression as if to say, "Why did you bring this child into the world? You really messed up." We had no idea that the society was so prejudiced against people with limitations until we had Shirley.

We tried early intervention by putting her in a special education class in preschool. She also saw a speech and language therapist on a regular basis. Shirley went to physical therapy because of her musculoskeletal weakness. One of the physical problems of having Down syndrome is muscle weakness. Shirley had a social worker and a psychiatrist who worked with her, our goal was to make sure that she could function at her best. Teaching Shirley social skills was a great challenge. Learning how to hold silverware and to eat without making too much of a mess was a tough challenge for her. Mealtime was a very messy time; she would spill her drink and have her food all over her face at age six. She would put her hands in her siblings' food, which was often very upsetting for her siblings. She would throw big temper tantrums whenever we set limits with her. Toilet training Shirley was also a big challenge for us. She was not out of diapers until age six. She would have a bowel movement on herself, and put her hand in the bowel movement and rub her hand everywhere in the house. It was very tough teaching her basic social skills, but with patience and perseverance, she got better everyday.

We tried to make sure the older siblings were not ignored because caring for Shirley was very demanding. We spent a lot of time talking to our older children so that they would understand the limitations of their younger sister. They were treated badly at times by their peers for having a sister with Down syndrome. Our oldest daughter came home one day crying that her friends at school were making fun of her because of her sister, saying her sister was an alien because of her funny appearance. She said none of her friends wanted to come and spend the night in her house anymore because of Shirley.

Surprisingly enough, we found that we felt the rejection even more from our family members. My nephew told my son that he was going to have a birthday party at his house, but his mom did not mention it to us. My nephew kept on asking my son if he was coming to his birthday party because they were very close buddies and playmates, and my son kept asking me if I was taking him to his cousin's birthday party. I finally asked my sister about the birthday party, and she was quick to tell me that her son was going to invite only his friends from school. She repeatedly tried to avoid inviting us to any social gathering or functions in her house because she did not want us to bring Shirley.

Shirley became very frustrated a lot because of her minimal speech and other limitations. She indulged in disruptive behavior and sometimes acted aggressively toward others. She had difficulty understanding social rules for a long time. With the help of the therapist, her school teachers in special education, and continuous reinforcement at home, Shirley continued to do very well. She was successful in her special education program at school.

Taking her to a public or social setting could be very stressful. We had to keep an eye on her to make sure she did not do anything that would be considered socially unacceptable. I remember taking Shirley to Rachel's birthday party; Rachel lived in our neighborhood, and this was one of the very few birthday parties that she was ever invited to. Shirley dipped her finger into Rachel's birthday cake before Rachel could blow out her birthday candles and her mother could cut the cake. The little birthday girl was very upset. She cried uncontrollably. I felt so bad, and I did not know what to do. I felt like running to the store and buying another birthday cake for Rachel, but it was a customized cake. One of the parents of the guests turned to another parent and said, "I cannot believe Rachel's mother would invite that child," and the other parent replied to her and said, "That was such a stupid thing to do! She probably invited her just to be nice, and now she is messing her daughter's party. It is obvious that the other kids don't want her around anyway." I felt so awful listening to the conversation, especially because of their insensitivity to my feelings. They did not care at all that I was right next to them. I turned around and told them that I was very sorry for what my child did. They could not even be bothered; they just turned around and looked down at me with a very unkind expression, as if to let me know I shouldn't have brought Shirley, even if she was invited. I thanked the celebrant's parents and apologized to the celebrant about Shirley's behavior. I took Shirley and left immediately, and you could see the relief on all of their faces as we were leaving.

The news would reach us through the grapevine all the time that our old friends would have a get-together and would not invite us because of Shirley. In fact, our two older siblings virtually lost most of their friends because their friends did not want to be around Shirley. We continued to live with the public rejection, but our love for Shirley was unconditional. We do not need the approval of the public to love our child. We were never ashamed of our child; we believed that she was specially created for a special purpose. Every day is a better day with Shirley. We have enjoyed some wonderful support from a few people who have accepted Shirley unconditionally and who treat our family with kindness. These kind people have shown us what true friendship means, and we pray we will take advantage of every opportunity presented to us to show the same unconditional acceptance to others. We have also enjoyed a good social support system in the community for Shirley. She has a neurologist, pediatrician, psychologist, psychiatrist, hearing and speech therapist, physical therapist, social worker, and wonderful school teachers. Shirley has improved tremendously in her social skills and communication skills. She is able to take care of herself now and is able to do little chores at home, even if she has to take her time. Shirley's communication skills have improved a whole lot. She is less anxious and less frustrated. Her aggression has decreased. Shirley realizes that she is different, but she also realizes that she is special, because she is surrounded by people who love her. We praise her for every little success, and she is also enrolled in Special Olympics. Her participation in sports has helped her self-esteem a lot.

Watching Shirley grow is full of mixed emotions for all of us in the family. Every single day is different because we experience joy, pain, frustrations, challenges, success, and failures with each day. Most of all, we are happy that there is hope. Shirley is very special, and we are very grateful to have her. Shirley has taught us a lot about life and living as a family, and we would not change anything about our lives or have it otherwise.

# Quotes of Encouragement...

As the wind blows harder and Shirley's story sounds familiar to you, remember the following:

*"Applaud us when we run, console us when we fall, cheer us when we recover."*

~ *Edmund Burke*

Living with Down syndrome is already a challenge for a child; the least you can do is to encourage and not discourage, build and not break down this special child. Put yourself in the child's shoes as you react to the child, and don't forget to be kind. Kindness is a choice you make, and it is free. Together we can all console, applaud, cheer, and encourage; together we can all make the world a better place for these special people. *(LB)*

*"Most of us swimming against tides of trouble the world knows nothing about, need only a bit of praise and encouragement – and we'll make the goal."*

~ *Jerome P. Fleishman*

Society can be very unkind to people with limitations due to lack of understanding; when you are around somebody with limitations, don't forget that you are part of the society. Watch your body language. Down syndrome is not a choice. These individuals may be physically different from us, but they experience the same emotions just like we do. They are different but they don't have a disease. Extend a simple act of kindness and make them feel that the world is not a horrible place just because they are different.*(LB)*

*"If human beings are perceived as potential rather than problems, as possessing strengths instead of weaknesses, as unlimited rather than dull and unresponsive, then they can thrive and grow to their capabilities."*

~ *Bob Conklin*

Having Down syndrome does not mean that these individuals should be written off and treated as nonentities. Get to know these special people personally, and you will be amazed at the strength they possess and their unique personal attributes. *(LB)*

*Winds Against The Mind*

Conduct Disorder:

# Conduct Disorder:
# BASIC FACTS &
# UNDERSTANDING

Adolescents go through a lot of changes emotionally, physically, and intellectually. They are no longer children, but at the same time, they are not fully grown adults. They constantly struggle with trying to establish their own identity as adults by trying to prove to everybody that they are not children anymore. At the same time they find it difficult to do away with childish ways. The behavior of adolescents often becomes unpredictable and inconsistent. They go from being very sad to being very happy. While undergoing all these changes, some adolescents become defiant and oppositional. They become rebellious and aggressive, and constantly argue with authority figures and their parents or parental figures. Some adolescents can be very disobedient and hostile. They may test limits continuously. They always maintain that they are right all the time. In fact, they usually believe that they are the ones being violated and wronged by irrational adults who are making unreasonable demands from them. Some adolescents can be very annoying, stubborn, and extremely spiteful with their words.

These behaviors are usually observed at home at first. Many adolescents have two sides—the public side and the private side. At times, when a parent or a parental figure lodges a complaint about the unruly adolescent son or daughter to the teacher at school, the teacher may be totally shocked. The child may never show the troublesome side at school. Some adolescents, on the other hand, may exhibit the unruly behavior at home and also at school right from the start. Some of the unruly behavior could also start long before the pre-adolescent years, even before the age of eight. If a lot of oppositional characteristics is noticed in a child before the age of eight the child may be diagnosed with *oppositional defiant disorder.*

With oppositional defiant disorder, a child may go through a phase of insecurity, confusion, hostility, and resentment of authority. If he eventually outgrows these behaviors and does not carry them into the pre-adolescent years, the child would only get a definitive diagnosis of childhood oppositional defiant disorder. However, if a child continues with the unruly behavior as he grows older into the pre-adolescent years and into the teenage years, and begins to actually violate the rights of others, the child would be diagnosed with *conduct disorder.* Adolescents with conduct disorder may show absolutely no respect for societal norms and rules. They could be very impulsive and defiant. They may be physically and verbally aggressive to others, especially to authority figures. They usually get into frequent fights with peers and authority figures. They may be violent and possess weapons. They could be extremely critical of authority figures and their parents. They may be sexually active and even go into prostitution.

One of the hallmark characteristics of adolescents with conduct disorder is their lack of ability to accept responsibility for their actions. They perpetually play the blaming game, and whatever problem they are experiencing is the fault of somebody else, and they are just victims. They are convinced that other people are vicious and are out to get them. The feelings of being persecuted by others make it very easy for them to blame others for their unruly actions. They may be highly suicidal or homicidal toward other people, by frequently expressing the wish to kill themselves or others. They usually have failing grades in school and may eventually drop out of school.

Most adolescents with conduct disorder abuse drugs or alcohol or both. It is almost assumed that they should embrace the drug and alcohol culture to be accepted into the group of other adolescents with conduct disorder. They are not considered "cool" or good enough for the group if they are not using drugs or alcohol. They have a desperate and obsessive need to be approved and to be accepted by their peers. They crave fitting in with peers, so they try to keep up with the current fashion and style, even if it means stealing to be able to obtain the clothing. They usually idolize some people or become obsessed with hero worshipping. They may go into tumultuous or explosive relationships, and they fall in and out of love all the time.

Group stealing and group shoplifting are common with these adolescents. They may vandalize or set fires on properties. They tend to join a group or a gang, and their allegiance is usually to the gang or the group. They usually believe in the group or the gang to the extent that they would do anything for the group or the gang they belong to. They usually substitute the group or the gang for their families. Their emotional instability makes them highly suicidal. They must be watched closely for suicide. They may eventually become unmanageable by their parents, and may end up in the juvenile court system where they are referred to as juvenile delinquents. They may be in and out of the court systems, and may eventually have to be placed in an inpatient hospital or a juvenile delinquent home.

Age of onset for *conduct disorder* may be as early as ten or the teenage years. There may or may not be a prior history of childhood oppositional defiant behavior or disorder. The most shocking to accept by most parents or most parental figures are the children who develop conduct disorder but who showed no childhood trait of oppositional behavior while they were growing up. There are many children who grow from perfect little children to troubled teenagers. Such a scenario sometimes poses big challenges to some parents or parental figures. The parents never anticipate or prepare for the change. When adolescents are diagnosed with conduct disorder, it is considered a serious problem. Parents, parental figures, and authority figures always hope that these adolescents will outgrow these destructive behaviors and will become responsible adults.

There are oppositional defiant behavior and conduct disorder among younger children and adolescents in every culture. Wherever there are children, there will also be behavioral problems. Every culture definitely has its own fair share of childhood and adolescent problems. The severity of the manifestation of the behavioral problems may be influenced by the cultural values of each culture, and the level of flexibility or freedom that children have in that culture. In some cultures, children are not allowed to express their feelings freely. The adults may be exceptionally strict with the children. Adolescents in such cultures may not be able to form a gang or to join a group. They may also not have the support of anybody in the culture if they have behavioral problems. Children may manifest fewer behavioral problems in such a strict culture because of the limited or restricted freedom for children. Behavioral problems seem to be more prevalent in the cultures where children have a lot of freedom. Children may also have more behavioral problems in a culture where families and extended families are spread out. The spread-out family situation can usually minimize the extended family support and closer supervision for the children. Also, if both parents are away from home most of the time, working longer hours and spending less time with their children, such a void can make the children act out. It is understandable that some homes are single parent homes. Also in some two parent homes, both parents may have to work longer hours to improve the quality of life of the family. Unfortunately, less supervision of the children in single or two parents home may have tough consequences.

Other contributory factors to conduct disorder or oppositional defiant behavior may include but are not limited to: a major life event or stressor in the life of the child, family problems, organic or medical problems, hereditary (or inborn) characteristics of the child, as well as community, and environmental factors. If there is a sudden change in a child's family routine, the child may not understand what is going on. Such changes can come in the form of a divorce, death, or a chronic illness of a family member. Moving to another neighborhood could also be stressful for a child. Children may easily misinterpret a change or a difficult family situation. They may even turn to blaming themselves for the situation. For example, if the parents are getting a divorce, the children may internalize the anger, believe it was their fault, and revolt by acting out. Also the death of a sibling or a parent may be traumatic for a child and make the child act out. The birth of another child could be equally devastating for some children. Chronic illness of a parent or a sibling could also be very devastating for a child. Acting out could be a way for a child to express his or her frustrations in some situations.

Family structure may also influence a child's adjustment. The first set of people that a child is introduced to in the world is the child's nuclear family. Providing a nurturing environment in the early years of life could influence a child's adjustment later in life. Adequate emotional bonding, proper sensory stimulation such as playing with a child, adequate shelter, proper clothing, and proper nutrition would definitely influence a child's adjustment in life.

Reinforcing positive behavior, teaching concepts of right and wrong, and modeling good behavior are all factors that could affect a child's adjustment later in life. Children learn a lot from their parents or parental figures. Sibling interaction is also important to a child's adjustment. Children learn early social interaction such as sharing, caring, and healthy and unhealthy competition from their siblings. A home that is full of discord, fights, and constant arguments over money may also affect a child's adjustment. Parents who have a criminal history from constant struggles with the law, move a lot for dysfunctional reasons, and battle with drug and alcohol problems are likely to raise children with oppositional defiant behavior and conduct disorder. Also, parents with no steady job and an unstable life are likely to have children with oppositional defiant behavior and conduct disorder. It must also be mentioned that children with a stable family may also develop conduct disorder for no apparent reasons.

Children who grow up in foster care and move from one foster care to the other may also grow up with emotional problems. They may be diagnosed with childhood behavioral disorder. It will be very difficult if not almost impossible for a child to develop proper bonding if they have to be moved several times from one foster home to another. Since there is not a steady parental figure, they would not be able to develop any form of bonding or attachment with anybody. As a result of the instability in their lives, they can easily develop behavioral problems. Children who were abused physically, emotionally, and sexually may also develop conduct disorder.

The inborn or hereditary temperament factor may also influence a child's adjustment in life. Everybody is born with an inborn temperament. Most mothers can always tell the difference between the temperaments of their children as infants. Some children are fussy and inpatient, while some children are patient and quiet. Some infants with fussy temperaments may keep the same temperament into later years of life. Children born with physical and psychological or mental disability such as slow-learners may also react to their disability by acting out. Some of these children react out of frustration because they are labeled by the society. They could be easily labeled by their friends, parents, or even teachers who may call them stupid, bad, or slow. Such children may try to live up to the expectation of the labels given to them and may try to prove to the world that they are really bad kids by acting out.

Other undiagnosed mental illnesses may be responsible for possible acting out behavior of some children, especially the adolescents. For instance, adolescents who are experiencing depression (extreme sadness), bipolar disorder (mood swings), or psychosis (losing touch with reality) may not be able to express how they are feeling. They may not understand that some chemical changes going on in their brain and body are partly responsible for these feelings. They may choose to act out instead.

Community influence may also have a strong effect on a child's adjustment. It is very important for parents or parental figures to pay attention to what is going on with their children outside of the home. If a child is coming home to complain about certain peers in school or in the neighborhood very frequently, it is worth looking into it by the parents. Parents should check into or investigate their children's complaints instead of ignoring them. For children, school is like a full-time job, just as work is for parents. If parents can take time to fix a problem at work, they should try and take time to fix a problem their child may be experiencing at school or in the neighborhood.

The problem could sometimes be the child's teacher. It is not unusual for a teacher to lack the ability or maturity to get along with a particular child. A parent should not assume that teachers are perfect, or that every teacher is good for their child. If a child is complaining about a teacher on a regular basis, it is worth the parent's time to investigate this problem. This is especially necessary if the child has no history of having problems with teachers in the past. If a child is constantly exposed to a hostile environment involving a teacher, the child may become frustrated, hate school, and develop conduct disorder. Likewise, if a child is constantly complaining about some other children in the neighborhood or at school, especially if it is a bully situation, the child may develop behavioral problems in self-defense, if nothing is done about it. The child may go as far as joining a group or a gang to fight off another set of bullies.

Apart from environmental and situational factors, biological factors are also implicated in the development of conduct disorder. The biological factors attributed the cause of conduct disorder to dysregulation or abnormal regulation of certain naturally occurring chemical in the brain called neurotransmitters. The dysregulation or abnormal regulation of these neurotransmitters could increase aggression or anxiety in some children. So many changes are going on in the body and the brain of adolescents. Other biological factors may also be involved.

To help a child with conduct disorder, a qualified clinician who is specialized in treating behavioral problems in children must be contacted. Parents and parental figures must be aware that adolescent children do not usually ask for help. They are always in denial and unwilling to admit that there is a problem. They usually believe that they are just like many other adolescent children out there who are having a difficult time with their parents and authority figures. Adolescents compare notes, and they may have a communal sense of persecution by adults. It is very important to seek professional help for them. With professional help, an intense assessment will be done, and this usually includes family history, social history, psychological history, physical, and health assessment. The goal of the clinician is to get to the root of the child's problem. The child may require some one-to-one counseling with the clinician and also some group therapy with other troubled adolescents who are willing to make positive changes in their lives. Medication intervention may also be necessary to treat underlying mental problems like depression, anxiety, and aggression. It is important to work with the child to modify the child's behavior and ways of thinking. The child must learn personal responsibility and the importance of having a goal and vision in life. Children must understand that they are going to be children only for a season or a period of time, after which they become an adult. When they become adults, society will hold them to a different standard and will hold them accountable for their actions. Sometimes, the child may require long-term rehabilitation and hospitalization where they would have no access to drugs, alcohol, or weapons.

Family therapy sessions with a clinician are also very important. Family therapy includes the family and the child in family sessions. In some situations, the family is the root of the problem. The family will learn a more functional way of dealing with a youth with behavioral problems during family therapy. Some families adopt the wrong approach in dealing with behavioral problems of adolescent and younger children. They get into power struggles with them, which are exactly what these disturbed youths want. These clashes usually do not work.

A family support group allows family members of adolescents with behavioral problems to come together and to help one another by sharing with each other about the best possible way to deal with the troubled youth. It is always helpful for people to know that they are not alone. Talking about what works and what is not working in different families could be beneficial.

Many troubled children turn their lives around and become success stories. Unfortunately, some youth follow the troubled road to destruction and usually end up in the adult prison system. Early intervention is the key to achieving greater success with troubled children. The goal is not to give up. Some youth may need more than one chance to wake up from their deep slumber and to turn their lives around. A parent should be able to say, "I gave my child every possible opportunity to help him to succeed in life."

## Attention Deficit Hyperactivity Disorder:
# BASIC FACTS & UNDERSTANDING

A*ttention deficit hyperactivity disorder (ADHD)* is characterized by excessive hyperactivity, difficulty paying attention, restlessness, and excessive impulsivity in children. It is believed to be more common in boys than in girls. Children with ADHD experience difficulty in paying attention to very simple tasks. Playing with peers becomes difficult because of the short attention span. They are unable to sit still in school and to finish their school work. Parents may have noticed that their child had been restless before the age of three. Most parents may attribute the restlessness to normal hyperactivity that is typical of some children at that age, especially if the child is a boy.

Children with ADHD are constantly on the move. They jump from one activity to the other and find it impossible to pay attention to details. They could be very destructive because of their restlessness. They may break things in the house such as dishes, glasses, and even their toys. They sometimes act as if they have zoned out the rest of the world around them when it comes to following instructions. They simply do not follow directions. They are very forgetful, and they have difficulty with organizational skills. As a result, they are usually disorganized. They may also show some motor skills coordination problems, or left and right confusion. This may be due to their restlessness and impatience.

Children with ADHD get easily frustrated because they lose things very easily. They may climb and run excessively. They have difficulty waiting for their turn in a line. They also move excessively while sleeping. They may be labeled as "bad kids" by their teachers and other adults. This may affect their self-esteem and their self-confidence. They may actually internalize the stigma and truly believe that they are bad kids. This is very unfortunate, but it does happen. Children with

ADHD have a low tolerance for frustration. They have problem with temper tantrums and may be quick to strike other children. They can be very intrusive. They may interrupt other children in socialized play-like games, and frequently interrupt other people's conversations. They may have difficulty making friends because of their poor social skills.

The school performance of ADHD children is always very poor. As a result, they may be labeled as underachievers because of their inability to complete their assignments or organize their work. They may act out their frustrations by resulting to stealing, telling lies, and becoming verbally and physically aggressive. They are a handful for teachers because they require a lot more supervision and attention than other children in the classroom. Their behavior often stands out in the group. They may require frequent correction by the teacher. There is the tendency for them to be labeled as bad kids by their peers because they stand out as the children who are always getting into trouble with the teacher.

Coping with ADHD children on a daily basis is emotionally very draining for the parents, the teachers, and other primary caregivers. With inappropriate intervention or no intervention at all, they may turn to drugs and alcohol as adolescents and also develop conduct disorder. ADHD is present in most cultures. Children with ADHD in a poorly informed society where there is no public education about the disorder stand a chance of being labeled forever as bad children in that culture. No treatment or help may be sought for them because of a lack of knowledge about this mental illness.

Several reasons are attributed to the cause of ADHD, and these include neurological damage, maternal deprivation (non-nurturing mother), parental abuse, environmental toxins (such as lead poisoning), malnutrition in early years of life, excessive consumption of chocolates and sugar, food dyes, postnatal (after birth) or intrauterine (during pregnancy) brain damage. There is not enough conclusive evidence to justify most of the reasons given for the cause of ADHD. The good news is, with appropriate intervention, many children do outgrow it. On the other hand, if there is no structure in the child's life or a good support system, the ADHD child that develops into an adolescent with severe behavioral problems may eventually become a felon as an adult.

Diagnosis is usually made when the child starts school. Most teachers can very easily tell the difference between a child with ADHD and other children. Teachers have a large comparison group, and the difference is always very obvious. Teachers are trained to know the age-appropriate behavior and developmental skills of the children in their classrooms. A marked deviation from the norm on the developmental skills is always a red flag to the teacher.

It is important to get professional help for a child with ADHD. A certified clinician in the community who is knowledgeable in the treatment of ADHD must be consulted. In the United States this could be a psychiatrist, a pediatrician, a family physician, a psychiatric nurse practitioner, a pediatric nurse, a family nurse practitioner, a psychologist, or any licensed clinician certified to treat ADHD. The pediatrician or the primary care physician may be the first to make the diagnosis from assessment during a routine visit.

An extensive medical history and family history are usually taken, and several tests are carried out, including psychological and neurological tests. Intelligent quotient test (IQ) could also be done to determine if there is any disability. Intervention and treatment for a child with ADHD should be multidisciplinary, and this would require a combination of different specialists coming together to work towards the common goal of helping a child with ADHD reach his potential. A joint effort is needed between the family, the school teacher, and the clinician in order to have a good outcome with the child. Lack of education and poor understanding of the illness will significantly affect the outcome. Family members and the caregivers must be educated extensively about ADHD. Extensive knowledge of the disorder would promote the parental understanding of the child. Increased understanding would decrease frustration and would allow the family to have a realistic expectation of the child. Knowing that the child may not always be like every other child could help to decrease the strife and the stress on the family. This would increase the family's ability to cope and function with a child with ADHD in the house.

Acceptance is important to be able to work with ADHD children and to have a good outcome. Acceptance does not mean abandoning appropriate interventions. It means accepting the child for who he or she is, and knowing that it is not the child's fault for having ADHD. At the same time, the parents can help the child to reach his or her full potential despite the limitations. For example, it is important to reduce sensory stimulation for him because he is already hyper-stimulated. It is good to provide a quiet environment and a personal space for him without necessarily isolating him from other children, at least until that child learns how to interact with his peers without being disruptive. It is also important for the parent or the caregiver to work with the school teacher to provide structure for the child. He may need to be in a small classroom to prevent sensory overload. He may also need to sit closer to the teacher in the classroom to keep him from disrupting other children in the class.

Positive reinforcement is also helpful to children with ADHD. Whenever they sit through a task, they must be rewarded for it. At the same time, firm limits must be set for inappropriate behavior without being punitive (without punishing the child). A good example is having the child sit in a quiet corner when disruptive. The goal is to allow the child to associate his inappropriate behavior with the consequences of sitting in a quiet corner. On the other hand, if the child receives a new pencil, toy, coloring book, or an extra snack for following directions or completing a task, the child will be able to associate positive rewards with good behavior. Corporal punishment such as excessive spanking has not been shown to work well in modifying the behavior of children with ADHD.

The behavior modification approach must be a continuous process. It must not be limited to the classroom. At home, parents must carry on the process of reward for good behavior and limit-setting for disruptive behavior. The behavior modification process must be continuous to be effective. Some children with ADHD may need to be placed in a special education program. The goal is not to stereotype them, but to put them in an environment where the teacher-student ratio is very low, and the academic program is tailored to meet the need of the child. Having several ADHD children in a regular classroom could be overwhelming for a teacher. It could compromise the quality of education given to other children in the classroom. Children with ADHD are usually academic underachievers. This is not due to their lack of intelligence, but primarily due to their poor concentration and inability to complete tasks. They can perform effectively in an academic setting tailored to work with their limitations.

The problems of low self-esteem, lack of self-confidence, rejection, depression, and poor social skills must be addressed. They are factors that affect the way the child with ADHD sees and interprets the world around him. A child should not grow up internalizing all the negative views of self and the world around him. All these problems must be dealt with in therapy sessions.

Medication intervention may also be necessary to treat some of the symptoms of

ADHD. Proper education should be given to caregivers; they should not rely on medication intervention alone. Behavior modification is equally important. There is no one "magic fix" or pill out there for all the problems that come with ADHD. There are several medications available in the market. The choice of medication should be determined by a qualified clinician working with the child, based on the thorough assessment of the child. Some of the medications used for the treatment of ADHD have some side effects that must be carefully monitored. Parents and caregivers must show interest in understanding the side effects of the medications that the children are taking. They must quickly report the unusual signs and symptoms to the clinicians. Children should be carefully monitored when on medication for the treatment of ADHD in order to avoid long-term physical and psychological or mental damage from the poor management of the side effects of the medications.

In addition to family counseling with the child, family members or caregivers of the child with ADHD need to join a family support group. The purpose is to learn how to manage and cope with the disorder better. It is also good to know that other families are dealing with the same issues. Different families coming together could be a great source of support for one another by providing information about what works and what does not work for different families.

## Autism:
# BASIC FACTS & UNDERSTANDING

*Autism* is a childhood disorder affecting the brain. It is characterized by distorted functioning in the area of communications, socialization, perception, movement, behavior, and reality testing. It is a disturbing illness for the parents and the caregivers. Autistic children may not show any attachment toward their parents and caregivers. They are usually locked up in their own world and are not concerned about the outside world. They may not show any interest in people around them, or sometimes may attach to only one person. They have serious impairments in communication skills, and some may have no language at all. They lack emotion and affect. As a child, cuddling them may be like cuddling an object. They may even resent physical contact and fight it. Interaction with peers is almost impossible for autistic children. They enjoy solitary play and usually stay away from cooperative play.

Change is stressful for them. They want things the same way all the time. For instance, they like the same seat in the classroom, the same food every day, or the same clothes every day. Autistic children may act out some self-destructive behavior by banging their heads on the floor or the wall. They seem to get a relief from such self-destructive behavior, and they show no visible signs of sensitivity to pain by their actions. They may show unusual fascination with certain motions such as spinning objects like the wheel of a bike or a fan. Ritualistic behavior is very common with them. They may rock in a chair for hours, clap their hands on and off all day long, walk on their toes, or spin and dance in circles for hours. They may not make any eye contact with people or show any facial expression toward another human face. The brains of autistic children may not register the human faces of people whom they encounter or come in contact with.

Language problems are always profound in autistic children. They may totally lack the ability to communicate or have delayed speech. Their grammatical structure is usually immature. They may also reverse their pronouns. They may not be able to name an object. For instance, if they are thirsty and see a cup, they may not be able to say "I want a cup of water." They may take a cup and call it an orange. The language of an autistic child may be repetitive. They may also mimic or repeat what others are saying (echolalia). They may also giggle, babble, and use inappropriate pitch or tone.

There is totally no spark and spontaneity with some autistic children, which is emotionally very painful for the caregiver. Their motor and developmental milestones may be delayed. As a result, they may not show any manifestation of certain behaviors that a child is supposed to show at a certain age. They may develop exceptional ability in certain areas. For instance, they may be exceptionally good with numbers and have the ability to solve almost any mathematical problem. They may show exceptional ability with memorization and be able to memorize the map of the world.

The cause of autism is still widely unknown, but there is a common scientific agreement that autism is a brain disorder. It is believed that in the early months of life, something went dramatically wrong in the brain development of an autistic child. Genetic factors are also implicated in the cause of autism. A family may have more than one autistic child. This may speak greatly to the authenticity of the genetic component that children with autism usually have a strong family history of relatives with autism. It is also believed that when mothers contact certain infections such as rubella, meningitis, encephalitis, or are exposed to certain toxins during pregnancy, the child may develop autism. There is currently a public ongoing debate about certain childhood vaccines and the possibility that children could develop autism after receiving these vaccines. This discussion is generating a lot of public attention, and more research and public studies are going into it.

Autism has not been associated in any way with poor parenting. This is good for parents to know in order to prevent the possible guilt or self-blame about having a child with autism. A fairly good number of autistic children develop seizure disorder in pre-adolescent or adolescent years. The reason for the development of the seizure disorder is poorly understood. Autism affects millions of children all over the world. It is a disturbing illness for the parents and the caregivers.

The diagnosis of autism may not be made until a child is around age two. There may be early cues in the first few months of life that may be missed by the parents or parental figure. Nobody wants to see anything different or unusual about her child. There is the natural tendency for parents or parental figures to play down any of the earlier signs and symptoms of autism. The older the child grows, the more pronounced the disorder. At the latest, by age three, the diagnosis should clearly be made. The ultimate goal in healthcare is to be able to make the diagnosis of autism in the first few months of life, with the hope of improving the prognosis or the outcome of this disorder. With an earlier diagnosis, the primary goal of keeping the child from shutting out the rest of the world may be better achieved or at least significantly reduced.

The diagnosis should be made by a qualified, knowledgeable, and licensed clinician who is certified to make such diagnosis in the community. In the United States, this could be a primary care physician, a family physician, a psychiatrist, a psychiatric nurse practitioner, a pediatric nurse practitioner, a psychologist, or a family nurse practitioner. There is no magic formula or one particularly recommended treatment for autism. What works for one child to increase the child's level of functioning may not necessarily work for another child. There are different types of treatments and interventions out there for the treatment of this disorder. In their efforts to find a cure, parents of autistic children may get drained financially. The cost of getting treatment for an autistic child could be astronomical. Families may have limited coverage or no coverage at all from health insurance companies. Unfortunately, autism is a chronic illness. Some autistic children make relatively fair adjustment into the adult life and they are able to hold down a job and live a semi-independent life. For some, it is a life long challenge. They may constantly need care and supervision with no hope for independent living.

The prognosis or outcome is better for autistic children in more informed societies like the Western world. Unfortunately, in the less informed societies where the disorder is poorly understood, autistic children may be treated like social outcasts. It must be emphasized that only a knowledgeable clinician in the field of autism should determine or recommend the best treatment approach for an autistic child. This must be based on the extensive history of the child. The child's limitations and level of functioning at the time of the diagnosis must also be taken into consideration. Most interventions are primarily focused on behavior modification. The main focus is to promote interaction with others and to improve social skills. Building and improving verbal communication is also an important part of the intervention.

Medication management is essential to treat some of the behavioral problems associated with autism. Some of the common problems may include hyperactivity, which is usually manifest by an inability to stay still. Obsessive and repetitive behaviors must also be addressed. Common examples are walking in circles or rocking all day long. Low tolerance for frustration and aggressive behavior are also very common. For instance, an autistic child may turn violent and hit another child for taking his usual seat at the dining room table because he or she cannot tolerate change. Medication is also used to treat seizure disorder if a child with autism develops seizure disorder late in life. Many factors are taken into consideration to determine the best medication for each autistic child. The medication decision must be made by a certified clinician only.

It is important for parents, parental figures, and caregivers of autistic children to be in support groups. When a child is affected with autism, the entire family is affected. One child with autism or any other chronic illness in the family totally changes the family dynamics. Unfortunately, some families have more than one child with autism. It may be more expensive and more financially draining for such families to pay for most of the recommended treatments and medications for their children. Most parents in search of cure would probably do whatever it takes to try every recommended treatment out there out of desperation. They want to be able to go to sleep at night knowing that they have done everything they could possibly do to help their child. Joining a support group could provide an avenue for families to vent their frustration and to learn about what is new and working out there in terms of treatment. Families in support groups could also learn how other families cope with the day-to-day emotional and financial pressure of living with autistic children.

There is a high tendency for the other children in the family to be ignored because a child with autism requires a lot of attention. It is important to pay attention to the siblings of an autistic child, and to involve them in a support group as well if they are old enough to understand what is going on. A neutral environment like a support group could help to provide an avenue for the siblings to express their frustrations. The goal of everybody affected by autism — such as parents, teachers, researchers, clinicians, therapist, caregivers, and family members — is to one day have the magic or miracle key to unlock the mind of every autistic child in the world.

## Down Syndrome:
# BASIC FACTS & UNDERSTANDING

Down *own syndrome* is not a mental illness; it is a genetic disorder. Down syndrome is discussed in this book because some children with abnormal developmental problems such as Down syndrome or cerebral palsy or other similar developmental anomaly may have behavioral problems which may require psychological help. Some children with Down syndrome may also have autism or ADHD. Clinicians such as a psychiatrist, a psychologist, a psychiatric nurse practitioner, or any licensed clinician in the medical field or the field of mental health who is specialized in the behavioral management of such special children should be consulted. The goal of the discussion is to provide awareness to the parents, parental figures, and caregivers that specialized help could help to improve the outcome with the children. The quality of life of the child and the family members could be greatly enhanced with good management of the disorder. Furthermore, Down syndrome is discussed to increase the awareness of the society to treat a child or a person who is different or limited in certain areas with human kindness, dignity and respect.

Down syndrome is the most common cause of mental retardation in newborns. The term Down syndrome was taken from the name of Dr. John Langdon Down, an English physician who happened to be the first to describe this condition in 1866. In 1959, Dr. Jerome Lejuene discovered the abnormal chromosome that is responsible for babies to have Down syndrome. The disorder occurs in every culture and every socioeconomic group, irrespective of color, race, or religion.

Children with Down syndrome usually have some health problems such as heart problems, intestinal problems, visual problems such as crossed eyes (amblyopia), near or far sightedness and cataracts. Down syndrome babies are at a higher risk of developing infections, especially ear infections. They may also have pneumonia and bronchitis. Other common health problems include thyroid disease and hearing loss. They also have a higher risk of developing leukemia(a form of blood disorder) and abnormal heart conditions. A pediatric cardiologist (a doctor who is specialized in the treatment of heart disease of children), must be consulted in the early weeks of life of the child to determine if such defects exist. The defects could be corrected by surgery.

Another common problem is the problem with the digestion of their food. The problem can interfere with the baby's milk digestion, causing the baby to have a low weight and also to vomit forcefully after feeding. This condition could also be corrected by surgery. Visual problems are common, and this could also be corrected with glasses or surgery by a pediatric ophthalmologist (a doctor who is specialized in the treatment of the eye of children). Infections such as pneumonia, bronchitis, and ear infection could be easily treated with antibiotics by a pediatrician. It is important for children with Down syndrome to have vision and hearing examinations on a regular basis. This would allow for early detection of any problem that may hinder the development of language and other skills needed in life.

Other possible health problems that usually increase with age in people with Down syndrome are the development of Alzheimer dementia, diabetes, thyroid, and seizure problems. Alzheimer dementia is a disease of senility or forgetfulness that results from a shrinkage and breakdown of some brain cells, causing the brain to gradually lose its functions. The memory functions in a faulty manner, and the body coordination may gradually get worse. The recent memory is the first to go. For instance these individuals may remember a family wedding twenty years ago, but have no recollection of what they ate for lunch. (See the discussion on Alzheimer dementia.) Despite all the health problems that an individual with Down syndrome is likely to face, the average life expectancy is fifty-five years or older because of advance knowledge in science and medicine. The prognosis (chances of living longer) is far better than it has ever been. At one time in history most children with Down syndrome did not live past infancy or childhood; they would usually die from infection and other medical complications. Advances in medicine have helped to treat the majority of the health problems associated with Down syndrome.

It is important for the public to understand that Down syndrome is not infectious or contagious. Some people are scared of touching or being touched by a child with Down syndrome. They feel uncomfortable around children with Down syndrome because they look different. The truth is that people with Down syndrome are more like us than they are different from us. With the wrong attitude, the public could make growing up very difficult for them. The constant rejection and humiliation they face from some people could also contribute to the development of some behavioral problems sometimes experienced by these special children. People with Down syndrome may have some impairments and limitations, but they are not stupid. They have talents and gifts to benefit their community. Several years ago, they were considered not useful to society, and they were usually put in a long-term institution. This position has changed because people with Down syndrome are now mainstreamed into the community. They live in their own homes with their families. Society needs to be more understanding and accommodating. Again, it is important to remember that people with Down syndrome have feelings, rights, needs, emotions, and similar desires just like the rest of us. It is not by choice that they have Down syndrome; it could have been any of us.

Down syndrome occurs in one in every eight hundred to a thousand births, and it affects boys and girls equally. The chromosomal abnormality that causes most cases of Down syndrome occurs as a result of the extra chromosome from the egg of the mother as opposed to an extra chromosome from the sperm of the father during conception or the making of the baby. More detailed understanding of the chromosomal abnormality may require consulting a clinician who is knowledgeable about Down syndrome. The risk of having a Down syndrome baby also increases significantly with the age of the mother. It must be noted that after the age of thirty-five, the risk of having a baby with Down syndrome increases by one in every four hundred births, and goes higher with advancing age. It must be mentioned, however, that eighty percent of children with Down syndrome are born to women under thirty-five years of age, despite the increasing risk with maternal age.

Down syndrome could be diagnosed before a baby is born. If a family has a strong history of Down syndrome or genetic birth defects or the woman is over thirty-five years of age, it may be advisable for her to get tested during pregnancy. Sonogram or ultrasound is used to take the picture of the baby in the womb during pregnancy. Down syndrome may be suspected with ultrasound, but it is not conclusive. There is the need to carry out other tests in addition to ultrasound, and this should be determined by a physician.

Down syndrome is usually identified at birth through the observation of some of the distinct physical characteristics of the babies. They tend to be very quiet babies with weak muscles. They are usually less responsive than other newborns. Other physical characteristics may include a small or flattened head, flattened face, depressed nasal bridge, small nose, small ears, small mouth (which causes the tongue to stick out and appear to be very large), and slanting eyes with skin folds at the inner corner of the eyes near the nose (this is called epicanthal fold). More physical characteristics may show wide and small hands, round cheeks, malformed fifth finger, atypical or unusual creases on the sole of the feet, excess skin at the back of the neck at birth, wide spaces between the big and the second toes, shorter than normal height, extremely flexible joints, loose ligaments, and reduced muscle strength and tone. If Down syndrome is not tested for or discovered during pregnancy, it could be tested after birth. If the physical characteristics of the baby at birth show that the baby could have Down syndrome, the physician will test for Down syndrome. The physician would be the one to recommend the conclusive test.

Developmental milestones may be different for children with Down syndrome. It may take longer time for them to walk, talk, toilet train, or learn other social skills. It may be difficult for the family to adjust to the child's special needs initially. With time and patience on the part of everybody involved with the care of the child, the child will eventually master all or most of the skills. Part of the goal is to teach her independence so that she can eventually carry out activities of daily living such as brushing her teeth, combing her hair, taking a bath, and eating on her own. Although some people with Down syndrome may have difficulty with abstract thinking, forming some basic concepts, and learning complex skills, with continuous family and community support, they may overcome some of these obstacles and at least learn appropriate basic social skills. A structured program of physical activities and a weight maintenance program can help to improve the poor muscle tone, and the gross and fine motor skills. Language therapy can also help to improve language development. An early intervention in a center-based setting outside of the home and in the home is the key to helping them achieve their developmental milestone sooner.

People with Down syndrome may experience some mental retardation. The severity of the mental retardation varies. It is usually mild to moderate for most. Very few people with Down syndrome have severe mental retardation. However, each case must be treated independently, depending on the presenting symptoms and the extent of the complications resulting from the disorder. Unfortunately, there is no way to formally predict the mental development of a child with Down syndrome by simply looking at the physical features. The ultimate goal is to work with each child and to help him or her reach the best possible potential as we take these limitations into consideration.

Some children with Down syndrome go to regular schools and attend regular classes. If a child has special needs in some areas, special classes are available in some communities to help the child. It is important to encourage active participation in sports and play. Socialized play teaches social skills, and sports promote physical health and self-esteem. Children with Down syndrome should also be encouraged to participate in other recreational activities such as dance and music. A Down syndrome child with mild mental retardation can read and write and participate in other activities outside of the school. Some children with Down syndrome grow up to be responsible adults. They become gainfully employed, and some are very enthusiastic about their jobs. They work in the community in places such as grocery stores, restaurants, fabrics stores, or large departmental stores.

Some of them have also pursued other goals, depending on their level of limitation. They can be very dedicated, responsible, and hardworking.

Mild to moderate medication may be needed to treat some noticeable behavioral problems associated with Down syndrome. The medications must be strictly prescribed by a licensed clinician who is knowledgeable in the management of people with special needs like Down syndrome. The child must be carefully monitored while on medication, especially for the side effects of the medication.

Genetic counseling may be necessary if a couple has a child with Down syndrome and plans to have another baby. Some people with Down syndrome also get married and may plan to have children. A woman with Down syndrome has a fifty percent chance of having a baby with Down syndrome. With rare exceptions, most men with Down syndrome are believed to be uniformly sterile. This means they cannot father a child. It is very important to seek genetic counseling if people with Down syndrome plan to have children.

The importance of support groups cannot be overemphasized for families with Down syndrome babies. Having a child with this disorder is a life-changing event and a life-long journey. Going to a support group will help families learn how to deal with the physical and the emotional strain of raising these special children. Families can learn how to deal with each developmental stage of their children as it presents itself by listening to other families who have been through it. Families could also make better plans for their children's future and learn about available resources in the community. There are also national organizations that provide help and literature on raising a child with Down syndrome.

Unfortunately there is no cure for Down syndrome, and the chromosomal accident or the genetic problem that causes Down syndrome cannot be medically prevented either. A lot of research is going into the studies of the chromosomal or genetic accident that causes the disorder to occur when a baby is being conceived. Several studies are going into the possible prevention of other genetic birth defects as well. More knowledge and understanding from research will continue to improve the treatment and outcome of Down syndrome and will hopefully improve our attitude toward people with Down syndrome.

Finally, it cannot be overemphasized that growing up with Down syndrome may be very difficult for the individual and their family members. Other children may tease children with Down syndrome, call them names, and bully them because they are afraid of their difference. Unfortunately, some adults also treat people with disability or certain limitations with unkindness. It is important for parents to educate their children that children with Down syndrome have feelings, too, and they should not behave in an unkind way to them. Parents should teach their children that all people deserve to be treated with respect, regardless of physical appearance, ability, or distinguishing features. Parents should also communicate to their children that Down syndrome is not contagious or infectious. They cannot contract Down syndrome by playing with a child with Down syndrome. Parents can also be a big help by setting a good example of role-modeling kindness to other people in the presence of their children. Children learn a lot from their parents. Children learn more from what they see than what they are told. With scientific research, we can hope that the day will come in the near future when no child will be born with Down syndrome or any other form of genetic or physical abnormality.

PART X

# THE ROLE OF SUPPORT GROUPS

# THE ROLE OF SUPPORT GROUPS IN MENTAL ILLNESS

Much has been said throughout the book about the importance of joining a support group for people living with mental illness and their families. They can all benefit tremendously from joining a support group.

Dealing with mental illness is emotionally draining for everybody involved. There is usually a lot of guilt and self-blame on the part of the victim, the significant others, and their family members. Support groups usually provide a nonjudgmental and accepting atmosphere. Everybody in the group is usually transparent and honest because they are all dealing with the same or similar issues. Nobody feels like an outsider. Most people in support groups have worked past the denial stage and have accepted that they have an illness. The illness is real, and it is a mental illness. People come to realize that they are not alone, and they are not the only human beings dealing with a mental illness. People in support groups can freely discuss their day-to-day struggles with their illness. They can discuss their successes and their failures without feeling any sense of embarrassment.

Going to support group can be especially beneficial for a person newly diagnosed with mental illness. It could provide a forum for the newly diagnosed to learn how those who have been living with the illness for a long time have dealt with it daily. They can also learn how other people managed the different stages of the illness. Newly diagnosed people can learn how to deal with failures and relapses, which can be especially frustrating. Some support groups also offer a mentorship program for their new members. The new member will be assigned a mentor who has been through the program and succeeded. The mentor could be called at any time if the new member is having some difficulty. This is especially helpful in addiction-related issues. For example if a new member dealing with addiction is having a craving for the substance of addiction, instead of giving in to the craving, he could call the mentor. The mentor could help him work through his difficult time and provide the support needed to prevent a relapse.

The majority of the people with mental illness always have a very low self-esteem and poor self-confidence, because they have been looked down on and talked down to all of their lives. Going to a good support group could help to build their self-esteem and self-confidence and also help them to realize that living with mental illness is not the end of the world. They could be empowered and encouraged to learn to develop to their full potential. They could learn to be independent as much as possible by listening to other members of the group with success stories.

Many people with mental illness are abandoned or avoided by their family members and significant others because family members and significant others may not know how to act around the mentally ill. They may not want to be bothered with this illness that they cannot understand. As a result, isolation could be a problem for people with mental illness. A support group usually provides the nuclear support. Members grow to see each other as family members. People have formed long-lasting and positive relationships with people they meet at their support group. Making friends who understand what you are going through can make a lot of difference in your recovery.

Members could learn new information from support groups as well. Different members may bring different sets of information to the group on what is current in the treatment of that particular illness. Some members are very aggressive about researching new information, and are always willing to share it with the rest of the group. For instance, information on newer medications in the market and newer therapies for the treatment of that particular mental illness may be discussed in support groups.

Family members, caregivers, or significant others of people with mental illness could also benefit tremendously from attending support groups for families of the mentally ill. Mental illness is emotionally, physically, and financially draining to the family members of the victims. To be in an environment where you can easily voice your frustration without being judged, can be very therapeutic. Talking about the mental and physical stress of taking care of a family member with mental illness can be viewed as whining or complaining to people who cannot relate to that situation. Some family members, caregivers, and significant others just want to talk about what they are experiencing. They feel better, verbalizing their feelings, and feel ready to face new challenges each day.

Family members can learn how other families cope with having somebody in the house with mental illness. They also learn how to blend the special care of the special family member into the family routines. They also learn how to balance the care of the mentally ill with the care of other members of the family. For instance, it could be especially difficult if a mentally ill child has other siblings. It is so easy for the parents to neglect the other siblings and not even realize that they are doing it. The parents could be totally consumed with taking care of the sick child only. Another good example is the care of a family member with Alzheimer's dementia; this could also be a tough daily challenge. Family members could advise each other on what works and what does not work in their individual homes whenever they come to the group.

Some of the support groups are spiritual and very insightful. Being able to get the problem off your chest and not allow it to burden you can help lighten the load. Venting may help, and looking to a higher power for help can provide strength. This is very much needed in the area of forgiveness. Some people with mental illness struggle with forgiving themselves for the mistakes they made when their illness was active. Family members with poor understanding of some of these illnesses may feel responsible for the illness and blame themselves.

Family members can also work out arrangements for group babysitting or adult sitting in order to provide relief for each other. For instance, family A could keep the mentally ill individual for family B for a day to allow family B a day off without worrying about the mentally ill person in the family. Likewise, family B could do the same or provide the same relief for family A on a later date. Opportunity to have some time away from around -the-clock care of a mentally ill person could provide a great mental or psychological relief for the caregivers.

The financial issue is always a pressing issue for families of mentally ill people. Mental illness can throw a hardworking family into poverty. A good example is Alzheimer's dementia. It is important for family members to talk to other families and to find out how they handle the financial aspect of the illness. It is also important to know what is available in terms of aid in the community that could directly or indirectly provide financial relief. For instance, there could be a volunteer group that provides free house-sitting or free meals to the victims and their family members.

Medication compliance has always been another pressing issue for people with mental illness because of the side effects. A support group could provide a forum for people with mental illness and their family members to talk about what to expect in terms of side effects of their medications and how to manage the side effects when they occur. If several people are on similar medications, they may have similar or close to similar experiences in side effects.

Support groups can be open or closed. An **open support group** allows people to attend the group even if they are not dealing with the illness. Some people may attend out of curiosity, they may just want to sit watch and learn. Students may sometimes be required to go to support groups for educational purposes and listen to how people cope with mental illness. An open group will always accommodate non-members. On the other hand, a **closed support group** will not allow anybody to sit in the group unless he or she is a member. Everyone in attendance must be dealing with the same or similar issues. Some people join closed support groups because they feel very free to discuss their problems because of the privacy of the group. Members could be more open and honest with one another without being guarded once they know that everybody is there for a common purpose. They have no fear of been judged by people who cannot identify with their illness. Members know exactly who is coming, unless a new member is joining the group. They do not have to worry about the surprise of seeing somebody they do not want to expose their illness or their struggle to just walk into the group unexpectedly. Many people struggling with mental illness are still likely to lean toward keeping it a secret because of the stigma. Such people will obviously prefer a closed group to an open group. No one should be judged based on the type of group they join, the choice of open or closed group is a personal decision that must be respected.

A group could be productive and counterproductive. If a group focuses on the purpose for which it was established, the group will be productive. If the group does not focus on the purpose for which it was established, the group could become counterproductive. It is important to find a group that fits your schedule and your time, and also serves a productive purpose in your life. People go to support group in between work, at their lunch time, on weekends, and in the evenings. Groups are usually held at different times of the day.

It is advisable to have an identifiable group leader to keep the group focused and in check. No one person should be allowed to dominate a group. Every one in the group should have a chance to talk, contribute, or seek advice from the group. For instance, everybody could be limited to five minutes only when he or she talks. This is to avoid a situation where some people may continuously monopolize the group without any consideration for other members of the group. People play different roles in groups. They come together to give the group its identity or character. Here are some of the different roles played by group members:

- An initiator would bring new ideas to the group and suggest ways to implement the ideas.
- An orienter will help new members to get familiarized with the group, and also state the goal of the group to newcomers.
- An opinion seeker would seek clarification about personal issues or issues affecting the group or the group members.
- An energizer motivates and empowers other members in the group. This person also helps others work through decision-making process.
- A recorder is the note taker or bookkeeper of the group.
- An encourager praises others for their big or little successes and builds their self-esteem.
- A gatekeeper encourages others to participate, making sure no one person is dominating the group.
- A group harmonizer will promote peace in the group and bring people together. He or she tries to make sure there is no tension in the group.
- A follower wants to be everybody's friend. He or she usually goes along with the crowd and have no personal opinion.
- A blocker brings negativity to the group. He may be unreasonable and always have a contrary opinion to the group.
- A dominator may be unnecessarily assertive and manipulative, seeking to have his or her way with the group all the time.
- A recognition seeker is focused on himself. He or she may boast about personal achievements, and make up stories so to look good or better than others.

A group must have a system in place to vote out a group member who is continuously disruptive to the group and is not willing to grow, change, or learn from the group. The system to remove a group member must be fair. The group must keep it in mind that the disruptive behavior manifest by a group member may be the result of his or her mental illness. Patience must be exercised before banning or voting a group member out of the group. Such a decision must be made only in situations where the persistent disruptive behavior of that member gets to the point of possibly destroying the group.

Anybody can start a support group by seeking the help of an existing or similar group. A very common group which has been used as a model in starting a support group is the twelve-step group of Alcohol Anonymous or AA. This is a group for people recovering from alcohol addiction. Every group may not be able to use the Alcohol Anonymous model. The goal is to research and to find the model that would work best for the members when starting a group. An individual or a family may have to visit different support groups before they find the one that would work best for them.

*Winds Against The Mind*

<u>PART XI</u>

# THE IMPORTANCE OF SUPERVISED MEDICATION MANAGEMENT

# THE IMPORTANCE OF SUPERVISED MEDICATION MANAGEMENT IN THE TREATMENT OF MENTAL ILLNESS

**M**edication management in the treatment of mental illnesses should be **strictly prescribed and supervised by a licensed clinician** who has undergone the training to prescribe psychotropic medications (medication used in the treatment of mental illnesses). In the United State of America, it could be a psychiatrist, a psychiatric nurse practitioner, or any credentialed and licensed clinician who could prescribe psychotropic medication in that community. Usually the initial diagnosis could also be made by a primary care provider, such as a family physician, an internist, a nurse practitioner, or any licensed clinician in that community who may be the first or initial contact with the client. A clinician must be very knowledgeable to be able to treat mental illness. The mind is very delicate, and it is the center of our being. Licensed clinicians take several factors into consideration in prescribing psychotropic medications. Medication mismanagement in the treatment of a mental illness could have unfavorable and tragic results. Every case or every suspicion of **a mental illness must be referred to a licensed clinician.** There are several reasons why a specialized clinician must be consulted in the management of a mental illness. Some of the factors include but are not limited to the following:

- To discourage people from self-medicating and trying to treat mental illnesses on their own without appropriate training and education.

- To encourage people to strictly seek professional help in the diagnosis and management of mental illness whenever they observe unusual signs and symptoms that arouse their suspicion.
- To promote the understanding that trained clinicians who diagnose and treat mental illnesses take a lot of factors into consideration based on their knowledge, experience and expertise. They evaluate signs and symptoms manifested by the client, before prescribing any medication for the treatment of the particular mental disorder.

Some of the factors considered by a clinician before prescribing a medication include allergy history, the interaction of one drug with other medications, family history, availability of the drug in the market, side effects, costs of the medication, the extent to which the drug has been tested, individual comprehensive health history, and several other factors. Most of these factors would be clearly explained to enhance the understanding of the public, and to clarify the importance of consulting a knowledgeable and licensed clinician in medication management.

Most trained clinicians usually take a very **comprehensive medical and health history** from their clients at the initial interview. The information collected is used to determine the plan of care for the clients. Some clients may require only therapy and counseling, while some may require a combination of medication and therapeutic management.

A clinician would definitely require the information about the **allergy history of a client.** At times, the client may not know all of the medications that could give him or her allergic reaction. A clinician may elicit or get this information indirectly out of the client by asking him a simple question such as the food he is allergic to, in order to collect information on the client's medication allergy history. For instance, somebody allergic to shellfish and seafood may not be able to take certain types of medications. If a client is accidentally given a medication that could cause an allergic reaction, she could develop or have a serious anaphylactic (severe allergic reaction that could be life threatening) reaction, and develop serious complications. If a person tries to self-medicate without a good knowledge of the action of the medication and the interference with her allergy, she could run into serious health complications.

A clinician would also require **the list of medications that a person is currently on** at the time of the initial contact with the client. There are some medications that **must not** be taken together. Drug interaction between some medications that are not supposed to be taken together may render all or some of the medication taken ineffective. The person then wonders why there is no change or improvement in his or her health condition while on the medications. He or she may later find out that the ineffectiveness is the direct result of the drug interaction.

**A comprehensive family history** is usually taken by a clinician in the treatment and diagnosis of mental illness. For instance, if a client has a strong family history of clinical depression, what worked and what did not work for other family members could be taken into consideration in prescribing a medication for that client. This does not change the fact that every individual is treated differently. However, knowing the family history should be helpful rather than harmful. Side effects and treatment response could be partially determined by gathering family information from the client. A particular antidepressant medication that worked effectively for the father of a depressed person may first be tried for the son in the treatment of his depression before any other medication is tried.

A clinician also takes into consideration the **availability of the medication that is being prescribed in the market.** Many psychotropic medications or medication used in the treatment of mental illness is used by clients for a long time. To maintain its therapeutic effect, it is important to make sure that the prescribed medication will be readily available when needed. A clinician is not likely to prescribe a medication that may not be easily available for purchase, especially if the medication will be needed for a long time.

**The side effects of a medication** are an important consideration in prescribing a medication to a client. For instance, it may not be wise to prescribe a medication with a sedative or sleeping effect as the early morning pill for somebody who drives a vehicle all day long. The person could fall asleep at the steering wheel and have a wreck. Such medication could be prescribed as an evening or night pill when the person goes to bed. The **safety** of the client is taken very seriously in medication management. Also, if the side effects of certain medications are very unpleasant and unbearable, a clinician will know to look for alternative ones with fewer side effects. **It must be noted,** however, that almost every medication has a side effect. Some side effects could be very frightening to the client. Client education about the side effects from the clinician could help to alleviate the client's fear when it occurs. A clinician will have to weigh the risk of not treating the patient versus the discomfort of the side effects. In addition, a clinician could recommend the use of some adjunctive or other medication for the relief of some side effects. For instance, some side effects from antipsychotic medications could be relieved by the use of some antiparkinsonian medication.

A clinician would not always rush into medication intervention especially **if the psychiatric or mental illness appears like one that could be self-limiting** and the signs and symptoms are most likely to disappear with time. For instance, a person may have a psychosis or confusion that was induced from the use of a medication that is not for the treatment of a mental illness. This could be caused by accidental overdose of that particular medication. The client's reaction from taking the medication may resemble a mental illness. The clinician would know not to prescribe any more medication to treat such confusion or psychosis. A clinician would also know that this confusion or psychosis was caused or induced by a medication. Allowing the effect of the medication that is causing the psychosis to wear off could be the best decision in this type of situation. A routine medical support such as hydration and allowing the situation to run its course could be the best intervention for the client. A person with no vast medication knowledge may not be able to take such a decision.

**Cost** is another important consideration in prescribing a medication. Clients have different social economic status and different insurance plans. As much as clinicians advocate wellness, they do not want to put their clients in a situation in which they have to make a choice between buying their medication and their food. The most expensive medication may not necessarily be the most effective medication. It is a common knowledge, however, that newer medications are usually more expensive. Clinicians try to work with affordability for their clients. If cost is an issue, medications that are available in the **generic form** (not a name brand) may be prescribed by the clinician. Generic brands are usually less expensive than name brands, and they have the exact, same chemical composition. A clinician can also prescribe a medication that has been in use for a long time, but equally effective as a newer brand and much cheaper with few side effects.

Drugs have been marketed as miracle drugs and later recalled from the market as a very dangerous drug because of the side effects. Clinicians may be reluctant to put their clients on **medications that are not widely tested for safety,** or medications that are not well known. If a clinician is not very familiar with a medication, he may not want to risk prescribing it. This is very important because some medications have been known to cause irreversible damage to the body and some vital organs before they were recalled from the market.

**Comprehensive history of the individual** is also taken into consideration in prescribing a medication. Having a thorough knowledge of a client's medical and psychological history would help the clinician to determine the medication that is likely to work best for that person. Family members could help in supplying the data on the client's history. Questions such as previous symptoms, treatments, and responses must be asked. History of drug and alcohol use must also be asked or elicited. Clients sometimes may not be forthcoming in giving their history to the clinician. This could be a barrier in picking the right medication for them.

Another important factor for eliciting or collecting a client's history is the **potential lethal (deadly) effect of the medication when taken in overdose.** Emotional and psychological or mental stability of the client is seriously considered by the clinician in prescribing medications. For instance, a clinician would likely stay away from prescribing a medication that is highly lethal when taken in overdose to a person who is very **suicidal** at the time of treatment or has a strong suicidal history. Also if a client is **confused** and is more likely to make mistakes when taking the medications, the clinician will be careful by possibly not prescribing a medication that could be highly lethal if taken in overdose. The only exception would be a situation where the confused or the suicidal person is properly supervised.

A thorough assessment of the **client's physical health** must be done in order to **rule out** any other underlying medical condition that could mimic a mental illness. For instance, signs and symptoms of a low thyroid level (hypothyrodism) may mimic depression. Once the thyroid level is corrected, the signs and symptoms that mimic depression may disappear. Such a client could be wrongly treated for depression instead of being treated for thyroid problems. If the clinician did not take a thorough medical and physical health history, the client's problem could be compounded instead of getting solved.

A clinician would usually **order a routine laboratory work up** for the client to **rule out** other organic or non-psychiatric causes that may be responsible for some of the signs and symptoms that are observed. For instance, a diabetic person may manifest signs and symptoms that could mimic psychotic illness and confusion if the blood sugar is too high (hyperglycemia) or too low (hypoglycemia). A laboratory blood test or a simple accucheck (using a blood sugar machine to test the blood sugar level), may reveal the blood sugar imbalance. Once this is corrected, the confusion that may mimic a psychosis or mental problem will usually disappear.

**A clinician is expected to be very knowledgeable about the medication** that is being prescribed to a client. As a result, a clinician can advise a client on the specific symptoms that the medication is targeting and the specific symptoms that the medication may not be able to provide relief for. A clinician could also educate clients on the common side effects and signs and symptoms of medication toxicity. Symptoms such as nausea, vomiting, and diarrhea may be indicative of drug toxicity to some medications. If it is not addressed immediately, it could lead to electrolyte imbalance (losing water and some essential minerals in the body) and this can cause serious complications.

**The primary rule in medication management is to use one pill at a time,** if it is possible. **However,** there are so many situations which require the use of combination medications in treating some signs and symptoms of some mental illnesses. A knowledgeable clinician would be able to make such a determination. A knowledgeable clinician would also know what medications to combine and not to combine. Furthermore, there may be situations where a medication dosage would have to be adjusted either by increasing or decreasing the dosage. This should only be done by a licensed clinician. When it is also necessary to change a client's medication, a trained clinician should be the one to take that decision. All of the above judgment calls must be strictly made by a licensed clinician with thorough medication knowledge in order for a client to have a good outcome. The ultimate rule is this: nobody should try to manage a mental illness with medication on their own.

*Winds Against The Mind*

## National Alliance For The Mentally Ill (NAMI):

# CONTACT LIST

For more information on Mental Illness and Mental Health Related Issues, contact:

**NATIONAL ALLIANCE FOR THE MENTALLY ILL (NAMI)**
200 North Glebe Road, Suite 1015
Arlington, VA 22203-3754
1-800-950-NAMI
*http://www.nami.org*

Listed on the next few pages is the contact information for State NAMI locations that can help individuals to find other local NAMI organizations closer to them:

### Alabama
NAMI Alabama
4122 Wall St
Montgomery, AL 36106-2861
(334)3963-4797
(800)626-4199
FAX: (334)396-4794
*www.namialabama.org*

### Alaska
NAMI Alaska
144 W 15 Ave
Anchorage, AK 99501-5106
(907)277-1300
(800)478-4462
FAX: (907)-277-1400
*www.nami.org/sites/alaska*

### Arizona
NAMI Arizona
2210 N 7th St
Phoenix, AZ 85006-1604
(602)244-8166
(800)626-5022
FAX: (602)244-9264
*www.namiaz.org*

### Arkansas
NAMI Arkansas
712 W 3rd Street
Suite 200
Little Rock AR 72201-2222
(501)661-1548
(800)844-0381
FAX: (501)664-0264
*ar.nami.org*

### California
NAMI California
1010 Hurley Way
Ste 195
Sacremento, CA 95825-3218
(915)567-0163
FAX: (916)567-1757
*www.namicalifornia.org*

### Colorado
NAMI Colorado
1100 Filmore Street
Ste 201
Denver, CO 80206-3334
(303)321-3104
(888)566-6264
*www.namicolorado.org*

### Connecticut
NAMI Connecticut
242 Main St 5th Floor
Hartford, CT 06106
(860)882-0236
(800)215-3021
FAX: (860)882-0240
*www.namict.org*

### Delaware
NAMI Delaware
2400 W 4th St
Wilmington, DE 19805-3306
(302)427-0787
(888)427-2643
FAX: (302)427-2075
*www.namide.org*

## District of Columbia
NAMI District of Columbia
422 8th St SE
2nd Floor
Washington DC, 20003-2832
(202)546-0646
FAX: (202)546-6817
*www.nami.dc.org*

## Florida
NAMI Florida
1615 Village Square Blvd
Suite 6
Tallahassee, FL 32309
(850) 671-4445
(877)626-4352
FAX: (850)671-5272
*www.namifl.org*

## Georgia
NAMI Georgia
3050 Presidential Drive
Suite 202
Atlanta, GA 30340-3916
(770)234-0855
(800)728-1052
FAX: (770)234-0237
*www.namiga.org*

## Hawaii
NAMI Hawaii
770 Kapiolani Blvd
#613
Honolulu, HI 96813-5212
(808)591-1297
FAX: (808)591-2058
*namihawaii.org*

## Idaho
NAMI Idaho
PO Box 68
Albion, ID 83311-0068
(208)673-6672
(800)572-9940
FAX: (208)673-6685
*www.namiorg/sites/NAMIIDAHO*

## Illinois
NAMI Illinois
218 W Lawrence Ave
Springfield, IL 62704-2612
(217)522-1403
(800)346-4572
FAX: (217)522-3598
*il.nami.org*

## Indiana
NAMI Indiana
Po Box 22697
Indianapolis, IN 46222-0697
(317)925-9399
FAX: (317)925-9398
*www.namiindiana.org*

## Iowa
NAMI Iowa
Attn: Margaret Stout 5911 Meredith Drive,
Ste E
Des Moines, IA 50322-1903
(515)254-0417
(800)417-0417
FAX: (515)254-1103
*www.namiiowa.com*

367

## Kansas

NAMI Kansas
112 SW 6th Ave, Suite 505 Po Box 657
Topeka, KS 66601-0675
(785)233-0755
(800)539-2660
FAX: (785)233-4804
*www.namikansas.org*

## Kentucky

NAMI Kentucky
10510 Lagrange Rd
Bld 103
Louisville, KY 40223-1277
(502)245-5284
(800)257-5081
FAX: (502)245-6390
*ky.nami.org*

## Louisiana

NAMI Louisiana
PO Box 40517
Batton Rouge, LA 70835-0517
(225)926-8770
(866)851-6264
FAX: (225)926-8773
*www.namilouisiana.org*

## Maine

NAMI Maine
1 Bangor St
Augusta, ME 04330-4701
(207)622-5767
(800)464-5767
FAX: (207)621-8430
*www.namimain.org*

## Maryland

NAMI Maryland
804 Landmark Dr
Suite 122
Glen Burnie, MD 21061-4486
(410)863-0470
(800)467-0075
FAX: (410)863-0474
*md.nami.org*

## Massachusettes

NAMI Massachusettes
400 West Cummings Park
Suite 6650
Woburn, MA 01801-6528
(781)938-4048
(800)370-9085
FAX: (781)938-4069
*www.namimass.org*

## Michigan

NAMI Michigan
921 N Washington Ave
Langsing, MI 48906-5137
(517)485-4049
(800)331-4264
FAX: (517)485-2333
*mi.nami.org*

## Minnesota

NAMI Minnesota
800 Transfer Rd
Suite 7A
Saint Paul, MN 55114-1414
(651)645-2948
(888)473-0237
FAX: (651)645-7379
*www.namimn.org*

## Mississippi

NAMI Mississippi
411 Briarwood Dr
Ste 401
Jackson, MS 39206-3058
(601)899-9058
(800)357-0388
FAX: (601)956-6380
*www.nami.org/sites/NAMIMississipii*

## Missouri

NAMI Missouri
1001 Southwest Blvd Ste E
Jefferson City, MO 65109-2501
(573)634-7727
(800)374-2138
FAX: (573)761-5636

## Montana

NAMI Montana
Mihelish's Residence
554 Toole Ct
Helena, MT 59602-6946
(406)443-7871
(888)280-6264
FAX: (406)862-6357
*www.namimt.org*

## Nebraska

NAMI Nebraska
1941 S 42nd St
Ste 517 -Center Mall
Omaha, NE 68105-2986
(877)463-6264
(402)345-8101
FAX: (402)346-4070
*www.nami.org/sites/ne*

## Nevada

NAMI Nevada
1170 Curti Drive
Reno, NV 89502
(775)329-3260
(775)688-3317
FAX: (775)329-1618
*www.nami-nevada.org*

## New Hampshire

NAMI New Hampshire
15 Green St
Concord, NH 03301-4020
(603)225-5359
(800)242-6264
FAX: (603)228-8848
*www.naminh.org*

## New Jersey

NAMI New Jersey
1562 US Highway 130
North Brunswick, NJ 08902-3004
(732)940-0991
FAX: (732)940-0355
*www.naminj.org*

## New Mexico

NAMI New Mexico
PO Box 3080
6001 Marble NE Suite 8
Albuquerque, NM 87190-3086
(505)260-0154
FAX: (505)260-0342
*nm.nami.org*

**New York**
NAMI New York
260 Washington Ave
Albany, NY 12210-1312
(518)-462-2000
(800)950-3228
FAX: (518)462-3811
*www.naminys.org*

**North Carolina**
NAMI North Carolina
309 W Millbrook Rd Ste 121
Raleigh, NC 27609-4394
(919)788-0801
(800)451-9682
FAX: (919)788-0906
*www.naminc.org*

**North Dakota**
NAMI North Dakota
PO Box 3215
Minot, ND 58702-3215
(701)852-8202

**Ohio**
NAMI Ohio
747 East Broad Street
Columbus, OH 43205
(614)224-2700
(800)686-2646
FAX: (614)224-5400
*www.namiohio.org*

**Oklahoma**
NAMI Oklahoma
500 N Broadway Ave
Suite 100
Oklahoma City, OK 73102-6200
(405)230-1900
(800)583-1264
FAX: (405)230-1903
*ok.nami.org*

**Oregon**
NAMI Oregon
3350 SE Woodwar St
Portland, OR 97202-1552
(503)230-8009
(800)343-6264
FAX: (503)230-2751
*www.nami.org/sites/NAMIOregon*

**Pennslyvannia**
NAMI Pennslyvannia
2149 North 2nd Street
Harrisuburg, PA 17110-1005
(717)238-1514
(800)223-0500
FAX: (717)238-4390
*namipa.nami.org*

**Rhode Island**
NAMI Rhode Island
154 Waterman St
Suite 5B
Providence, RI 02906-3116
(401)331-3060
(800)749-3197
FAX: (401)274-3020
*www.namirhodeisland.org*

## South Carolina
NAMI South Carolina
PO Box 1267
Columbia SC 2920-1267
(800)788-5131
(803)733-9592
FAX: (803)733-9593
*www.namisc.org*

## South Dakota
NAMI South Dakota
PO Box 88808
Sioux Falls, SD 57109-8808
(605)271-1871
(800)551-2531
FAX: (605)271-1871
*www.nami.org/sites/NAMISouthDakota*

## Tenessee
NAMI Tennessee
1101 Kermit Drive
Suite 605
Nashville, TN 37217-2126
(615)-361-6608
(800)467-3589
FAX: (615)361-6698
*www.namitn.org*

## Texas
NAMI Texas
Fountain Park Plaza III
2800 South Ih35, Suite 140
Austin, TX 78704
(512)-693-2000
(800)633-3760
FAX: (512)693-8000
*www.namitexas.org*

## Utah
NAMI Utah
4005 S 900 E
Suite 160
Salt Lake City, UT 84102-2981
(801)323-9900
FAX: (801)323-9799
*www.namiut.org*

## Vermont
NAMI Vermont
132 South Main street
Waterbury,VT 05676-1519
(802)244-1396
(800)639-6480
FAX: (800)639-6480
*www.namivt.org*

## Viriginia
NAMI Viriginia
PO Box 8260
Richmond, VA 23226-0260
(804)285-8264
(888)486-8264
FAX: (804)285-8464
*www.manivirginia.org*

## Washington
NAMI Washington
500 108TH Ave NE
Suite 800
Bellevue, Wa 98004-5580
(425)990-6404
(800)782-9264
*www.namiwa.org*

## West Virginia

NAMI West Virginia
600 Westmoreland Office Park
Dunbar, WV 25064-2719
(304)342-0497
(800)598-5653
FAX: (304)342-0499
*charityadvantage.com/namiwv/home.asp*

## Wisconsin

NAMI Wisconsin
4233 W Beltline Hwy
Madison, WI 53711-3814
(608)268-6000
(800)236-2988
FAX: (608)268-6004
*www.namiwisconsin.org*

## Wyoming

NAMI Wyoming
133 W 6th Street
Casper, WY 82601-3124
(307)234-0440
(888)882-4968
FAX: (307)265-0968
*www.nami.org/sites/*
*namiwyoming*

# About the Author

**Lola Bamigboye** received her law degree from the University of Lagos and Nigerian Law School. She later attended Tennessee State University in Nashville, where she received an Associate of Science in Nursing degree. She proceeded to attend Vanderbilt University School of Nursing in Nashville, where she received a Master of Science in Nursing, with a specialty in psychiatric nursing. She has worked for more than seventeen years as a psychiatric nurse in various roles. Her areas of experience include child and adolescent psychiatry, adult psychiatry, geriatric psychiatry, and substance abuse. She is currently an instructor at Vanderbilt University School of Nursing and an adjunct faculty member at Belmont University School of Nursing, both in Nashville, Tennessee. She has more than seven years of experience as a clinical instructor, alternately teaching nursing students at both schools. She also has a private practice with a focus on individual, marriage, and family counseling. She is married with three children.

*Lola.bts51@yahoo.com*

# Building Towards Success L.L.C.

## Our Publishing Mission:

To produce publications that would have a positive influence on the life of the reader, by promoting psychological and emotional well being, and to enable the reader to strive to reach his or her optimum potential.

To contact us or order the book:

BUILDING TOWARDS SUCCESS
P.O. BOX 275
BRENTWOOD
TENNESSEE, 37024
U.S.A.
Tel: 615-469-5076
Fax: 615-661-9535
*www.windsagainstthemind.com*

# Acknowledgements

With deepest appreciation I thank my creator for giving me the inspiration to write this book. I felt the presence of my creator throughout my journey of putting this book together.

To all the authors whose work I read or to whom I am indebted for their ideas, I thank you for your good work and perpetuation of knowledge. I am especially grateful to the author of the Best of Success, a book of hope and inspiration for me.

To my spiritual mother in Canada, Mummy Winifred O. Oyelese, I thank you very much for your help. You are a reservoir of knowledge and wisdom; only the wise can tap into it. Thank you for many hours and sleepless nights of helping me to edit and rearrange the book.

To Beth and Michael Robertson, thank you for your friendship and support as I completed this book. Thank you for your encouragement and hours of editing. Thank you for searching for a publisher and for introducing me to Sarah Davis, who has been a great help.

Thank you, Sarah Davis, for all of your help. God's blessings to you.

To Marylou and Jim Parrish, I cannot thank you enough for your encouragement; I thank God for putting both of you in my life.

To Henry and Queen Okafor, I am grateful for your encouragement and support as I completed this book.

To my friend Caroline Cone, who introduced me to teaching and who always believed in me, I thank you very much.

To my friend and my colleague Joyce Alexander, I am very grateful for your encouragement. You went out of your way for me to see that I completed this book.

# Winds Against The Mind

*To Leslie Folds, thank you for believing in me. Your encouragement and outstanding support in promoting this book will always be appreciated. You are a true friend. God's blessings to you always.*

*To Susie Adams, you are the best. Thank you for your unwavering support and friendship. You went out of your way to promote this book. Your kindness and humility is an inspiration. I will always be grateful to you.*

*To Lynn Myrick, I thank you very much for taking the time out of your busy schedule to edit this book.*

*To Scherie Lammert, Dennis, and Patty Huffer, my neighbors, I thank you so much for your support. Everyone should have neighbors like you.*

*To my inquisitive students at Belmont University School of Nursing and at Vanderbilt University School of Nursing, who richly bless my life and are also a source of encouragement to write this book, I say thank you.*

*To my colleagues, faculty members and staff at Vanderbilt University School of Nursing and Belmont University School of Nursing, I thank you all for your support.*

*To the memory of three special people who influenced my life positively but are no longer here, Dr. Robert Hardy, a mentor and a good physician, Tom Armstrong, a talented poet and a good friend of my family, and Dr. Michael Omotosho, a noble soul and a very kind cousin to me, I thank God that you were all in my life, even if it was for a short time.*

*To many others who have blessed me enormously, who stood by me in time of need, who supported me through tough and good times, who have been true friends and family to me, especially during the transition of my parents, I thank you and express my deepest appreciation. Even if I did not mention your names, I am very grateful. God's blessings to all of you.*

# Glossary

**Abstract thinking** the ability to conceptualize ideas (*e.g.*, finding meaning in proverbs).

**Acrophobia** Fear of high places.

**Activities of daily living** For a person with a chronic mental illness, this term refers to the skills necessary to live independently as an adult.

**Addiction** Addiction incorporates the concepts of loss of control with respect to use of a drug (*e.g.*, alcohol), taking the drug despite related problems, and a tendency to relapse. *Addiction* is an older term that has been replaced by the term *drug dependence*.

**Affect** An objective manifestation of an experience or emotion accompanying an idea or feeling. The observations one would make on assessment. For example, a client may be said to have a flat affect, meaning that there is an absence or a near absence of facial expression. Some people, however, use the term loosely to mean a feeling, emotion, or mood.

**Aggression** Any verbal or nonverbal (actual or attempted, conscious or unconscious) forceful means to harm or abuse another person or object.

**Agnosia** Loss of the ability to recognize familiar objects. For example, a person may be unable to identify familiar sounds, such as the ringing of a doorbell (auditory agnosia), or familiar objects, such as a toothbrush or keys (visual agnosia).

**Alcoholism** The end stage of the continuum that includes addiction to and dependence on the drug alcohol.

**Amnesia** Loss of memory for events within a specific period of time; may be temporary or permanent.

**Anergia** Lack of energy; passivity.

**Anger** An emotional response to the perception of frustration of desires or threat to one's needs.

**Anorexia** A medical term that signifies a loss of appetite. A person with anorexia nervosa, however, may not have any loss of appetite and often is preoccupied with food and eating. A person with this condition may suppress the desire for food in order to control his or her eating.

**Antidepressants** Drugs predominantly used to elevate mood in people who are depressed.

**Antipsychotic drugs (neuroleptics, major tranquilizers)** Drugs that have the ability to decrease psychotic paranoid, and disorganized thinking and positively alter bizarre behaviors, they are thought to reduce the effects of certain neurotransmitters that is believed to be responsible for psychosis.

**Anxiety** A state of feeling apprehension, uneasiness, uncertainty, or dread resulting from a real or perceived threat whose actual source is unknown or unrecognized.

**Aphasia** Difficulty in the formulation of words; loss of language ability. In extreme cases, a person may be limited to a few words, may babble, or may become mute.

**Apraxia** Loss of purposeful motor movements. For example, a person may be unable to shave, to dress, or to do other once-familiar and purposeful tasks.

**Assault** An intentional act that is designed to make the victim fearful and that produces reasonable apprehension or harm.

**Assertiveness** Asking for what one wants or acting to get what one wants in a way that respects the rights and feelings of others.

**Attention-deficit hyperactivity disorder** a behavioral disorder usually manifested before the age of 7 that includes over-activity, chronic inattention, and difficulty dealing with multiple stimuli.

**Bipolar disorders** Mood disorders that include one or more manic episodes and usually one or more depressive episodes.

**Blocking** A sudden obstruction or interruption in the spontaneous flow of thinking or speaking that is perceived as an absence or deprivation of thought.

**Boundaries** Those functions that maintain a clear distinction among individuals within a family or group and with the outside world. Boundaries may be clear, diffuse, rigid, or inconsistent.

**Bulimia** An eating disorder characterized by the excessive and uncontrollable intake of large amounts of food (binges), alternating with purging activities such as self-induced vomiting; use of cathartics, diuretics, or both; and self-starvation. These alternating behaviors characterize the eating disorder *bulimia nervosa*.

**Character** The sum of a person's relatively fixed personality traits and habitual modes of response.

**Child abuse-neglect** This abuse can be physical (e.g., failure to provide medical care), *developmental* (e.g., failure to provide emotional nurturing and cognitive stimulation), *educational* (failure to provide educational opportunities to the child according to the state's education laws), or a combination.

**Chronic illness** An illness that has persisted over a long period of time and that generally involves progressive deterioration, with a resulting increase in functional impairment symptoms, and disability.

**Co-dependent** Coping behaviors that prevent individuals from taking care of their own needs and have as their core a preoccupation with the thoughts and feelings of another or others. It usually refers to the dependence of one person on another person who is addicted in one form or another.

**Compulsions** Repetitive, seemingly purposeless behaviors performed according to certain rules known to the client in order to temporarily reduce escalating anxiety.

**Confabulation** Filling in a memory gap with a detailed fantasy believed by the teller. The purpose is to maintain self-esteem. This is seen in organic conditions, such as Korsakoff's psychosis.

**Culture** The total life style of a people, the social legacy the individual acquires from his or her group, or the environment that is the creation of humankind.

**Delirium** An acute, usually reversible brain syndrome with multiple causes.

**Dementia** A progressive and usually irreversible deterioration of cognitive and intellectual functions and memory without impairment in consciousness.

**Denial** Escaping of unpleasant realities by ignoring their existence.

**Desensitization** The reduction of intense reactions of a stimulus (e.g., phobia) by repeated exposure to the stimulus in a weaker or milder form.

**Disorientation** Confusion and impaired ability to identify time, place, and person.

**Drug abuse** Defined by the American Psychiatric Association as the maladaptive and consistent use of a drug despite social, occupational, psychological or physical problems exacerbated by the drug; or recurrent use in situations that are physically hazardous, such as driving while intoxicated.

**Dysthymia** A depression that is; mild to moderate in degrees and is characterized by a chronic depressive syndrome that is usually present for many years. The depressive mood disturbance is hard to distinguish from the person's usual pattern of functioning and the person has minimal social or occupational impairment.

**Echolalia** Mimicking or imitating the speech of another person.

**Emotional abuse** Essentially, emotional abuse is depriving an individual of a nurturing atmosphere in which the he or she can thrive, learn, and develop. This takes many forms (e.g., terrorizing, demeaning, consistently belittling, withholding warmth).

**Empathy** The ability of one person to get inside another's world and see things from the other person's perspective and to communicate this understanding to the other person.

**Enabling** Helping a chemically dependent individual avoid experiencing the consequences of his or her drinking or drug use. It is one component of a person in co-dependency role.

**Family therapy** A treatment modality that focuses on the relationships within the family system.

**Fantasy** A retreat from reality and an attempt to solve problems in a private world. The difference between a healthy person and a schizophrenic, for example, is that a schizophrenic may not know where fantasy leaves off and reality begins.

**Fear** A reaction to a specific danger.

**Flight of ideas** A continuous flow of speech in which the person jumps rapidly from one topic to another. Sometimes the listener can keep up with the changes; at other times, it is necessary to listen for themes in the incessant talking. Themes often include grandiose and fantasized estimation of personal sexual prowess, business ability, artistic talents, and so on.

**Frustration** Curtailment of personal goals, satisfaction, or security by conditions of external reality or by internal controls.

**Grandiosity** Exaggerated belief in or claims about one's importance or identity.

**Grief** The subjective feelings and affect that are precipitated by a loss.

**Group** Two or more individuals who have a relationship with one another, are interdependent, and may share some norms.

**Group therapy** Psychotherapy based on the examination of group interaction with a view toward understanding and eventually changing the ways in which clients interact with others.

**Hallucination** A sense perception (seeing, hearing, tasting, smelling, or touching) for which no external stimulus exists (e.g., hearing voices when none are present).

**Hopelessness** The belief by a person that no one can help him or her; extreme pessimism about the future.

**Hostility** Anger that is destructive in nature and purpose.

**Hypomania** An elevated mood with symptoms less severe than those of mania. A person in hypomania does not experience impairment in reality testing, nor do the symptoms markedly repair the person's social, occupational, or interpersonal functioning.

**Ideas of reference** False impressions that outside events have special meaning for oneself.

**Illusion** An error in the perception of a sensory stimulus. For example, a person may mistake polka dots on a pillow for hairy spiders.

**Insomnia** Inability to fall asleep or to stay asleep, early morning awakening, or both.

**Intimacy** Emotional closeness.

**Labile** Having rapidly shifting emotions; unstable.

**Limit setting** The reasonable and rational setting of parameters for client behavior that provide control and safety.

**Looseness of association** A state in which thinking is haphazard, illogical, and confused, and connections in thought are interrupted; it is seen mostly in schizophrenic disorders.

**Magical thinking** The belief that thinking something can make it happen; it is seen in children and psychotic clients.

**Mania** An unstable elevated mood in which delusions, poor judgment, and other signs of impaired reality testing are evident. During a manic episode, clients have marked impairment in their social, occupational, and interpersonal functioning.

**Manipulation** Purposeful behavior directed at getting needs met. According to Chitty and Maynard (1986), manipulation is maladaptive when (1) it is the primary method used for getting needs met., (2) the needs, goals, and feelings of others are disregarded, and (3) others are treated as objects in order to fulfill the needs of the manipulator.

**Mental status exam** A formal assessment of cognitive functions such as intelligence, thought processes, and capacity for insight.

**Modeling** A technique in which desired behaviors are demonstrated. The client learns to imitate these behaviors in appropriate situations.

**Mood** Defined by the American Psychiatric Association as a pervasive and sustained emotion that, when extreme, can markedly colors the person's perception of the world.

**Mourning** The processes by which grief is resolved.

**Neurons** Specialized cells in the central nervous system. Each neuron has a cell body, an axon, and a dendrite.

**Neurotransmitter** A chemical substance that functions as a neural messenger. Neurotransmitters are released from the axon terminal of the presynaptic neuron when stimulated by an electrical impulse.

**Nursing** The diagnosis and treatment of human responses to actual or potential health problems.

**Obesity** A weight gain of at least 20% over the acceptable standard or ideal weight.

**Obsession** An idea, impulse, or emotion that a person cannot put out of his or her consciousness, it can be mild or severe.

**Orientation** The ability to relate the self correctly to time, place, and person.

**Organic mental disorder** As defined by the American psychiatric association, a specific brain syndrome for which a cause is known, for example, alcohol withdrawal delirium or Alzheimer's disease.

**Panic** Sudden, overwhelming anxiety of such intensity that it produces disorganization of the personality, loss of rational thought, and inability to communicate, along with specific physiological changes.

**Paranoia** Any intense and strongly defended irrational suspicion. These ideas cannot be corrected by experiences and cannot be modified by facts or reality.

**Perception** Mental processes by which intellectual, sensory, and emotional data are organized logically or meaningfully.

**Perseveration** The involuntary repetition of the same thought, phrase, or motor response (e.g., brushing teeth, walking); it is associated with brain damage.

**Personality** Deeply ingrained personal patterns of behavior, traits, and thoughts that evolve, both consciously and unconsciously, as a person's style and way of adapting to the environment.

**Phobia** An intense irrational fear of an object, situation, or place. The fear persists even though the object of the fear is harmless and the person is aware of the irrationality.

**Poverty of speech** Speech that is brief and uncommunicative.

**Primary depression** A depressive mood episode that is not due to a known organic factor and is not part of another psychotic disorder, such as schizophrenia (APA 1987).

**Psychiatry** The science of teaching clients and their families of their disorders, treatments, coping techniques, and resources. It helps empower clients and families by having them become more involved and prepares them to participate in their own care once they have the knowledge.

**Psychomotor Agitation** The constant involved in some tension-relieving activity, such as constantly pacing, biting one's nails, smoking, or tapping one's finger on a tabletop.

**Psychomotor retardation** Extremely slow and difficult movements that in the extreme can entail complete inactivity and incontinence.

**Psychosis** An extreme response to psychological or physical stressors that affects a person's affective, psychomotor, and physical behavior. Evidence of impairment in reality testing is evident by hallucinations or delusions.

**Psychotherapy** A treatment modality based on the development of a trusting relationship between clients and therapist for the purpose of exploring and modifying the client's behavior in a satisfying direction.

**Psychotropic** Affecting the mind.

**Relapse** The process of becoming dysfunctional in sobriety that ends in a return to chemical use.

**Rituals** – Repetitive actions that a person must do over and over until he or she is exhausted or anxiety is decreased; they are often done to lessen the anxiety trigged by an obsession.

**Schizophrenia** A severe disturbance of thought or association, characterized by impaired reality testing, hallucinations, delusions, and limited socialization.

**Seclusion** The last step in a process to maximize safety to a client and others whereby a client is placed alone in a specially designed room for protection and close observation.

**Self-esteem** Feelings individuals have about their own worth and self value.

**Self help group** An organization of people who share similar problems who meet to receive peer support and encouragement and work together using their strengths to gain control over their lives.

**Splitting** A primitive defense in which persons see themselves or others as all good or all bad, failing to integrate the positive and negative qualities of the self and others into a cohesive whole.

**Stress** The body's arousal response to any demand, change, or perceived threat.

**Stupor** A state in which a person is dazed and awareness of reality in his or her environment appears deadened. For example, a person may sit motionless for long periods of time and in extreme cases may appear to be in a coma.

**Support groups** Groups that help people during stressful periods using a variety of modalities in order to overcome overwhelming situations or unwanted behaviors.

**Tolerance** – A need for higher and higher doses of a drug in order to achieve intoxication or the desired effect.

**Unconscious** Repressed memories, feelings, thoughts, or wishes that are not available to the conscious mind. Usually, these unconscious memories, feelings, thoughts, or wishes harbor intense anxiety and can greatly; affect an individual's behavior.

**Word salad** A mixture of phrases meaningless to the listener and to the speaker as well.

# References

Alcohol Anonymous, New York: AA World Service Inc.

American Psychiatric Association (2000). *Diagnostic and Statistical Manual of Mental Health Disorders* (DSM IV T-R) (4th ed., rev.) Washington, D.C.

Anabolics.com, Inc. (2005) *Anabolic Steroids Side Effects.* Retrieved October 14, 2005. http://www.steroids.org/side-effects.htm.

Anabolic Steroids and Their Use by Athletes in Competition (2005). *Steroid in Athletic Competition Becoming More Widespread.,* Retrieved October 14, 2005. http://www.collegesportsscholarship.com/steroids-athletic-competition.htm.

Davis, W. (1992). *The Best of Success* Illinois: Celebrating Excellence, Inc.

Drug-Rehabs.org (2005). *Huffing Despite Death of Two Teens Last Year, Inhalant Abuse Among Youth Rises in Bay County, Michigan,* Retrieved October 21, 2005, http://www.drug-rehabs.org/articles.php?aid=347

Grandin, T. (2005) *Center for the study of Autism—An inside View of Autism.* Retrieved December 4, 2004, http://www.autism.org/temple/inside.html.

HealthAtoZ.com (2005). *Down Syndrome,* Retrieved October 21, 2005, http://www.healthatoz.com/healthatoz/Atoz/ency/down_syndrome.jsp

Inhalant Abuse (2005) *Inhalants,* Retrieved October 21, 2005, http://www.alb2c3.com/drugs/inh01.htm

*Winds Against The Mind*

Kidshealth.org (2005). *Down Syndrome*, Retrieved October 21, 2005,from http://kidshealth.org/kid/health_problems/birth_defect/down_syndrome.html

LB. Lola Bamigboye (author).

March of Dimes.com (2005). *Down Syndrome*, Retrieved October 21, 2005. http://www.marchofdijmes.com/professionals/681_1214.asp.

Mathias, R (2005). *National Institute of Drug Abuse Notes on Steroid Prevention Program Scores with High School Athletes*. Retrieved October 14, 2005, http://www.drugabuse.gov/NIDA_Notes?NNV0112N4/steroid.html.

Mikkelson, B, and D.P Mikkelson. (2005). *Dusted Off*. Retrieved October 14, 2005, from http://www.snopes.com/toxins/dustoff.asp.

Moiltra, A(2005). *Anabolic Steroids: Is It Worth It?* Retrieved October 14, 2005, from http://www.vanderbilt.edu/AnS/psychology/health_psychology/anabolic-steroids.html.

National Association for Down Syndrome (2005). *Down Syndrome Facts*. Retrieved October 21, 2005, from http://www.naads.org/pages/facts.htm.

Student Health Services, Oregon State University (2005). *Steroid Abuse*. Retrieved October 14, 2005, from http://studenthealth.oregonstate.edu/topcis/steroid-abuse.php.

Varcarloris, E.M. (2002). *Foundations of Psychiatric Mental Health Nursing*. Philadelphia: WB Saunders.

Waldinger, R.J. (1997). *Psychiatry for Medical Students*, Washington, D.C.: American Psychiatric Press, Inc.

CPSIA information can be obtained at www.ICGtesting.com
Printed in the USA
LVOW13s0327110714

393623LV00004B/8/P